D1440712

Osteoporosis:
Genetics, Prevention and Treatment

ENDOCRINE UPDATES

Shlomo Melmed, M.D., Series Editor

1. E.R. Levin and J.L. Nadler (eds.): Endocrinology of Cardiovascular Function. 1998. ISBN: 0-7923-8217-X
2. J.A. Fagin (ed.): Thyroid Cancer. 1998. ISBN: 0-7923-8326-5
3. J.S. Adams and B.P. Lukert (eds.): Osteoporosis: Genetics, Prevention and Treatment. 1998. ISBN: 0-7923-8366-4

Osteoporosis: Genetics, Prevention and Treatment

edited by

JOHN S. ADAMS, M.D.
Cedars-Sinai Medical Center
Los Angeles, California, USA

and

BARBARA P. LUKERT, M.D.
University of Kansas Medical School
Kansas City, Missouri, USA

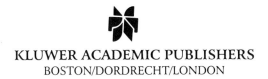

KLUWER ACADEMIC PUBLISHERS
BOSTON/DORDRECHT/LONDON

Distributors for North, Central and South America:
Kluwer Academic Publishers
101 Philip Drive
Assinippi Park
Norwell, Massachusetts 02061 USA
Telephone (781) 871-6600
Fax (781) 871-6528
E-Mail <kluwer@wkap.com>

Distributors for all other countries:
Kluwer Academic Publishers Group
Distribution Centre
Post Office Box 322
3300 AH Dordrecht, THE NETHERLANDS
Telephone 31 78 6392 392
Fax 31 78 6546 474
E-Mail <orderdept@wkap.nl>

 Electronic Services <http://www.wkap.nl>

Library of Congress Cataloging-in-Publication Data

A C.I.P. Catalogue record for this book is available
from the Library of Congress.

Printed on acid-free paper.

Printed in the United States of America

Table of Contents

vi

List of Contributors

Henry G. Bone, III, M.D.
Director
Michigan Bone and Mineral Clin
22201 Moross Ste 260
Detriot, MI 48236
Tel: 313/640-7700
Fax:313/640-4766

Michael Davies, MBBS, FRCP
Department of Medicine
Royal Infirmary
Oxford Road
Mancester, United Kingdom
Tel: 061/276-4060/4066
Fax:061/274-4833

Arnold J. Felsenfeld, M.D.
13493 Rand Drive
Sherman Oaks, CA 91423
Tel: 310/824-4334
Fax:310/824-6681 xt4334

Vicente Gilsanz, M.D.
Radiology MS #81
Childrens Hosp of Los Angeles
4650 Sunset Boulevard
Los Angeles, CA 90027
Tel: 213/669-4571
Fax:213/666-7816

Deborah E. Kipp
Associate Professor
Dept. of Dietetics & Nutrition
Univ. of Kansas Med. Center
3901 Rainbow Blvd.
Kansas City, KS 66160
Tel: 913/588-5356
Fax:913/588-5677

Michael R. McClung, M.D.
Oregon Osteoporosis Center
5050 NE Hoyt. Suite #651
Portland, OR 97213
Tel: 503/215-6586
Fax: 503/215-6428

Mark S. Nanes, M.D., Ph.D.
Medical Service (111E)
VAMC and Emory University
1670 Clairmont Avenue
Decatur, GA 30033
Tel: 404/321-6111 xt 2076
Fax: 404/235-3011

Eric S. Orwoll, M.D.
Chief, Endo & Metab
Portland VA Medical Center
P.O. Box 1034
Portland, OR 97207
Tel: 503/273-5015
Fax: 503/721-7807

Munro Peacock, M.D.
Professor of Medicine
General Clinical Res Center
Indiana Univ Medical Center
550 N. University Blvd.
Room 5595
Indianapolis, IN 46202-5250
Tel: 317/274-4356
Fax: 317/274-7346

Lawrence G. Raisz, M.D.
Endocrinology MC 1850
Connecticut Health Center
Farmington, CT 06030
Tel: 860/679-3851
Fax: 860/679-1258

List of Contributors (con't.)

Robert F. Klein, M.D.
Research Med Services-111P
VA Medical Center
3710 SW US Veterans Hosp Road
Portland, OR 97201
Tel: 503/273-5015
Fax:503/721-7807

Clinton T. Rubin, Ph.D.
Professor
Dept of Orthopaedics T18-030
State Univ of NY - Stony Brook
Musculo-Skeletal Research Lab
Stony Brook, NY 11794-8181
Tel: 516/444-2215
Fax:516/444-7671

Elizabeth Shane, M.D.
Assoc. Prof. Of Clinical Med
Dept of Medicine.PH 8 West
Columbia University
College Physicians & Surgeons
630 West 168th Street
New York, NY 10032
Tel: 212/305-6289
Fax:212/305-6486

Stuart L. Silverman, M.D.
8641 Wilshire Blvd. #301
Beverly Hills, CA 90211
Tel: 310/358-2234
Fax:310/659-2841

Vicki Rosen, Ph.D.
Laura W. Gamer, Ph.D.
Genetics Institute, Inc.
87 Cambridge Park Drive
Cambridge, MA 02140
Tel: 617/498-8365
Fax: 617/498-8875

Janet Rubin, M.D.
VA Medical Center, 111
1670 Clairmont Road
Decatur, GA 30033
Tel: 404/321-6111 xt 2080
Fax: 404/728-7750

Dean Yamaguchi, M.D., Ph.D.
Assoc. Dir, Deputy ACOS
Research and Development
Geriatrics Res Education and
   Clinical Center
VAMC West Los Angeles
11301 Wilshire Blvd.
Los Angeles, CA 90073
Tel: 310/268-4122
Fax: 310/478-4538

Osteoporosis:
Genetics, Prevention and Treatment

This volume is dedicated to the memory of Bayard DeWolfe "Skip" Catherwood, M.D.

Skip Catherwood was a fine scientist, who made important contributions to our understanding of signaling pathways, particularly those involving calcitropic hormones. He was a knowledgeable and perceptive physician whose clinical acumen was informed by deep biological understanding. As a teacher he communicated not just information and insight, but a way of thinking and working that has served his trainees well. His intellectual discipline led to a rational, although not always fashionable, understanding of the world. He was reserved in his manner, but possessed a wry sense of humor. He was a caring husband and father and exceptional friend. His personal and professional integrity were absolute. These are all admirable qualities of our friend's character, and they cause us to miss him grievously, especially since he left us long before his work was done, long before we could bear to let him go.

It is not simply because of these qualities of his character that we dedicate this book to Skip's memory. The extraordinary thing about him was the integration of these qualities into his work. He was an insightful biologist and biochemist, always mindful of the relationship between the molecular, cellular, systemic and medical levels of a problem. Thoroughness and solidity were Skip's hallmarks. He approached any problem with perception, patience and a fundamentally positive approach that expressed his basic optimism. He believed in the ultimate solubility of problems and communicated his persevering, steady approach to his colleagues and trainees. On more than one occasion, a discouraged colleague, describing an apparent scientific impasse, got a fresh start when Skip asked "Have you tried...?" or "What if...?" followed by a cogent exposition of why "...?" just might work. These suggestions, low-keyed and often made after a reflective pause, have been extraordinarily helpful to many who knew him, not only because of their specific scientific content, but also because they restored confidence that a discouraging problem could be attacked. In this way, he expressed a sense of collegiality which was far more than social. His belief in cooperation and sharing of ideas and effort was central to his character as a scientist and as a person. He expected no less from his colleagues, whom he brought together in many different settings, challenging them to integrate their ideas and efforts, in order to enhance their understanding of problems and to reach deeper insights into their solutions. Skip's interest in the problems and projects of others and his responsiveness to them were expressions of the good nature, good will and inquiring intelligence that bound us to him not only as colleagues but, forever, as friends.

Henry G. Bone, M.D.

and Louisa Titus, Ph.D.

1 Osteoporosis: Understanding and Managing a Growing Health Care Problem

John S. Adams, M.D.

Barbara P. Lukert, M.D.

The Scope of the Problem

Current estimates are that 13-17 million American women have osteoporosis (1) as defined by the World Health Organization (2). If one applies the same criteria to men, then 8-10 million American males also have this disease (1). There are approximately 300,000 hip fractures annually in the United States with another 6% of this total going unreported (3). The case fatality rate at year one post fracture is 24% (4) with most victims never being able to regain their premorbid lifestyle (5, 6). In 1995 (3) it was estimated that 93.8 billion dollars were expended for the care of osteoporotic fractures. Sixty two percent of the total, or 58.2 billion dollars, was expended for in-hospital care of fractures, primarily hip fractures. The combination of the cost of in-patient care and that of nursing home care for hip fracture victims accounts for >90% of the total expenditure for osteoporosis fracture syndromes or $84 billion annually. At the current growth rate of hip fracture incidence in the United States, estimates are that cost of caring for hip fractures alone may exceed $240 billion by the middle of the next century (7). Obviously, there is neither the desire or the financial where-with-all to deal with a clinical predicament of this magnitude.

How Could a Problem of this Magnitude Arise?

The simple answer to this question is that modern society is altering the lifestyle and longevity of its constituents much more quickly than evolutionary adaptation to these changes can take place. For example, the current required calcium intake for carniverous non-human primate species as well as primitive human hunter-gatherers is in the range of 2.0 nmol/100 kCal or 200-400% greater than that provided by most Western diets (8). This suggests that modern man is chronically and severely calcium deprived. The problem of calcium deficiency in the population is compounded by the growing percentage of aged individuals with relatively fragile, less massive skeletons; the average age in Western societies is expected to reach 85 within the next 20 years (9). Clearly, current-day civilizations are much more effective in prolonging human life in a state of relative debility than even a few decades ago. This reality is unlikely to change and mandates that we develop strategies to prevent aging-related diseases like osteoporosis before they become manifest.

As with other common diseases of an oligogenic nature, including atherosclerosis, diabetes mellitus, obesity, and hypertension, physicians and scientists alike have focused their attention and research on effective management of the outcomes of osteoporosis after the osteoporotic phenotype is already clearly established. This approach makes sense when one considers the following two realities. First, the diagnosis of a susceptible phenotype is always easier in the later stages of a disease. For example, it is relatively easy to identify a patient at risk for heart disease once they have experienced and survived a myocardial infarction. It is also relatively straight forward to predict osteoporotic fractures in a patient who has already lost height or experienced a fracture. The second important consideration is that the medical care establishment, including hospitals, insurance companies and the pharmaceutical industry, have prospered more from providing interventive therapy than from preventive care. This too is bound to change. We can no longer afford to just treat existing disease, because too many people will be suffering from osteoporosis.

Osteoporosis Management in the Near Future

How is the landscape in osteoporosis management going to change? First and probably foremost is the fact that age-related diseases like osteoporosis will bankrupt providers, including federal governments, that will have to pay for the morbid consequences of the disease in a rapidly aging population. This means that there will be huge economic pressure to prevent or delay the onset of disease rather than merely treating the disease once it develops. Second, medical science and technology are now making it possible to identify phenotypes which characterize those who are predisposed to a disease before the disease is fully manifest clinically; a good example of this is the use of bone mineral density measurements to determine those individuals that have a lower than normal peak bone mass. Technological advances in matching susceptible phenotypes with genotypes is the other major factor reshaping the way we care for patients with these oligogenic disorders (10). With a comprehensive map of the human genome now being a certainty in the near future and recent dramatic progress in mammalian cloning capabilities (11), it will be possible to identify the genes which collaborate in the causation of diseases like osteoporosis. Once the causative genes are identified, more directed therapy can be delivered to those at risk as well as those who already have the disease.

Text Content and Organization

In view of the rapid progress predicted for cloning major disease genes including osteoporosis susceptibility genes (12) and in contrast to other practical texts in the field, this book will place more emphasis on the 1] genetic predisposition 2] early recognition and 3] prevention of osteoporosis. Our intent is not to move the practitioner's attention away from intervention therapy of osteoporosis, but rather to expand their view of this disease as one beginning at birth and one in which susceptibility is manifest at the conclusion of adolescence not at menopause. The first section of the text will focus on the genetic aspects of osteoporosis. Dr. Rosen will review bone morphogenic proteins and how these and related proteins cooperate to legislate the shape and size of the skeleton. Peak bone mass is the major determinant of whether an individual will or will not develop osteoporosis, with genetics contributing up to 85% of the interindividual variability in peak bone mass. Dr. Adams and Dr. Klein will address the genetics of osteoporosis in man and syntenic animal models of the human disease, respectively. These authors will discuss state-of-the-art strategies for finding osteoporosis susceptibility genes and the utility of animal models in speeding up the search for human disease genes. Finally, Drs. Rubin will delve into the interplay of genetic and non-genetic (epigenetic or environmental) influences on bone structure and strength.

The second section of the book will center attention on the early diagnosis, prevention and treatment of osteoporosis. This section will be initiated by a discussion by Dr. Gilsanz of the best and most reliable methods for determining bone mass with special emphasis on bone mass measurement in children. Dr. Allen's chapter comprehensively reviews those non-genetic factors which influence peak bone mass and then presents strategies for optimizing peak bone mass during the period of adolescent growth and development. Because of its central role in maintaining as well as achieving bone mass, the contribution of physical exercise to overall skeletal health will be emphasized in chapter by Dr. Marcus. The role of nutritional facts is considered in chapters by Allen and Davies. The central section of the book will conclude with three chapters addressing postmenopausal osteoporosis. The chapter by Drs. Doran and Khosla will provide a general review of the diagnosis and treatment of postmenopausal osteoporosis, by far and away the most common of the osteoporotic syndromes. Dr. Silverman will focus on the individualization of those therapeutic regimens recommended by the FDA for the management and prevention of postmenopausal osteoporosis. Drs. Rigler and Studenski will speak to the often-overlooked issue of fall prevention and physical therapy in the overall management of osteoporosis.

The third part of the volume will be dedicated to a review of the pathophysiology and management of osteoporotic syndromes that are emerging as major problems facing clinicians caring for patients with metabolic bone disease. This includes a modern-day view of the diagnosis and treatment of male osteoporosis by Dr. Orwoll; of renal osteodystrophy by Drs. Yamaguchi and Felsenfeld, and of immunosuppression therapy-associated bone disease by Drs. Rodino and Shane. Dr. Davies covers the diagnosis and management of osteoporosis complicated by non-iatrogenic, commonly-occurring metabolic disturbances affecting the skeleton, including hyperparathyroidism, hyperthyroidism, vitamin D-deficiency, and intestinal malabsorption syndromes. The next contribution to the third section of the text comes from Drs. Nanes and

4

Titus. These authors address the ever-increasing realization that most cancer syndromes have an impact on the skeleton, either directly through metastasis or indirectly through endocrine, paracrine and autocrine signaling pathways. They also remind us of the many lessons we have learned about normal bone physiology by studying tumors that affect bone. The book concludes with the predictions of Dr. Raisz. We will provide his informed view of the future in terms of the recognition, prevention, and management of osteoporosis.

References

1. Looker AC, Orwoll ES, Johnston CC, Lindsay RL, Wahner HW, Dunn WL, Calvo MS, Harris TB, Heyse SP 1997 Prevalence of low femoral bone density in older U.S. adults from NHANES III. J Bone Miner Res 12:1761-1768.

2. Kanis JL, Melton LJ, Christiansen C, Johnston CC, Khaltaev N 1994 The diagnosis of osteoporosis. J Bone Miner Res 9:1137-1141.

3. Bacon WE 1996 Secular trends in hip fracture occurrence and survival: age and sex differences. J Aging Health 8:538-553.

4. Looker AC, Johnston CC, Wahner HW, Dunn WL, Calvo MS, Harris TB, Heyse SP, Lindsay RL 1995 Prevalence of low femoral bone density in older U.S. women from NHANES III. J Bone Miner Res 10:796-802.

5. Jones G, Nguyen T, Sambrook P, Kelly PJ, Eisman JA 1994 Progressive loss of bone in the femoral neck in elderly people: longitudinal findings from the dubbo osteoporosis epidemiology study. Br Med J 309:691-695.

6. Slemenda C, Longcope C, Peacock M, Hui S, Johnston CC 1996 Sex steroids, bone mass and bone loss: a prospective study of pre-peri-and postmenopausal women. J Clin Invest 97:14-21.

7. Lindsay R 1991 The burden of osteoporosis: cost. Am J Med 98:9s-11s.

8. Heaney RP 1993 Nutritional factors in osteoporosis. Annu Rev Nutr 13:287-316.

9. Wilmoth JR 1998 The future of human longevity: A demographer's perspective. Science 280:395-397.

10. Lander ES, Schork NJ 1994 Genetic dissection of complex traits. Science 265:2037-2048.

11. King M-C 1997 Leaving Kansas...finding genes in 1997. Nature Genet 15:8-11.

12. Kahn P 1996 Gene hunters close in on elusive prey. Science 271:1352-1354

I.   Genetics

2 Molecular Genetics of Skeletal Morphogenesis

Vicki Rosen, Ph.D.

Laura Gamer, M.D.

Introduction

Our understanding of the molecular mechanisms that control growth, patterning and repair of skeletal tissues has increased greatly in the past few years. An emerging paradigm is that signals important for embryonic skeletal formation are also utilized by adult organisms to regulate skeletal homeostasis. Current research has shown that bone morphogenetic proteins (BMPs) play an important role in these processes. BMPs are widely expressed in developing skeletal structures and mutations in individual BMP genes block early events in skeletal morphogenesis at specific anatomical sites. Based on available information, it seems likely that different members of the BMP gene family have evolved to control the formation of distinct sets of skeletal structures. This chapter will focus on BMPs because of their central role in bone formation. We will describe our current understanding of osteogenic BMP proteins, the BMP signaling pathway, and also discuss the interactions of BMPs with other developmental molecules that play important roles in skeletal morphogenesis. We will also speculate about the regulation of BMPs by agents that are known effectors of bone mass in adults, thus defining a potential role for BMPs in adult skeletal homeostasis.

Discovery of BMPs

The identification of a bone-inductive component resident in bone itself by Urist in 1965 lead to the cloning of the first osteogenic BMPs in 1988 (1-3). We now know that BMPs are part of a large multigene family, the TGF-ß gene superfamily, whose members have wide ranging biological activities. BMPs, like other members of this superfamily have seven conserved cysteine residues in the mature, carboxy-terminal portion of the protein where biological activity resides (4-6; **Figure 1A and B**) BMPs are synthesized as large precursor molecules that are then processed to dimers of approximately 30,000 MW before they are secreted from the cell (7). BMPs are able to form both homodimers and heterodimers, increasing the number of potential active proteins available to an organism (8,9).

Unlike other members of the TGF-ß superfamily, BMPs are active upon secretion and are thought to act locally in a paracrine and possibly autocrine manner (10).

BMP/TGF-β Family

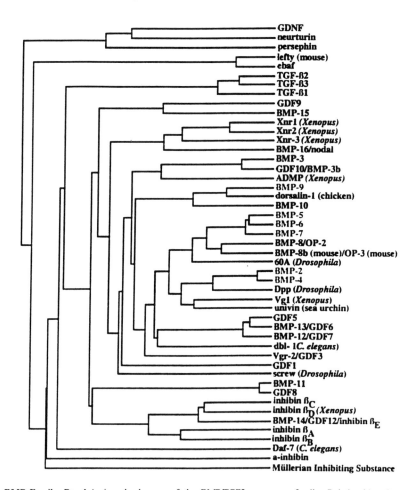

1. **BMP Family, Panel A:** is a dendogram of the BMP/TGFß gene superfamily. Relationship of family members is determined by comparing amino acid identities from the first conserved cysteine residue in each protein. The shorter the connecting line between proteins, the more alike the proteins are. **Panel B:** is a schematic representation of a BMP homodimer. Triangles denote possible N-linked glycosylation sites.

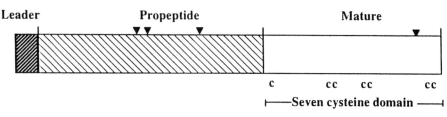

Many BMP family members have been shown to possess osteoinductive activity in vivo as either homodimers or heterodimers. Using a rat ectopic bone formation assay to measure osteoinductive potential, BMPs 2, 4, 5, 6, 7, and 9 have been shown to be osteogenic agents (8, 11-15). In adult animals, the target cell of osteogenic BMPs appears to be a mesenchymal precursor that upon stimulation with an osteogenic BMP begins the differentiation cascade whose end result is endochondral bone formation (16). During embryogenesis, BMPs appear to have multiple target cells and act in many different tissues. Osteogenic BMPs appear to influence multiple steps in both the endochondral and intramembranous bone formation pathways during embryonic skeletal development (see below).

Localization of BMPs During Embryonic Skeletal Formation

The most widely studied area of skeletogenesis is the developing limb, and in this model system localization of BMPs to developing skeletal structures provides primary evidence for the roles of these proteins in skeletal patterning and skeletal cell differentiation. Data obtained from in situ localization studies confirm that transcripts for BMPs 2, 3, 4, 5, 6, 7, GDF5, GDF6 and GDF7 are all present in the developing embryo at sites and times consistent with their involvement in mesenchymal condensation and cartilage differentiation (7; **Figure 2**). While many of the upstream signals that control the expression of individual BMPs at specific sites are still to be defined, data from many labs suggest that BMPs, fibroblast growth factors (FGFs), and sonic hedgehog (Shh) interact in a hierarchical way to pattern limb skeletal elements (17-19). In limb formation, BMP 2 and 4 transcripts are found in the apical ectodermal ridge (AER) and a region of posterior mesenchyme, the zone of polarizing activity (ZPA), two important signaling centers (20). At these locations, BMPs 2 and 4 are thought to act downstream of FGF and Shh signals. When BMP-2 or BMP-4 are inactivated by homologous recombination in ES cells, the resulting BMP-2 and BMP-4 null mice die early in embryogenesis before limb patterning occurs (21, 22). While these experiments highlight the global importance of BMPs during mouse development, they have not been useful in dissecting out specific roles for BMPs 2 and 4 in the early limb. Another osteogenic BMP, BMP-7 (also known as OP-1) is expressed in the early limb bud in a manner consistent with involvement in early limb formation. Mice lacking BMP-7 survive until birth and display only mild skeletal abnormalities in the limb (23, 24). The absence of a strong skeletal phenotype in the BMP-7 knockouts may be due to the ability of BMPs to compensate for each other (see receptor section), and BMPs 2 and 4 are still present in limbs of BMP7 null mice (25).

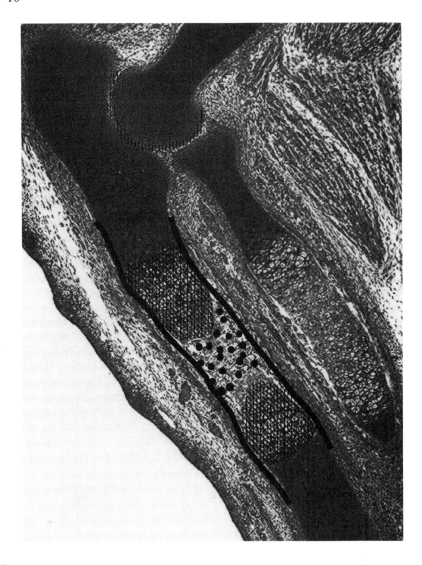

FIGURE 2. Expression of BMPs during limb development. An embryonic day 14
mouse forelimb is shown with schematized in situ hybridization patterns for several BMPs known
to be important in skeletogenesis. BMP6 (cross hatched) localizes to the hypertrophic
chondrocytes in the maturing bone. GDF5 (hatched) is expressed in the joint space and articular
surface of the elbow. BMP2 (black) is detected in the osteogenic zone adjacent to the hypertrophic
chondrocytes and the periosteum.

Later in limb formation, mesenchymal condensation and cartilage differentiation occur and osteogenic BMPs have been localized to sites of these activities. Transcripts for BMPs 2, 4, 5 and 7 are present in precondensing mesenchyme and in the cells surrounding early cartilage condensations. Recent data from the chick embryo limb has shown that misexpression of individual osteogenic BMPs results in changes in the morphogenesis of specific skeletal elements, but the ability of multiple BMPs to signal through the same receptor make some of these results hard to interpret (26). The most clear cut example of BMPs directing the differentiation of specific skeletal structures is in the GDF5 null mouse which exhibits a brachypodism phenotype, as evidenced by shortening of the long bones of the appendicular skeleton, reduction in the number of digits in the paws, and misshapen bones in both the front and hind feet (27, 28). In these mice, expression of GDF5 transcripts normally occurs at all sites where skeletal malformations take place. The lack of GDF5 signals results in failure of joint morphogenesis between individual bones and in alterations in the size and shape of the mesenchymal condensations themselves. Humans with mutations in the GDF5 gene display joint dysmorphogenesis at sites where GDF5 is normally expressed, and in this instance the skeletal anomalies can be directly related to the expression pattern of GDF5 (29,30).

Once endochondral bone formation progresses to the cartilage hypertrophy stage, BMP6 expression appears to mark chondrocytes actively undergoing hypertrophy. Data using misexpression of several BMPs and Shh in the embryonic chick have established a temporal relationship between the expression of these molecules and chondrocyte hypertrophy and replacement by bone (31). However, BMP6 null mice appear to have normal skeletons at birth, suggesting that BMP6 is not absolutely required for endochondral ossification to occur (7). As new bone begins to replace the calcified hypertrophic cartilage, localization of osteogenic BMPs appears confined to the periosteum and forming marrow spaces, areas that may contain mesenchymal stem cells. Addition of osteogenic BMPs at this time results in increases in bone formation at both sites.

In the craniofacial skeleton where much of the bone is formed through a combination of intramembranous and endochondral ossification, BMPs have been localized in precondensing mesenchyme of the skull and also in the precartilaginous elements of the mandible and nasal cartilages (32). Addition of exogenous BMPs during chick craniofacial development induces changes in skeletal patterning and also an overgrowth of bone at these sites. Tooth formation also appears to be BMP mediated, and specific BMPs have been localized in early dental epithelium, in dental mesenchyme, and finally during the terminal differentiation of both odontoblasts and ameloblasts (33-35).

In the axial skeleton, BMP5 appears to play a central role in formation of the skeletal structures of the outer ear, the sternum and the ribs. BMP5 transcripts have been found at each of these locations during organogenesis, and mice lacking a functional BMP5 gene display the short ear (SE) phenotype, with characteristic defects in each of these structures (36). These defects are evident early in skeletal development, as condensations that give rise to affected structures are altered in size and shape. BMP5 transcripts can also be found in other skeletal structures where no effect of the loss of BMP5 is observed (37). Here, the presence of other osteogenic BMPs may compensate for the absence of BMP5. Interestingly, SE mice also exhibit a reduced ability to heal fractures, suggesting a role for BMP5 protein in the adult skeleton (38).

BMP Signaling

BMPs induce a wide variety of biological responses in target tissues, including cell proliferation, apoptosis, differentiation and morphogenesis. How BMPs mediate these diverse effects has been a recent subject of intense study and major advances have been made in our understanding of how osteogenic BMPs exert their effects on target cells.

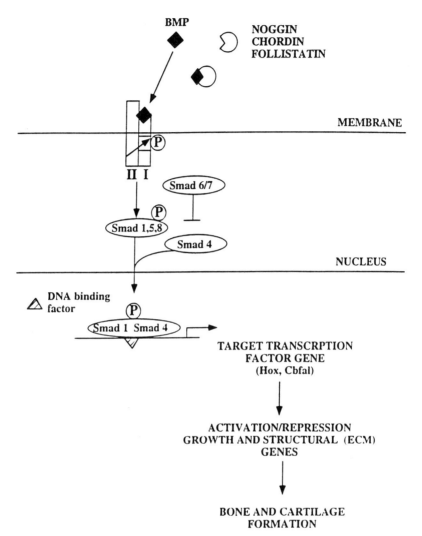

3. Generalized model of BMP signaling. BMPs bind to and activate distinct combinations of type I and type II serine threonine kinase receptors. Outside the cell, this binding can be blocked by association with secreted BMP antagonists such as noggin, chordin, or follistatin. BMP binding to its receptors results in a transient association with pathway specific SMADs and subsequent phosphorylation by the type I receptor. This leads to association with a co-SMAD and translocation of this complex into the nucleus. Inside the cell, signaling can be inhibited by anti-SMADs which act by blocking carboxy-terminal phosphorylation of receptor activated SMADs and/or by preventing association with co-SMADs. In the nucleus, the SMAD complex associates with DNA binding factors leading to the activation of target gene expression. These target transcription factors then activate or repress a specific subset of growth and structural genes, eventually resulting in bone and cartilage formation.

Members of the TGFß family initiate their cellular action by binding to transmembrane serine-threonine kinases known as the type I and type II receptors. These closely related receptors are composed of a short cysteine rich extracellular domain, a single transmembrane spanning domain, and an intracellular domain with serine and threonine kinase regions (39,40). The current model of how these receptors are activated comes from studies on signaling by TGFß. TGFß ligands initially bind the type II receptor and this interaction recruits a type I receptor into a heteromeric complex (41; **Figure 3**). Interestingly, TGFß can only bind type I receptor in the presence of type II receptor. Transphosphorylation of the type I receptor on a specific region (GS domain) by the type II receptor causes activation and initiation of downstream signaling events. The BMP receptor system appears to work in a slightly different manner. BMPs can bind both the type I and type II receptor alone with low affinity 42). High affinity binding of BMPs is only achieved when both receptors are present together. The same BMP can bind more than one type II receptor which in turn can interact with different type I receptors. The nature of the signal, therefore, depends on the composition of the receptor complex and in particular on the specificity of the type I receptor kinase. This system gives the ligand direct control over signal diversity.

Localization studies of BMP receptors have provided clues as to what cells in the developing skeleton are responding to signals from BMPs. In the developing chick limb, BMPR-1B is expressed in the precartilaginous condensations while BMPR-1A is expressed at low levels throughout the mesenchyme with highest levels in the posterior distal region where cell fate specification is occurring (43,44). At later stages, BMPR1A is highly expressed in the prehypertrophic chondrocytes (43). The type II BMP receptor is also found in precartilaginous condensations, as well as the AER and interdigital mesenchyme (44).

Studies with dominant negative and constitutively activated BMP receptors in chick embryos have revealed critical roles for BMP signaling in chondrogenesis and skeletal patterning. Interestingly, the two type I receptors appear to mediate distinct responses during limb formation. BMPR-1B signaling appears to be necessary for mesenchymal condensation and cartilage formation during the early steps of chondrogenesis (43). In addition, BMPR1-B also regulates the intracellular pathways that lead to cell death in the interdigital mesenchyme (43,45). In contrast, BMPR1-A appears to regulate the rate of chondrocyte differentiation during late stages of cartilage development. In similar studies using chick sternal chondrocytes, the type II receptor was shown to be required to maintain a differentiated phenotype and in the control of proliferation and terminal differentiation (46). BMP signaling appears to play a crucial role in multiple steps during endochondral bone formation. Each step in this process is critical for normal skeletal morphogenesis and alteration of BMP signaling may affect skeletogenesis at any given stage. It has been suggested that the temporally and spatially regulated expression of BMPs controls the formation of skeletal elements. The above data is evidence that further refinement of bone morphogenesis may also be controlled by the temporal and spatial expression and activity of the type I and type II BMP receptors.

Once a BMP has activated its receptor complex how is this signal relayed to the nucleus? A genetic approach to this question was undertaken in Drosophila and yielded the first member of the SMAD family of signaling molecules. Mad (mothers against decapentaplegic) was isolated in a screen to identify genes that were required for activity of the BMP related factor dpp (47). Homologues of Mad have been found in C. Elegans, Xenopus, mouse, and humans. The SMAD family has been divided into three subgroups based on structural and functional criteria (reviewed in 48,49). The first group are the receptor activated or pathway specific SMADs (Smad 1,2,3,5 and 8) which serve as direct and specific substrates for various ligand activated receptors and are therefore responsible for conveying specificity to the signaling pathway. The second group are the co-SMADs (Smad 4) which form a complex with the receptor activated SMADs upon their phosphorylation by receptors. Co-SMADs are required for transcriptional activational of target genes. The third group are the anti-SMADs (Smad 6 and Smad 7) which are the most divergent structurally and serve to inhibit specific SMAD signaling pathways.

Work in TGFß responsive cell lines and Xenopus embryos has generated the current model for intracellular signaling by SMADs (48,49). TGFß family growth factors bind to and activate receptor kinases leading to a transient association with specific receptor activatable SMADs. These SMADs become phosphorylated by type I receptor, associate with a co-SMAD, and move into the nucleus. In the nucleus, the SMAD complex associates with DNA binding transcription factors leading to active transcriptional complexes and stimulation of target gene expression. Therefore, SMAD proteins directly transmit TGFß family signals into the nucleus. This model shows that signaling specificity of a particular BMP is dictated at the cell surface by the receptors present and also in the target cell by the profile of SMADs present.

SMAD proteins have two regions of homology at the amino and carboxy terminals, termed mad homology domains MH1 and MH2, respectively, which are connected with a proline rich linker sequence (50). When SMADs are in an inactive configuration, the MH1 and MH2 domains make contact with each other (51). Upon phosphorylation of the C terminal MH2, these molecules open up, form hetero-oligomeric complexes and translocate into the nucleus. The MH1 domain is therefore, thought to be a negative regulatory region by initiating this inhibitory interaction with MH2 (51). The MH2 domain has been shown to be essential for positive regulation of SMADs via protein-protein interactions with receptor complexes, co-SMADs, and transcription factors (48,49).

The recent discovery of anti-SMADs has revealed another level of regulation of the BMP signaling system. Within the cell, the anti-SMADs function by blocking carboxy terminal phosphorylation by receptors and/or by inhibiting the association of receptor activated SMADs with co-SMADs (52-54). In contrast to the extracellular antagonists of BMPs like noggin, chordin, or follistatin (see below), the anti-SMADs may allow for a more precise regulation of different cells within the same microenvironment of a given organ. With multiple levels of control established inside and outside a cell, it seems reasonable that the same molecule, for example BMP4 in developing limb, could induce cell differentiation to form bone and cell death to form interdigital spaces.

BMP Gene Targets

A major question that still remains is once BMP signals reaches the nucleus what are the target genes for the genetic program responsible for skeletal morphogenesis. Candidates for BMP regulation include factors whose perturbation leads to skeletal abnormalities these include Hox, Msx and CBFA genes. Hox genes are members of a family of transcription factors that share a common DNA binding motif called the homeobox. Vertebrates have four clusters of homeobox containing genes HoxA, HoxB, HoxC, and HoxD. These molecules are critical for the anterior - posterior patterning in the embryo but also have important roles in skeletal pattern formation. Inactivation or overexpression of certain Hoxa and Hoxd genes in mouse results in deletion, addition, or transformation of skeletal elements. In humans, a mutation in the HOXD13 gene has been found recently in families affected by synpolydactyly, an inherited abnormality of the hands and feet which causes webbing and digit duplication (55). Misexpression experiments in chick have revealed roles for Hoxa genes in regulating cell adhesiveness in pre-cartilaginous condensations and for Hox d genes in regulating growth rates in developing bones (56,57). Homeobox genes that lie outside the four major clusters like msx1,2 and MHox also appear to play roles in skeletogenesis. Mice homozygous for a null mutation in the MHox gene have a range of skeletal defects involving loss or shortening of structures in the skull, face and limb which seem to reflect a perturbation of the process of mesenchymal condensation (58). In Drosophila, a direct genetic link has been established between BMPs and homeobox genes. In vertebrates, much correlative data exists to suggest that BMPs regulate Hox genes. For example, in the developing chick limb, BMP2 has been shown to play a role in inducing the expression of Hox d11-d13 in mesenchymal cells (59). The Cbfa1 gene has been shown to be critical for bone formation. Mice in which the Cbfa1 genes has been knocked out lack bone and have a calcified cartilaginous skeleton (60,61). Cbfa1 is a member of the core-binding factor family which regulates genes involved in osteoblast differentiation like osteocalcin (62). Although it is not known yet whether BMPs activate Cbfa1, if these factors are playing a critical upstream role in bone morphogenesis, Cbfa1 would be an important target for direct regulation by BMP signals.

What Regulates BMP Activity

Studies delineating the signals regulating embryogenesis in the African clawed frog, Xenopus, have led to the discovery of several diverse proteins that act as naturally occurring BMP antagonists. These proteins, noggin, chordin, follistatin, and members of the DAN gene family, act directly on BMP ligands, binding to specific BMPs with affinities approximating those of cellular BMP receptors (63-65). While roles of individual BMP antagonists have been assigned in Xenopus, the interactions of BMPs and these same antagonists during mammalian skeletal development and subsequent skeletal homeostasis are largely unknown (66). Since homologs for each of the Xenopus antagonists have been found in humans, and in some instances shown to be present in adult skeletal tissues or in the circulation, it will be important to understand this new dimension of BMP biology. Future research aimed at documenting BMP antagonist expression and BMP-antagonist interactions may allow us to determine if antagonists depress osteogenesis thereby reducing bone formation and repair. If so, regulation of BMP antagonists may provide a novel tool for controlling bone density in adults.

Few studies have focused on the regulation of BMPs by steroid hormones but this appears to be a theme of increasing interest for skeletal homeostasis. Estrogen is a potent anabolic agent, capable of increasing bone mass in the adult skeleton. The first convincing evidence that some of the actions of estrogen on bone and cartilage cells may be mediated through increased production of BMPs, and specifically, increases in BMP6 was recently provided by Richard et al (67). As bone remodeling in the adult skeleton involves the differentiation of progenitor cells into mature osteoblasts, the ability of BMPs to initiate osteogenesis from stem cells fits well with the observed phenotype changes. Glucocorticoids have also been shown to have profound effects on the skeleton both in vivo and in vitro. A possible link between glucocorticoid induced increases in osteogenesis and BMPs has been established in vitro by Boden et al who demonstrated that BMP6 mediates the glucocorticoid induced stimulation of bone nodule formation in a rat primary osteoblast culture system (68, 69). It will be interesting to examine effects of estrogen and glucocorticoids on bone formation and remodeling in BMP6 null mice who appear normal at birth but may develop osteopenias in later life. It will also be important to determine if the adult skeleton responds to steroid treatment in vivo by modulating levels of BMP6 and if this modulation results in corresponding changes in bone density. These areas present an exciting challenge for future investigations on the roles of BMPs in adult skeletal homeostasis.

Conclusions

BMPs have been identified as fundamental regulators of embryonic bone formation and preliminary data exists to link BMPs to bone formation and bone repair during adult life. Identification of the factors regulating osteogenic BMP expression will aid in our evaluation of how BMPs can be used to augment bone density. Understanding the downstream events of BMP action will be fundamental to our understanding of the mechanisms controlling endochondral bone formation both during embryogenesis and in the adult skeleton. Together research in these areas may provide us with additional ideas on how to design novel therapeutics that increase skeletal mass during adult life, helping to counterbalance the affects of bone loss during normal aging.

References

1.   Urist MR 1965 Bone: formation by autoinduction. Science 150:893-899.

18

2. Wang EA, Rosen V, Cordes P, Hewick RM, Kriz MJ, Luxenberg DP, Sibley BS, Wozney JM 1988 Purification and characterization of other distinct bone-inducing factors. Proc. Natl. Acad. Sci. USA 85:9484-9488.

3. Wozney JM, Rosen V, Celeste AJ, Mitsock LM, Whitters MJ, Kriz RW, Hewick RM, Wang EA 1988 Novel regulators of bone formation: molecular clones and activities. Science 242:1528-1534.

4. Hogan BLM 1996 Bone morphogenetic proteins in development. Curr. Opin. Genet. Dev. 6:432-438.

5. Hogan BLM 1996 Bone morphogenetic proteins: multifunctional regulators of vertebrate development. Genes Dev. 10:1580-1594.

6. Kingsley DM. 1994 What do BMPs do in mammals? Clues from the mouse short-ear mutation. trends Genet 10:16-21.

7. Rosen V, Cox K, Hattersley G, Bilezikian J, Raisz L, Rodan G 1996 Bone morphogenetic proteins. principles of bone Biology 661-670.

8. Aono A, Hazama M, Notoya K, Taketomi S, Yamasaki H, Tsukuda R, Sasaki S, Fujisawa Y 1995 Potent ectopic bone inducing activity of BMP-4/7 heterodimers. Biochem. Biophys. Res. Commun. 210:670-677.

9. Israel DI, Nove J, Kerns KM, Kaufman RJ, Rosen V, Cox K, Wozney JM 1996 Heterodimeric bone morphogenetic proteins show enhanced activity in vitro and in vivo. Growth Factors 13:291-300.

10. Kingsley DM 1994 The TGFß superfamily; new members, new receptors, and genetic tests of function in different organisms. Genes Dev. 8:133-146.

11. Wang EA, Rosen V, D'Alessandro JS, Bauduy M, Cordes P, Harada T, Israel DI, Hewick RM, Kerns KM, LaPan P, Luxenberg DP, McQuaid D, Moutsatsos IK, Nove J, Wozney JM 1990 Recombinant human bone morphogenetic protein induces bone formation. Proc. Natl. Acad. Sci 87:2220-2224.

12. Ozkaynak E, Rueger DC, Drier EA, Corbett C, Ridge RJ, Sampath TK, Opperman H 1990 OP-1 cDNA encodes an osteogenic protein in the TGFß family. EMBO J 9:2085-2093.

13. Gitelman SE, Kobrin MS, Ye JQ, Lopez AR, Lee A, Derynck R 1994 Recombinant Vgr-1/BMP-6 expressing tumors induce fibrosis and endochondral bone formation in vivo. J Cell Biol 126:1595-1609.

14. Celeste AJ, Song JJ, Cox K, Rosen V, Wozney JM 1994 Bone morphogenetic protein-9, a new member of the TGFß gene superfamily. J. Bone Miner. Res. 9:s137.

15. D'Alessandro JS, Cox K, Israel DI, LaPan P, Moutsatsos IK, Nove J, Rosen V, Ryan MC, Wozney JM, Wang EA 1991 Purification, characterization, and activities of recombinant BMP-5. J. Bone Miner. Res. 6: s153.

16. Reddi AH 1981 Cell Biology and Biochemistry of endochondral bone development. Col. Rel. Res. 1:209-226.

17. Bitgood MJ, McMahon AP 1995 Hedgehog and BMP genes are coexpressed at many sites of cell-cell interaction in the mouse embryo. Dev. Biol. 172:126-138.

18. Laufer E, Nelson CE, Johnson RL, Morgan BA, Tabin C 1994 Sonic hedgehog and FGF-4 act through a signalling cascade and feedback loop to integrate growth and patterning of the developing limb. Cell 79:993-1003.

19. Niswander L, Martin GR 1993 FGF-4 and BMP-2 have opposite effects on limb growth. Nature 361:68-71.

20. Lyons KM, Pelton RW, Hogan BLM 1990 Organogenesis and pattern formation in the mouse: RNA distribution patterns suggest a role for bone morphogenetic Protein-2A (BMP-2A). Develop. 109:833-844.

21. Winnier G, Blessing M, Labosky PA, Hogan BLM 1995 Bone morphogenetic protein-4 is required for mesoderm formation and patterning in the mouse. Genes Dev. 9:2105-2116.

22. Zhang H, Bradley A. 1996 Mice deficient for BMP2 are Nonviable and have defects in amnion/chorion and cardiac development. Develop. 122:2977-2986.

23. Dudley AT, Lyons KM, Robertson EJ 1995 A requirement for bone morphogenetic protein-7 during development of the mammalian eye. Genes Dev. 9:2795-2807.

24. Luo G, Hofmann C, Bronkers AL, Sohocki M, Bradley A, Karsenty G 1995 BMP-7 is an inducer of nephrogenesis, and is also required for eye development and skeletal patterning. Genes Dev. 9:2808-2830.

25. Dudley AJ, Robertson EJ 1977 Overlapping expression domains of bone morphogenetic protein family members potentially account for limited tissue defects in BMP7 deficient embryos. Dev. Dyn. 208:344-362.

26. Francis PH, Richardson MK, Brickell PM, Tickle C 1994 Bone morphogenetic proteins and a signalling pathway that controls patterning in the developing chick limb. Develop. 120:209-218.

27. Storm EE, Huynh TV, Copeland NG, Jenkins NA, Kinglsey DM, Lee S-J 1994 Limb alterations in brachypodism mice due to mutations in a new member of the TGFß-superfamily. Nature 368:639-642.

28. Gruneberg H, Lee AJ 1973 The anatomy and development of brachypodism in the mouse. J. Embryol. Exp. Morph. 30:119-141.

29. Thomas JT, Kilpatrick MW, Lin K, Erlacher L, Lembessis P, Costa T, Tsipouras P, Luyten, FP 1977 Disruption of human limb morphogenesis by a dominant negative mutation in CDMP1. Nature Genet 17:58-64.

30. Polinkovsky A., Robin NH, Thomas JT, Irons M, Lynn A, Goodman FR, Reardon W, Kant SG, Brunner HG, Van der Berg I, Chitayat D, McGaughran J, Donnai D, Luyten FP, Warman ML 1997 Mutations in CDMP1 cause autosomal dominant brachydactyly type C. Nature Genet 17:18-19.

31. Vortkamp A, Lee K, Lanske B, Segre GV, Kronenberg HM, Tabin CJ 1996 Regulation of rate of chondrocyte differentiation by indian hedgehog and PTH-related protein. Science 273:613-621.

32. Lyons K, Hogan BLM, Robertson E 1995 Colocalization of BMP7 and BMP2 mRNA suggests that these factors cooperatively mediate tissue interactions during murine development. 50:71-83.

33. Vainio S, Karavanova I, Jowett A, Thesleff, I 1993 Identification of BMP-4 as a signal mediating secondary induction between epithelial and mesenchymal tissues during early tooth development. Cell 75:45-58.

34. Thesleff I, Vaahtokari A, Partanen AM 1995 Regulation of organogenesis common molecular mechanisms regulating the development of teeth and other organs. Int. J. Dev. Biol. 39:35-50.

35. Thesleff I., Nieminen P 1996 Tooth morphogenesis and cell differentiation. Curr. Opin. Cell Biol. 8:844-850.

36. King AJ, Marker PC, Seung KJ, Kingsley DM 1994 BMP-5 and molecular, skeletal and soft-tissue alterations in short ear mice. Dev. Biol. 166:112-122.

37. Kingsley DM, Bland AE, Grubber JM, Marker PC, Russell LB, Copeland NG, Jenkins NA 1992 The mouse short ear skeletal morphogenesis locus is associated with defects in a bone morphogenetic member of the TGFß superfamily. cell 71:399-410.

38. Green MC 1958 Effects of the short ear gene in the mouse on cartilage formation in healing bone fractures. J. Exp. Zool. 137:75-88.

39. Lin HY, Wang XF, Ng-Eaton E, Weinberg RA, Lodish HF 1992 Expression cloning of the TGFß type II receptor, a functional transmembrane serine/Tthreonine kinase. Cell 68:775-785.

40. Franzen P, ten Dijke P, Ichijo H, Yamashita H, Schulz P, Heldin C-H, Miyazono K 1993 Cloning of a TGFß type I receptor that forms a heteromeric complex with TGFß type II receptor. Cell 75:681-692.

41. Wrana JL, Attisano L, Wieser R, Ventura F, Massague J 1994 Mechanism of activation of the TGFß receptor. Nature 370:341-347.

42. Liu F, Ventura F, Doody J, Massague J 1995 Human type II receptor for bone morphogenetic proteins (BMPs): Extension of the two-kinase receptor model to the BMPs. Mol Cell Biol 15:3479-3486.

43. Zou H, Wieser R, Massague J, Niswander L 1997 Distinct roles of type I bone morphogenetic protein receptors in the formation and differentiation of cartilage. Genes Dev. 11:2191-2203.

44. Kawakami Y, Ishikawa T, Shimbara M, Tanda N, Enomoto-Iwamoto M, Iwamoto M, Kuwana T, Ueki A, Noji S, Nohno T 1996 BMP signaling during bone pattern determination in the developing limb. Develop. 122:3557-3566.

45. Zhou H, Niswander L 1996 Requirement for BMP signaling in interdigital apoptosis and scale formation. Science 272:738-741.

46. Enomoto-Iwamoto M, Iwamoto M, Mukudai Y, Kawakami Y, Nohno T, Higuchi Y, Takemoto S, Ohuchi H, Noji S, Kurisu K 1998 Bone morphogenetic protein signaling is required for maintenance of differentiated phenotype, control of proliferation, and hypertrophy in chondrocytes. J. Cell Biol 140:409-418.

47. Newfeld SJ, Chartoff EH, Graff JM, Melton DA, Gelbart WM 1996 Mothers against dpp encodes a conserved cytoplasmic protein required in DPP/TGFß responsive cells. Develop. 124:2099-2108.

48. Heldin CH, Miyazono K, ten Dijke P 1997 TGF-ß signalling from cell membrane to nucleus through SMAD proteins. Nature 390:465-471.

49. Kretzchmar M, Massague J 1998 SMADs: mediators and regulators of TGF-ß signaling. Curr. Op. Gen. Dev. 8:103-111.

50. Massague J, Hata A, Liu F 1997 TGF-ß signalling through the Smad pathway. Trends Cell Biol. 7:187-192.

51. Hata A, Lo RS, Wotton D, Lagna G, Massague J 1997 Mutations increasing the auto-inhibition inactivate the tumor suppressors Smad2 and Smad4. Nature 388:82-87.

52. Nakao A, Afrakhte M, Moren A, Nakayama T, Christian JL, Heuchel R, Itoh S, Kawabata M, Heldin NE, Heldin CE, ten Dijke P 1997 Identification of Smad7, A TGFß-inducible antagonist of TGF-ß signaling. Nature 389:631-636.

53. Hayashi H, Abdollah S, Qiu Y, Cai J, Xu YY, Grinnell BW, Richardson MA, Topper JN, Gimbrone MA, Wrana JL, Falb D 1997 The MAD-related protein Smad7 associates with the TGFß receptor and functions as an antagonist of the TGFß signaling. Cell 89:1165-1173.

54. Imamura T, Takase M, Nishihara A, Oeda E, Hanai J, Kawabata M, Miyazono K 1997 Smad6 inhibits signalling by the TGF-ß superfamily. Nature 389:622-626.

55. Muragaki Y, Mundlos S, Upton J, Olsen BR 1996 Altered growth and branching patterns in synpolydactyly caused by mutations in HOXD13. Science 272:448-451.

56. Goff D, Tabin CJ 1997 Analysis of Hoxd-13 and Hoxd-11 misexpression in chick limb reveals that Hox genes affect both bone condensation and growth. Develop. 124: 627-636.

57. Yokouchi Y, Nakazato S, Yamamoto M, Goto Y, Kameda T, Iba H, Kuroiwa A 1995 Misexpression of Hoxa-13 induces cartilage homeotic transformation and changes cell adhesiveness in chick limb buds. Genes Dev. 9:2509-2522.

58. Martin JF, Bradley A, Olson E 1995 The paired-like homeobox gene MHox is required for early events of skeletogenesis in multiple lineages. Genes Dev. 9:1237-1249.

59. Duprez D, Kostakopoulou K, Francis-West PH, Tickle C, Brickell PM 1996 Activation of FGF-4 and HoxD gene expression by BMP-2 expressing cells in the developing chick limb. Develop. 122:1821-1828.

60. Komori T, Yagi H, Nomura S, Yamaguchi A, Sasaki K, Deguchi K, Shimizu Y, Bronson RT, Gao YH, Inada M, Sato M, Okamoto R, Kitamura Y, Yoshiki S, Kishimoto T 1997 Targeted disruption of Cbfa1 results in a complete lack of bone formation owing to maturational arrest of osteoblasts. Cell 89:755-764.

61. Otto F, Thornell AP, Crompton T, Denzel A, Gilmour KC, Rosewell IR, Stamp GWH, Beddington RSP, Mundlos S, Olsen BR, Selby PB, Owen MJ 1997 Cbfa1, a candidate gene for Cleidocranial Dysplasia Syndrome, is essential for osteoblast differentiation and bone development. Cell 89:765-771.

62. Ducy P, Zhang R, Geoffroy V, Ridall AL, Karsenty G 1997 Osf2/Cbfa1: A transcriptional activator of osteoblast differentiation. Cell 89:747-754.

63. Zimmerman LB, De Jesus-Escobar JM, Harland RM 1996 The Spemann organizer signal noggin binds and inactivates bone morphogenetic protein 4. Cell 86:599-606.

64. Piccolo S, Sasai Y, Lu B, De Robertis EM 1996 Dorsoventral patterning in Xenopus: inhibition of ventral signals by direct binding of chordin to BMP-4. Cell 86:589-598.

65. Holley SA, Neul JL, Attisano L, Wrana JL, Sasai Y, O'Connor MB, DeRobertis EM, Ferguson EL 1996 The Xenopus dorsalizing factor noggin ventralizes drosophila embryos by preventing dpp from activating its receptor. Cell 86:607-617.

66. Thomsen GH 1997 Antagonism within and around the organizer: BMP inhibitors in vertebrate body patterning. Trends Genet. 13:209-211.

67. Rickard DJ, Hofbauer LC, Bonde SK, Gori I, Spelsberg TC, Riggs BL 1998 Bone morphogenetic protein 6 production in human osteoblastic cell lines. Selective regulation by estrogen. J. Clin. Invest 101:413-422.

68. Boden SD, Hair G, Titus L, Racine M, McCuaig K, Wozney JM, Nanes MS 1997 Glucocorticoid-induced differentiation of fetal rat calvarial osteoblasts os mediated by bone morphogenetic protein 6. Endocrinol. 138:2820-2828.

69. Boden SD, McCuaig K, Hair G, Racine M, Titus L, Wozney JM, Nanes MS 1997 Differential effects and glucocorticoid potentiation of bone morphogenetic protein action during rat osteoblast differentiation in vitro. Endocrinol. 137:3401-3407.

Acknowledgments

We would like to thank Tony Celeste, Karen Cox and Helene George for their help with this manuscript.

3 Genetics of Osteoporosis

John S. Adams, M.D.

Introduction

Practitioners of clinical medicine in the Western World, whether primary care providers or subspecialists, are seeing more and more patients with osteoporosis. We propose two central explanations for this reality. As stated in the introductory chapter of this text, the first reason is that low bone mineral density (BMD) and resultant skeletal fragility is becoming more prevalent in our aging society. Using only dual energy x-ray absorptiometry (DEXA) measurements of femoral BMD from the third National Health and Nutrition Examination Survey (NHANES III, 1988-1994), the prevalence of osteoporosis (defined by the [WHO] as BMD>2.5 standard deviations [SD] below the mean of young, nonhispanic white females at peak bone mass) in women 50 years and older in the United States is 13-18% of the population or 4-6 million women (1). The prevalence of osteopenia (BMD>1.0 SD below peak bone mass) ranges from 37-50% of this population or 13-17 million women in the >50 age group (1). Furthermore, the percentage of currently osteopenic patients who will develop osteoporosis is projected to increase at a rate of 2% per year well into the 21rst century (2) if we do nothing to prolong the onset of this disease.

The second reason why practitioners are seeing more patients with osteoporosis is that awareness of the disease has increased dramatically in just the last few years. The genesis of this increase in disease awareness can be traced back to the female American public. When recently polled (NORA; 3), 5700 American women considered osteoporosis as the most worrisome accompaniment of menopause; on the other hand, in the same poll only 25% of the 100 physicians providing primary care for these 7500 women in the >50 age group were aware of the current WHO criteria for making the diagnosis of osteoporosis despite the fact that over 50% of these 7500 women had a BMD in the osteopenic or osteoporotic range (3). Increased awareness also resulted from the release by the FDA of three new drugs in the last three years for the treatment and prevention of osteoporosis. Advertising of these drugs has been very effective, with women often asking their physician about utility of these agents. In turn, the release of these drugs has led to a 6-fold increase in the number DEXA machines operating in the United States from 1995 to 1997 and a similar increase in the number of BMD evaluations performed on those machines (L. Sherwood, personal communication).

Genetics as a Critical Factor in Determining Susceptibility to Osteoporosis

As will be addressed in subsequent chapters in this book, there are a number of factors that contribute to the osteoporotic phenotype. Why is it then that genetic, and not environmental, factors are emerging as the most important predictors of who will develop osteoporosis? The first reason is a practical one. We simply can no longer afford to just treat this disease after it is manifest. At its current prevalence growth rate of greater than 2% per year in our population, it is estimated that by the year 2025 it will cost $62 billion dollars a year just to take care of the anticipated half million broken hips which will occur in our population (2). Therefore, financial necessity demands that we be able to predict those subjects who are most at risk for osteoporosis and then prevent or, at the very least, prolong the onset of the disease.

The second reason why knowing the genes for osteoporosis is important is that it will permit targeted drug development. Although they are superior to what we used to have at our disposal, all of the currently available drugs for treatment of osteoporosis are, relatively speaking, therapeutic 'sledgehammers' for the osteoclast. None were prospectively designed to interrupt a specific intracellular pathway in the bone-resorbing cell. Moreover, the dominant antiresorptive effect of the best of these drugs (4) appears to be relatively short-lived. In other words, these agents are a way of "buying some time". If one regards postmenopausal bone loss over time as a downward sloping line that eventually crosses the fracture threshold, current therapies can effect a transient increase in bone mass that will delay the time at which the patient crosses that fracture threshold. If this interval increase in BMD and skeletal stability does not keep pace with modern medicine's capacity to increase an individual's life-span, then we will still be losing ground to the disease. So, instead of relying solely on a temporary depression of bone resorption, it makes sense to initially or even coincidentally enhance bone formation, remembering that it is the relative balance between the numbers and activities of the major bone cell types, the bone-forming osteoblast and bone - resorbing osteoclast, that determines net bone mass over time.

Figure 1. Relationship Between Bone Cell Activity and Bone Mass Over Time

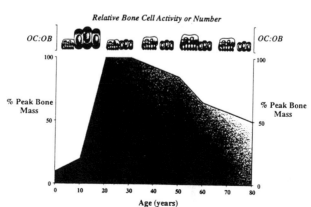

A schematic of this relationship in bone cell activity and bone mass over the human aging process is shown in **Figure 1**. Beginning in early adolescence there is a sizable relative increase in osteoblastic activity that translates into an 80% increase in bone mass in the span of just a few years. Peak bone mass is achieved near the end of the second decade (5,6). Osteoclast and osteoblast activities then stay in sink with one another, keeping bone mass relatively stable; this period of static bone mass varies somewhat depending on the skeletal site. However, thereafter osteoclast activity outstrips osteoblast activity, resulting in a decline in bone mass that can be accelerated by gonadal steroid withdrawal. The end result is that it requires an individual 50-60 years to loose 50% of the bone mass which was accumulated in just 5 or 6 years during adolescence. With the possible exception of prolonged immobilization and immunosuppressant (i.e glucocorticoid) administration, the major determinant of how much bone one has at age 80 is dependent on how much one has accumulated by the age of 20. In turn, the major determinant of how much bone we have at peak bone mass is genetic. Hence, identifying the genes responsible for acquisition of peak bone mass should eventually lead to the design of new drugs that target a specific, gene-directed pathway in the osteoblast, increasing osteoblast activity, numbers or both. Ideally then, genetically manipulating a specific pathway in the bone forming cell should permit either 1] an increase in the rate at which one acquires bone mass during adolescence and/or 2] prolongation of the period of bone mass development, providing any individual the opportunity to loose more bone before crossing the fracture threshold.

The third reason why genetics is becoming a principal focus in this disease is the extraordinarily rapid progress being made in sequencing the human genome. If it remains on target, the Human Genome Project will provide the requisite data base for identification by positional cloning strategies of each of 70,000 genes represented in the human genome. An example of extraordinary progress made possible by the Human Genome Project was recently pointed out by Mary-Claire King, co-discoverer of the first breast cancer-associated gene (7). It took her laboratory 17 years to succeed in cloning the first breast cancer-associated gene in the early 1990s. By comparison, using similar cloning strategies but with a much better genome map, only two years were required for investigators to identify the first prostate cancer-associated gene.

How Important, How Many, and Which Genes Are Involved in Determining Susceptibility to Osteoporosis?

The short answers to these questions are that: 1] genetics are the most important factor in determining susceptibility to this disease; 2] osteoporosis is likely to be a polygenic disorder (it is clearly not a monogenic, Mendelian disease like sickle cell anemia, nor is it likely to be a single-gene dominant disorder like breast cancer); and 3] despite the intense investigation of some candidates, we have not yet identified a single gene which is genetically linked to the osteoporosis phenotype.

The primary determinant of fracture risk at any site is the bone mineral content at that site (8), with a substantial upswing in relative risk of hip fracture once hip BMD approaches a value 2.5 SD below peak bone mass. The major determinant of BMD is peak bone mass, and peak bone mass is genetically determined. The contribution of genetics to peak bone mass is best illustrated by twin studies. The largest and most informative of these studies comes from the work of the late Charles Slemenda and his colleagues (9). They assessed the intraclass variation, or the fraction of the variance in BMD attributable to heredity alone, between 124 monozygotic and 47 dizygotic female twin pairs. They found that 85% and 81% of the variation in BMD at the spine and hip, respectively, was heritable. These extraordinarily high estimates of heritability could not be explained away on the basis of unequal environmental co-variance between monozygotic and dizygotic twins; when data were adjusted to control for height, weight, age and environment, estimates of heritability increased to near 100% or complete heritability of the trait. Importantly, the rate of bone loss in this and more recent studies was not heritable, suggesting that only the upslope of the BMD line shown in **Figure 1** is genetically-determined. This is not to say that some of the same gene products which control acquisition of bone mass may not be playing an important role in bone loss, only that their concerted expression is not genetically determined.

One would predict from this that the heritable nature of osteoporosis can also be borne out in family studies, where one looks at untwined same-sex siblings as well as their mothers and fathers and sons and daughters. In fact, from interviewing family members of patients with osteoporosis, one can develop empiric risk estimates for the disease. In our own survey (10) of more than 1000 family members of nearly 100 Caucasian subjects of Ashkenazi Jewish extraction, we found that if either parent has clinical osteoporosis, then female and male offspring harbor 25% and 5% life-long chance of developing an osteoporotic fracture, respectively. Furthermore, we found that age- and sex-normalized BMD values (at either hip or lumbar spine) of the female siblings of the probands as well as offspring of the probands at or near peak bone mass were significantly below normal. Although the phenotype of low BMD is relatively easily quantitated with considerable precision and BMD appears to be the major risk factor for fracture, the macroarchitecture or geometry of bone, the microarchitecture of bone, particularly in the femoral neck, as well as the propensity to fall are also heritable and contribute independently to fracture risk (11).

Finding Osteoporosis Genes

If this is a genetic disease, then how does one go about finding the 5-10 genes responsible for the osteoporosis phenotype among the 50,000-100,000 present in the human genome? There are two general approaches. The first is a candidate approach, and the second is a positional cloning approach; in either, the use of linkage analyses where one demonstrates coinheritance of a genotype and a phenotype in highly-related populations (i.e twins or sib-pairs) of the same ethnic descent (i.e. the Amish or Mormons) is considered to be more powerful and informative than so-called association studies, where the study population is unrelated and hence more genetically heterogeneous (12). In the positional cloning approach one tries to prove that a genomic locus, not a necessarily a specific gene, is in linkage disequilibrium with the phenotype. This is accomplished by surveying several hundred polymorphic (highly variable) genetic markers that are distributed throughout the human genome. Because of positional conservation of genes, if one of these markers is statistically-linked to the osteoporosis phenotype, then the marker will describe an area of the genome which harbors the disease-causing gene(s). In the candidate gene approach, the polymorphic marker and the disease-associated gene locus are one in the same. Hence, if the phenotype is more highly statistically-linked to this than any other neighboring locus, then the polymorphism will describe the genomic region harboring one or more of the disease-causing genes. The obvious advantage to the candidate gene approach is that a "good guess" for a disease-causing gene will narrow considerably the region of genome that must be searched for the gene of interest. In fact, a highly informative polymorphism in the disease-causing gene may actually lead one directly to the gene on interest.

Table I. Candidate Osteoporosis Genes

Bone Formation	*Bone Resorption*
• VDR	• VDR
• ER & AR	• ER & AR
• IGFs, IGFBPs & IGFr	• cathepsin K
• type I collagen	• integrin family
• SOX gene family	• LIF/IL-6 family
• BMP/TGF family	• TGFß
• gla protein family	• CSF family
• PTH & PTHr	• osteoprotegrin/TNFr family
• core-binding factor	
• *11q12-13 trait**	

* high bone mineral density trait

Candidate Approach to Finding Osteoporosis Genes. As demonstrated in **Table I**, there are a number of candidate genes that have been proposed to be associated with the phenotype of low or high bone mass. Some are involved with the process of bone formation and others with osteoclastic bone resorption. Some of these candidates, like the vitamin D receptor (VDR), the estrogen receptor, and the col1A1 gene have been shown to be associated with the osteoporotic phenotype (13); in cross sectional population studies all three of these genes have been shown to be statistically significantly associated with the phenotype of low bone density. However, this association has not held up (14,15) or not yet been performed in more rigorous linkage studies where large numbers of highly-related family members have been studied. The most intensively-studied candidate gene is, of course, the VDR. Current evidence (16) suggests that it is not itself one of disease-causing genes, but rather that it is in linkage disequilibrium with a nearby gene which is responsible for part of the osteoporosis phenotype. As the density of informative markers in this area of the genome increases, it can be anticipated that linkage of the VDR and the gene responsible for disease can be more precisely defined.

Another candidate-like approach to finding osteoporosis genes is the use of expressed sequence tags or ESTs. This method, designed by Drs. Hazeltine and Ventner (17), is based on high through-put, random sequencing of cDNAs from a pre-selected or candidate cell that is considered to be important in the disease process. In this method a cDNA library from the cell of interest is prepared. Clones from the library are randomly selected, and 300-500 bp of sequence is obtained from each of the clones. Those sequences are then analyzed in a sequence data base, looking for novel or conserved sequences that are particularly enriched in the cDNA library for that cell; unique and/or highly-expressed cDNAs are likely to be particularly important to the function of that cell.

The research group at SmithKline (18) has used this approach to identify what may be an osteoporosis-associated gene. These investigators targeted cells from a human osteoclastoma as a source of RNA. This tumor is highly enriched in cells that display the phenotype of a mature osteoclast. 9300 ESTs were generated from the osteoclastoma cDNA library. About 300 or 4% of those ESTs were found to be homologous with cDNAs coding for proteins in the cathepsin family. These same ESTs were shown to be rarely expressed in cDNA libraries from human tissues. The most abundant EST was determined to be cathepsin K. Cathepsin K is a cystiene protease that acts as a collagenase at low pH as is found under the ruffled border of bone-resorbing osteoclasts, and inhibitors of cathepsin K have recently been shown to inhibit bone resorption in vitro and in animals. As a result of these studies, SmithKline is targeting cathepsin K inhibitors as therapeutic agents for osteoporosis. While the EST approach may be useful in drug development, it is biased in terms of gene discovery. It targets the active osteoclast but ignores the osteoblast lineage as well as the critical steps of osteoclast stem cell maturation and osteoclast apoptosis, both of which may as or more important than osteoclast activity per se in determining bone loss.

Positional Cloning Approach to Finding Osteoporosis Genes. Because of the failure of the candidate approach to provide definitive proof of an osteoporosis-causing gene, it is the view of a growing number of investigators (15) that a better genetic study would not be biased by a candidate approach. Such a study would instead rely on performance of a high-density (i.e. ~500 markers) whole genome scan in genetically homogeneous study populations with the use of more specific phenotyping tools (i.e. quantitative computed tomography of specific bones in young adults at or near peak bone mass; 19). Human linkage studies like these, seeking to identify genomic loci statistically linked to the osteoporosis phenotype, are underway in a number of institutions, but no low BMD-linked genes have yet been identified. A locus on chromosome 11 (11q12-13) associated with high, not low, bone mass has recently been identified in a large kindred (20). Mapping of this genomic region is underway, but no gene responsible for the phenotype of high BMD in this family has been identified.

One way to speed up the positional cloning process is to do the linkage studies in species other than Homo sapiens. As will be discussed more thoroughly in the following chapter by Klein, there are several advantages to this approach, particularly in the mouse. First, unlike humans, environmental factors for mice can be strictly controlled. Second, among mouse strains, there is great variability in the phenotype of interest (i.e. bone mass) despite similarity in size and weight. Third, like that of the human, 80% of BMD in the mouse is heritable. Fourth, the mouse genome map is currently more dense than the human map. And fifth, mice are more efficiently bred than humans and most other mammals.

Such an experiment in the quantitative trait locus (QTL) mapping of mouse genes associated with high and low bone density is currently underway at the Jackson Labs (21). There investigators have performed an inbred strain cross with a mouse of low and another with relatively high peak bone mass. At 12 weeks, or the time of maximum total body bone mass, the F1 generation of this cross had BMDs that were intermediate between parents, while the F2 generation BMD was normally distributed through the parental range of BMD. A genome scan of mice with the lowest BMD identified a number of significantly-associated QTLs, one of which on mouse chromosome 3 was estimated to account for 11% of the variability in BMD. Another advantage of proceeding with positional cloning in mice instead of man is the ability to "Mendelize" an osteoporosis locus. For example, once a phenotype of interest has been identified in the F2 generation, with repeated backcrosses of this mouse with low BMD and the background strain, it becomes possible to separate and isolate in a single mouse the various osteoporosis-associated loci that are responsible for the phenotype of low BMD. In essence this process of "Mendelizing" the trait converts a multiple-locus problem into a series of single locus or single gene solutions for the cause of low BMD. Because there is a high degree positional conservation of genes in mouse and man, the syntenic human loci bearing these genes can be easily identified and searched for the human homolog of the mouse osteoporosis gene. This notion will be reinforced by Dr. Klein in the following chapter in his discussion of animal models of this human disease.

References

1. Looker AC, Orwoll ES, Johnston CC Jr., Lindsay RL, Wahner HW, Dunn WL, Calvo MS, Harris TB, Heyse SP 1997 Prevalence of low femoral bone density in older U.S. adults from NHANES III. J Bone Miner Res 12(11):1761-1768.

2. Ray NF, Chan JK, Thamer M, Melton III LJ 1997 Medical expenditures for the treatment of osteoporotic fractures in the United States in 1995: report from the National Osteoporosis Foundation. J Bone Miner Res 12(1):24-35.

3. Epstein RS, Sherwood LM 1996 From outcomes research to disease management: a guide for the perplexed. Ann Int Med 124(9):838-842.

4. Liberman UA, Weiss SR, Broll J, Minne HW, Quan H, Bell NH, Rodriquez-Portales J, Downs RW Jr., Dequeker J, Favus M, Seeman E, Recker RR, Capizzi T, Santora AC II, Lombardi A,

Shah RV, Hirsch LJ, Karpf DB 1995 Effect of oral alendronate on bone mineral density and the incidence of fractures in postmenopausal osteoporosis. N Engl J Med 22:1437-1443.

5. Matkovic V, Jelic T, Wardlaw GM, Llich JZ, Goel PK, Wright JK, Andon MB, Smith KT, Heaney RP 1994 Timing of peak bone mass in Caucasian females and its implication for the prevention of osteoporosis. J Clin Invest 93:799-808.

6. Teegarden D, Proulx WR, Martin BR, Zhao J, McCabe GP, Lyle RM, Peacock M, Slemenda C, Johnston CC, Weaver CM 1995 Peak bone mass in young women. J Bone Miner Res. 10:711-715.

7. King MC. 1997 Leaving Kansas...finding genes in 1997. Nat Genetics 15:8-11.

8. Cummings SR, Black D 1995 Bone mass measurements and risk of fracture in Caucasian women: a review of findings from prospective studies. Am J Med 98(suppl 2A):24-28.

9. Slemenda CW, Christian JC, Williams CJ, Norton JA, Johnston CC Jr 1991 Genetic determinants of bone mass in adult women: a reevaluation of the twin model and the potential importance of gene interaction on heritability estimates. J Bone Miner Res 6:561-567.

10. Henderson LB, Scheuner MT, Goldstein DR, Martin L, Adams J, Rotter JI 1997 Emperic risk estimates for osteoporosis. J Invest Med 45:94A.

11. Slemenda CW, Turner CH, Peacock M, Christian JC, Sorbel J, Hui SL, Johnston CC 1996 The genetics of proximal femur geometry, distribution of bone mass and bone mineral density. Osteoporosis Int 6:178-182.

12. Econs MJ, Speer MC 1996 Genetic studies of complex diseases: let the reader beware. J Bone Miner Res 11(12):1835-1839.

13. Ralston SH 1997 The genetics of osteoporosis. Oxford Univ Press 90:247-251.

14. Hustmeyer FG, Peacock M, Hui S, Johnston CC, Christian J 1994 Bone mineral density in relation to polymorphism at the vitamin D receptor gene locus. J Clin Invest 94:2130-2134.

15. Peacock M 1995 Vitamin D receptor genes alleles and osteoporosis: a contrasting view. J Bone Miner Res 10:1294-1297.

16. Cooper GS, Umbach DM 1996 Are vitamin D receptor polymorphisms associated with bone mineral density? A meta-analysis. J Bone Miner Res 11(12):1841-1849.

17. Haseltine WA 1997 Discovering genes for new medicines. Scient Am 92-97.

18. Drake FH, Dodds RA, James, IE, Connor JR, Debouck C, Richardson S, Lee-Rykaczewski E, Coleman L, Rieman D, Barthlow R, Hastings G, Gowen M 1996 Cathepsin K, but not cathepsins B, L, or S, is abundantly expressed in human ospteoclasts. J Biol Chem 271:12511-12516.

19. Gilsanz V, Kovanlinkaya A, Costin G, Roe TF, Sayre J, Kaufman F 1997 Differential effect of gender on the sizes of the bones in the axial and appendicular skeletons. J Clin Endocrinol Metab 82:1603-1607.

20. Johnson ML, Gong G, Kimberling W, Recker SM, Kimmel DB, Recker RR 1997 Linkage of a gene causing high bone mass to human chromosome 11 (11q12-13). Am J Hum Genet 60:1326-1332.

21. Rosen CJ, Dimai HP, Vereault D, Donahue LR, Beamer WG, Farley J, Linkhart S, Linkhart T, Mohan S, Baylink DJ 1997 Circulating and skeletal insulin-like growth factor-I (IGF-I) concentrations in two inbred strains of mice with different bone mineral densities. Bone 21:217-223.

4 Genetic Strategies in Preclinical Osteoporosis Research

Robert F. Klein, M.D.

Introduction

Osteoporosis is a disease characterized by an inadequate amount and/or faulty structure of bone, which increases the susceptibility to fracture with minimal trauma. Osteoporotic fractures are most commonly observed among the elderly. Yet the pathogenesis of osteoporosis starts early in life, leading some researchers to view osteoporosis as a pediatric disease (1). Susceptibility to osteoporosis appears to involve the interaction of multiple environmental and genetic factors. Considerable past research has centered on the influence of reproductive, nutritional and/or life-style factors on the development of osteoporosis. With the advent of new molecular genetic approaches, the focus of research has recently shifted towards genetic factors. Genetic epidemiological studies provide convincing descriptive data including population and ethnic differences, studies of familial aggregation, familial transmission patterns, and comparisons of twin concordance rates that a significant part of the vulnerability to developing osteoporosis is inherited. Almost certainly, the development of osteoporosis will be found to involve a complex interplay between both genetic and environmental factors that are difficult to control in complex populations.

Low bone mineral density (BMD), independent of other factors such as falls and aging, is the strongest known determinant of osteoporotic fracture risk (2-4). Bone mineral density (BMD) behaves as a quantitative (polygenic) trait. That is BMD *per se* shows continuous variation, and discrete phenotypes are not generally discernible by studying the frequency distributions for bone density. Continuous variation is the consequence of the additive effects of genes (alleles) at multiple genetic loci that influence bone mass. Polygenic inheritance for bone density makes sense, since bone mass is known to be influenced by multiple biochemical, mechanical and physiological systems, each of which may have its own genetic inputs. The challenge is to characterize these multiple genetic inputs (5). Quantitative traits pose new problems for gene cloning experiments. The DNA sequence variants that are responsible for them are unlikely to be immediately recognizable. In contrast to many qualitative traits where a discrete phenotypic difference is often the consequence of an inactivating mutation, the allelic variation responsible for quantitative traits probably has a subtler basis.

There are two general approaches to the genetic basis of individuality in complex traits: candidate gene analysis and quantitative trait locus (QTL) analysis. Candidate gene analysis seeks to test the association between a particular genetic variant (i.e., allele) and a specific trait. If the variant is more frequent in subjects with the trait than those without it, one can infer that either there is a causal relationship between the genetic variant and the trait or the variant is in linkage disequilibrium with a responsible gene residing near the locus in question. Although a straightforward enterprise, osteoporosis researchers employing candidate gene analysis face a dilemma. Given the complexity of skeletal physiology, there are likely to be an incredibly large number of candidate genes responsible for the acquisition and maintenance of bone mass. Analysis of each one of these candidates, in isolation of the others, is likely to be prohibitive and difficult to interpret statistically and biologically (6,7). In contrast, QTL analysis involves a true search for genes at different chromosomal locations without any assumptions about the candidacy of particular genes or genomic regions. A QTL is defined as a site on a chromosome whose alleles influence a quantitative trait. The overall genetic control of a quantitative trait generally results from the collective influence of many genes, each of which may contribute only a small amount to the genotypic variance, making their identification difficult. This previously daunting task has been made feasible through the recent implementation of technologies to identify genetic variation (polymorphisms) at landmark spots along the human genome (marker loci) and the development of statistical methods to detect and genetically map the chromosomal locations of QTLs (6,8-12). QTL analyses typically involve gathering a large number of related subjects thought to be segregating for genes that influence a given trait, and then following the transmission of allelic variants of marker loci from one relative to another. If polymorphisms at a particular marker locus segregate with genes apparently influencing the presence of the trait in question, then one can infer that a gene actually influencing the trait resides near, or is linked to, the marker locus. QTL mapping can be a powerful strategy for the study of inherited diseases in humans: genes are localized by linkage analysis and then cloned based on chromosomal position (13). The approach has proved successful for a variety of human diseases having simple Mendelian inheritance (14,15). However, the approach is more problematic for human diseases with complex inheritance patterns (16). Most human QTL analyses have, thus far, failed to detect genes with small to moderate effects and rarely, if ever, are designed to simultaneously assess multiple gene and environmental effects (17-20). Moreover, analyses designed to refine the chromosomal position of QTLs may require finding a large number of families each with individuals possessing the disease of interest. This is likely to be extremely costly, and may also create other problems. Families with different environmental exposures and genetic and ethnic backgrounds may enter into the sample, creating heterogeneity, and thereby increase the amount of noise obscuring the signal of a given QTL effect (21).

To overcome problems plaguing genome-wide searches for complex disease, it is necessary to reduce the impact of other factors surrounding the effect of individual genes. Workers investigating determinants of bone mass in humans have limited ability to intervene in the genetics, personal environment, or skeletal biology of their subjects. In a complex disorder such as osteoporosis, experimental approaches that can either manipulate or hold constant biological variables that determine BMD provide a crucial opportunity to systematically examine the pathophysiologic processes that contribute to osteoporosis vulnerability. Animal research can help to elucidate possible roles of genetic and environmental constituents in the regulation of bone mass that might be otherwise difficult to untangle. While the genetic basis for some extreme phenotypes might be due to the deletion of a gene or to an inactivating mutation, it is much more likely that extremes of BMD are due to subtle changes in gene expression, perhaps developmental genes early in life or possibly arising from allelic differences in untranslated regions of the genome that contain sequences controlling gene expression. Consequently, it will be very hard to devise a way of proving that a candidate gene really does underlie the phenotype. There may be no discernible sequence or expression difference to identify the gene, and even if there is, its presence does not prove etiological significance. While association studies can go some way to implicating a particular genetic locus, they can never be proof of a causal relation. For this a functional assay is needed: a way to alter the genetic sequence and see whether this modification results in a different phenotype. Such experiments are possible only in animals and may be the sole way to understand how genetic differences result in individual variation in bone mass (22). This chapter deals with preclinical research and entirely with genetic animal models. The intent is to indicate strategies that have been productive in recent years, and highlight future applications in the area.

Genetic Animal Models of Osteoporosis

Animal models are clearly limited in their ability to precisely mimic all aspects of the human condition. However, such studies do provide the experimental control of genetic and physiological manipulations essential to thoroughly explore mechanisms that contribute to vulnerability. Animal studies can thus serve to define the limits of possible genetic contributions to human osteoporosis. A number of *in vivo* animal models have been shown to emulate many of the most important clinical features of the developing and aging human skeleton.

An ideal model that can be used for all studies in bone research does not exist. Whether or not an animal model is useful depends largely on the specific objectives of the study and frequently involves tradeoffs between such factors as realism, reproducibility of results and feasibility. Birds, mice, rats, rabbits, dogs, sheep, pigs, and nonhuman primates have all been the subject of experimental osteoporosis research (23-25). Each of these animal systems has its own advantages and disadvantages in regard to the following parameters: the similarity of skeletal metabolism and experimental bone disease to human processes, the time needed for breeding and for skeletal development, the cost of acquiring and maintaining the animals, and the ability to take advantage of both classical genetic techniques and the more recently developed molecular genetic techniques to introduce or eliminate specific genes. The obvious requirement for a reasonably detailed knowledge of basic genomic structure currently limits the choice for genetic animal models of osteoporosis to mice, rats and nonhuman primates.

Mice and rats are by far the most commonly used animals in bone research. Both mice and rats reach peak bone mass early in their life span and then undergo bone loss with aging (26-30). Following ovariectomy, a reduction in bone mass and strength occurs, that can be prevented by estrogen replacement (31-36). The SAM/P6 (senescence accelerated mouse/prone) mouse has low peak bone mass and develops fractures in middle and old age (37-44). It is the *only* experimental animal model with documented fragility fractures of aging. Histomorphometric studies of primates and humans yield very similar values (45). The nonhuman primate has both growing and adult skeletal phases. Peak bone mass occurs around age 9 years in cynomologus macaques (46) and around 10-11 years in rhesus monkeys (47,48). Nonhuman primates experience decreased bone mass after ovariectomy (49-51), but the response to estrogen replacement has not been well-characterized. Nonhuman primates experience bone loss with age (52,53) but older animals also develop osteoarthritis with spinal osteophyte formation (54-56) that can obscure the accurate radiographic assessment of spinal bone mass (57). The extreme requirements for housing and care of nonhuman primates limit their use to a relatively small number of facilities.

Of the three currently available options, the mouse is arguably the model of choice because: (1) mice are much cheaper to house and easier to handle; (2) mouse genetic resources are quite extensive; and (3) once candidate genes are identified, the ability to manipulate them in mice and to deduce unambiguously their role in disease is unparalleled (58,59). Moreover, gene targeting has reached new heights in mice, but is barely on the horizon in other animals. With gene targeting perhaps as the ultimate arbiter for establishing cause-and-effect relationships between a candidate gene and osteoporosis susceptibility, the mouse is apt to remain the primary experimental model system for the foreseeable future (59). However, nonhuman primates maintained in controlled environments are excellent subjects for extended family pedigree analysis (60,61), the most powerful method of establishing genetic linkage to phenotypic traits (6). Combining mouse and nonhuman primate studies to dissect the genetic regulation of bone mass may offer the most expeditious way of identifying relevant hypotheses that are likely to prove fruitful for future exploration in humans.

Current Research: Inbred Strains

A strain of a species is inbred when virtually every genetic locus is homozygous. What this means is that all individuals within an inbred strain share a set of characteristics that uniquely define them compared to other strains. Typically, inbred strains are derived from 20 or more consecutive generations that have been brother x sister mated; the strain can then be maintained with this same pattern of propagation. Individual animals within an inbred strain are as identical as monozygotic twins. There are several qualities of inbred strains that make them especially valuable for research. The first is their long-term relative genetic stability. This is important because it allows researchers to build on previous investigations. Genetic change can occur only as a result of mutation within an inbred strain. A second important quality of inbred animals is their homozygosity because inbred strains will breed true. Once the characteristics of a strain are known they can be reproduced repeatedly allowing for replicate experimentation as well as for studies by other investigators. The influence of genotype upon a particular characteristic can be investigated by placing mice from several inbred strains in a common environment. Observed differences must then be, within limits, the consequence of genetic factors. By reversing this strategy, and placing mice from a single inbred strain in a variety of environments, it is possible to estimate the importance of environmental influences upon a parameter of interest. Thus, inbred animals can be used to determine whether genetic variation in the expression of a characteristic exists and the environmental malleability of the characteristic. Experiments with inbred strains also have some limitations. While strain differences are easily demonstrated, it is often very difficult to attach much meaning to these differences, because the genes and gene products involved are usually unknown. Because comparisons of mice from two or more strains do not usually provide any information about the nature of the genetic differences, crosses between genotypes must be used to analyze patterns of genetic influence. Additionally, when using an inbred strain to investigate any type of phenomenon, it is important to be aware that the observations may be relevant only to that strain. Because an inbred strain differs from all others, there will be characteristics unique to it. It is therefore, important to use more than one strain to confirm that any observation obtained pertains to the species and not just to the strain studied.

Inbred mice of different strains exhibit marked differences in parameters of skeletal integrity. Kaye and Kusy (62) examined bone tissue from five inbred mouse strains (A/J, BALB/CByJ, C57BL/6J, DBA/2J and PL/J). Although body weight was similar in all five strains, tibial bone mass, composition and biomechanical strength varied considerably. Using peripheral quantitative computed tomography, Beamer et al (63) surveyed female mice from 11 inbred strains (AKR/J, BALB/cByJ, C3H/HeJ, C57BL/6J, C57L/J, DBA/2J, NZB/B1NJ, SM/J, SJL/BmJ, SWR/BmJ and 129/J). This postmortem study found that phenotypically normal inbred strains of mice possess remarkable differences in total femoral BMD that were detectable as early as two months of age. Since these genetically distinct strains of mice were raised in the same controlled environment the observed differences are, in all likelihood, the result of genetic variation. Subsequent endocrinologic studies of F_2 progeny from a cross between C3H/HeJ and C57BL/6J found that those mice with the highest BMD also had the highest serum insulin-like growth factor-I (IGF-I) levels, whereas the F_2 progeny with the lowest BMD had low IGF-I levels (64). Although more than 35% of the variance in BMD for the F_2 mice could be attributed to serum IGF-I levels, definitive evidence of a causal relationship between circulating IGF-I and BMD will require more extensive functional studies using the two progenitor strains. These preliminary investigations clearly indicate substantial genetic regulation of BMD in mice. Modern genetic methods, such as selective breeding and QTL analysis, can exploit these heritable strain differences to find and more directly evaluate the genetic linkage of osteoporosis-related traits (*vide infra*).

Single Gene Mutations

As described above, the study of inbred strains usually provides very little information about specific mechanisms of gene action. The analysis of single mutant vs. normal genes is often a more effective approach. Comparisons between homozygous mutant mice and their "normal" homozygous wild-type and heterozygous litter mates may provide considerable information on cellular mechanisms critical for discrete aspects of bone biology. Mouse enthusiasts have been breeding mice for centuries, thus maintaining spontaneous mutations. More than 140 spontaneous mutations affecting mouse bone morphology have been summarized by Green (65). For example, the short ear (se/se) mutation is associated with a number of skeletal defects, including reductions in long bone length and width, and the size of several vertebral processes, the absence of several small sesamoid bones and a pair of ribs, and impaired fracture healing (66-68). Recently, investigators discovered that the gene for bone morphogenetic protein-5 is disrupted in short-ear mice (69). There is also an expanding list of induced mutations in mice that cause recognizable skeletal pathology. Several lines of mice with mutations in type I collagen genes have been shown to develop a phenotype of skeletal fragility with extensive fractures of long bones and ribs (70-73). Mutations of a number of genes necessary for normal osteoclast development and/or function have been shown to result in osteopetrosis in mice (74-77).

Recombinant Inbred Strains

Independently inbred strains of mice frequently exhibit numerous phenotypic differences reflecting the substantial allelic variability that can exist between laboratory strains. These differences have been accentuated further by the introduction of recombinant inbred (RI) strains, which are derived by systematic inbreeding starting from a cross between two inbred strains known to differ at some characteristic of interest (**Figure 1**). They are called RI strains because the parental chromosomes are recombined several times per chromosome during their development, resulting in a unique pattern of recombinations of the two initial parental genomes in each RI strain. The starting points are two inbred genotypes that are used to produce a group of F_1 hybrids. Brother x sister pairs of F_1 hybrids are mated to create an F_2 generation, in which all genes now segregate independently. Following the production of an F_2 generation from this interstrain cross, 20 or more different brother-sister pairs of F_2 individuals are mated. In each subsequent generation, only a single male and female from each pair are mated. After 20 generations, one has many inbred lines that differ from each other due to random differences in gene segregation, a process begun with the F_2. All the RI lines contain only those genes that were present in one or another of the parental strains. RI lines have been very useful in genetic mapping of traits that differ between inbred strains

The RI strains were originally developed as a tool for detecting and mapping major gene loci (78). Over the years, the RI strains have been characterized in respect to many genetic markers with known location on different chromosomes.

The influence of a single major gene on a given trait can be inferred when RI strain means for the trait are found to fall in a bimodal distribution (i.e., all the RI strains with one allele are in one phenotypic group and all those with the other allele are in the other group).

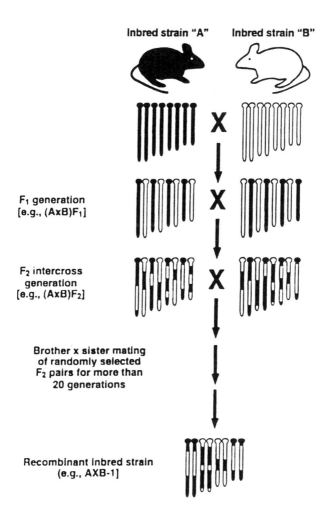

Inbred strain "A"   Inbred strain "B"

F_1 generation
[e.g., (AxB)F_1]

F_2 intercross
generation
[e.g., (AxB)F_2]

Brother x sister mating
of randomly selected
F_2 pairs for more than
20 generations

Recombinant inbred strain
(e.g., AXB-1]

Figure 1. Generation of recombinant inbred strains. Only four of the 19 autosome pairs from parental inbred strains "A" and "B", and the assortment of chromosomes in the subsequent crosses derived from these strains, are shown. F_1 hybrids are genetically identical to each other, but individuals in the subsequent F_2 generation are not because of recombination events. RI strains also harbor recombinations but are homozygous at all loci as a result of the extensive inbreeding involved in their production.

Comparison of the strain distribution pattern (SDP) for that trait can be made with the SDP's for known marker loci previously mapped to a particular chromosome region. A close match in SDP's between the unknown locus and a marker locus would thus allow provisional mapping to a chromosome region of the latter (78,79). Recent advances in statistics have succeeded in tailoring this experimental approach to a broader range of phenotypes, including continuously distributed traits without apparent major gene effects (80-82).

The SAM/P6 mouse strain and the control strain SAM/R1 (senescence accelerated mouse/resistant) were developed by the RI strain technique, though only one of the parental strains (AKR/J) is known (83). Weinstein and Jilka (43) have recently developed a method for BMD determination in live mice by dual-energy X-ray absorptiometry (DEXA). Compared to SAM/R1 mice, SAM/P6 mice undergo progressive bone loss between 3 and 15 months of age (43). Based on a survey of allelic differences in microsatellite markers distributed across the genome, SAM/P6 mice differ from SAM/R1 mice at 39% of their 20 chromosomes (84).

Using similar DEXA technology, Klein *et al* (85) examined peak whole body BMD in female mice from a panel of 24 RI BXD strains, derived from a cross between C57BL/6J and DBA/2J progenitors (79). C57BL/6J and DBA/2J strains have very diverse genetic origins. C57BL/6J mice had their origins in the colony of a mouse fancier, Ms. Abby Lathrop, in the early 1920s. DBA mice came from colonies established by Clarence Cook Little when he was an undergraduate student at Harvard in 1909 (86). Body weights for the two progenitor strains were very similar, but C57BL/6J animals exhibited considerably greater bone mass than their DBA/2J counterparts (63.2 ± 3.3 vs. 55.3 ± 3.3 mg/cm^2, p<0.0001). The distribution of BMD values among the BXD RI strains clearly indicated the presence of strong genetic influences, with an estimated narrow sense heritability of 35%. The pattern of differences in peak whole body BMD in the BXD strains were integrated with a large database of genetic markers previously defined in the RI BXD strains to generate chromosome map sites for trait locations. After correction for redundancy among the significant correlations, analysis of the BXD RI strain series provisionally identified 10 chromosomal sites linked to peak bone mass development in the female. Several of the identified sites map near candidate genes of interest in skeletal biology. The presence of an association between bone density and a site on mouse chromosome 7 is particularly interesting in view of a similar association recently reported between bone density and the syntenic region on chromosome 11 in humans (87).

An especially important feature of the RI method is the fixed nature of the genotypes of each of the RI strains. This means that any new hypothesis about a physiological mechanism underlying a trait can be assessed by making only observations on the new variable, and relating the outcome to the data base already established (88). For example, epidemiological studies have clearly demonstrated that body weight is a very strong predictor of BMD (89-92). However, the mechanism underlying the strong association of weight with BMD is poorly understood. The coincidence of increased body weight with increased BMD could stem from environmental factors such as complementary nutritional effects on body composition and skeletal mass or the association could largely be the result of mechanical loading (93). In addition to environmental causes, body weight and BMD may be modulated by linked genes or perhaps even the same genes. In the BXD RI experiment performed by Klein et al (85), 4 genetic loci for body weight were identified. All 4 of these loci had been previously identified by Keightley et al (94) in a prior analysis of mouse lines divergently selected for body weight from a base population derived from C57BL/6J and DBA/2J parental strains. Interestingly, one locus that was linked to body weight was also strongly linked to inherited variation in BMD. These findings raise the intriguing possibility that body weight and peak BMD may be influenced by linked genes or perhaps by common genes with pleiotropic effects. Furthermore, they demonstrate the increasing value of an RI series as data, both about phenotypes and about genotypes, are gathered from all of the laboratories utilizing them.

There are two additional aspects of the RI approach which deserve comment. First, only a few inbred strains are represented in the existing RI sets (e.g., the BXD RI set is the largest and it currently is composed of only 26 separate strains) and it is not easy to construct new sets. Inasmuch as the strain means are the units of analysis, the statistical power of the RI method is directly related to the number of RI strains within a given set. Thus, genetic associations only above a certain effect size will be discernible with this experimental method. For osteoporosis research purposes, this limitation is only a modest one, as the current objective is simply to identify any relevant genetic associations in either animal models or humans. A second, and perhaps more serious, disadvantage of the RI method is that some genetic correlations of marker and phenotype are likely to be fortuitous. Because of the large number of statistical tests performed (e.g., over 1500 informative genetic markers have been genotyped in the BXD RI strains), the type I error rate relative to a single correlation similarly increases. One way to reduce the chance of such errors is to increase the required significance level and consider only those correlations that are significant at a very high probability (95). However, in choosing this level of stringency, one risks not considering QTLs that may be important (i.e., type II error). A useful compromise is to use a moderately stringent alpha level and regard correlational analysis in RI strains as a preliminary screen for genetic associations to be confirmed using other techniques, such as verification in an F2 population.

QTL Analysis

For a number of reasons, the laboratory mouse has proven to be an especially powerful tool for the identification and mapping of QTLs affecting complex polygenic traits (96). First, there is a wide range of phenotypic variation in genetically characterized animals (97), which is a prerequisite for QTL analysis. Second, factors such as short generation interval, ability to make designed matings and raise very large populations relatively inexpensively, and capacity to control or experimentally alter environmental factors enable QTL experiments in mice to have increased power, precision and flexibility. Third, the mouse has an extensively developed and well-organized molecular marker map, consisting of over 6500 easily typed PCR-based microsatellite markers (98) that exhibit allelic variation between lines. And fourth, the mouse is an anchor species in comparative genome maps representing homology among mammalian species (99). Once a chromosomal region harboring a murine QTL is identified, candidate chromosomal regions in humans where homologous QTLs may reside will be immediately apparent. Based on these attributes, research groups have successfully used mice in QTL detection studies for a number of quantitative traits, including obesity (100), body weight (94), and drug-seeking behavior (101).

Osteoporosis researchers are just now embarking on QTL analyses in large populations of mice in the hopes of obtaining a more complete picture of the polygenic control of bone mass and an improved understanding of the complex interactions and physiological mechanisms involved. The basic strategy of such QTL mapping experiments is outlined in **Figure 2.** Beamer and colleagues examined femoral cortical bone density in 700 F2 progeny from a C57BL/6J and CAST/EiJ cross (102). Significant QTL associations ($p < 0.0001$) were found on three separate chromosomes and five other sites revealed suggestive correlations ($p < 0.01$) worthy of additional investigation. Similar sized projects examining skeletal phenotypes in the F2 progeny of crosses between AKR/J and SAM/P6 and SAM/P6 and SAM/R1 (84) as well as between C57BL/6J and DBA/2J (85) are also currently in progress. Results from these complementary studies should begin to define the landscape of the genetic regulation of BMD and help partition this quantitative trait into separate genetic components amenable for more detailed evaluation.

Studies of Non-human Primates

Captive populations of baboons are another useful resource for genetic studies of common human diseases. The fundamental rationale for using nonhuman primates is their phylogenetic proximity to humans. Chromosomal banding patterns (103) and even gene order (104) is highly conserved between baboons and humans. Just as with rodents, colony mating structures can be arranged to produce optimal pedigree structures for statistical genetic analysis, and prospective matings can be planned to test hypotheses about the inheritance of certain traits or examine interactions between environmental and genetic effects.

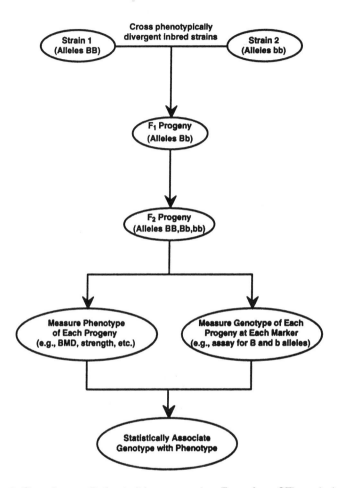

Figure 2 Steps in quantitative trait locus mapping. To perform QTL analysis two different inbred strains are first crossed to produce genetically heterogeneous F_2 progeny. All of the progeny undergo phenotype assessment and then DNA samples are obtained to allow genotyping of each individual at multiple marker loci distributed throughout the genome. Statistical associations of markers and phenotypes are then performed to identify putative QTLs underlying the trait(s) of interest.

The Southwest Foundation for Biomedical Research (SFBR) in San Antonio, Texas presently maintains more than 3000 baboons (Papio hamadryas), with nearly two-thirds of these linked into large pedigrees developed by breeding single males with harems of 10 – 30 females. Some of these pedigrees have already reached five generations, and some sires have yielded over 100 progeny. These extended pedigrees provide the substantial statistical power required for multifactorial genetic analyses of complex, quantitative traits, such as bone density. Moreover, all of these animals are easily accessible for phenotype assessment and genetic sampling, in contrast to large human pedigrees, in which the members are frequently scattered over broad geographic areas.

An initial study utilized radiographic morphometry of the second metacarpal to assess bone mass in 219 baboons from the pedigreed colony at SFBR. Kammerer et al (105) found significant heritabilities for the measures of medullary canal diameter (h2=0.64), the ratio of compact bone width (h2=0.67), and compact bone width (h2=0.40). Subsequently, DEXA technology was used to more directly evaluate BMD in 679 baboons at three spinal sites (thoraco-lumbar vertebrae 15, 16, and 17) and three forearm sites (the ulna and ultra-distal and diaphyseal regions of the radius) (106,107). The heritabilities for these phenotypic measures ranged between 0.3 and 0.5, indicating a significant role of genetic factors in the determination of BMD in baboons (106). Interestingly, modest linkage between BMD and a region on baboon chromosome 11 was recently identified. A similar association exists in humans at a homologous region on human chromosome 11 (87). Estimates of the effect of this QTL on BMD (h2) ranged from 0.13 to 0.20 depending upon the specific skeletal site. These preliminary results indicate that the baboon model is likely to be of considerable use in the ongoing search for genes influencing osteoporosis vulnerability. However, baboon researchers face a significant obstacle. The successful identification of genes that influence a complex multifactorial phenotype (e.g., BMD) requires a relatively dense map of chromosomal markers. The gene map of the baboon (as well as for other nonhuman primates) is rudimentary at best and until lately little effort was being invested to improve the situation (61). Rogers and colleagues at SFBR are in the process of constructing a panel of >300 polymorphic loci distributed across the baboon genome. The chromosomal markers are amplified from baboon DNA by using human PCR primers under slightly modified PCR conditions (104,108). Once the baboon chromosomal map is resolved to 10 – 15cM with those markers, the baboon model should prove to be an invaluable tool for quantitative trait linkage analysis.

Future Directions

QTL analysis promises to identify the chromosomal position of many genes influencing osteoporosis-related traits. However, the ultimate goals of complex trait analysis - to identify coding sequences and to understand their biological roles at a molecular level - remain the major challenge. Initial QTL analyses on an adequately-sized F2 intercross rarely succeed in narrowing map positions to less than 10 - 20cM. This is because the phenotypes of individual animals are easily swayed by the influence of unlinked or environmental noise (59). Positional cloning of human disease genes has demonstrated that even when the position of a gene has been defined within one or two million base pairs and all the DNA sequences within that region have been isolated, identification of the relevant gene can still be a formidable task. Fortunately, new experimental strategies for fine QTL mapping, development of transgenic technologies, and more traditional approaches employing congenic strains, promise to eventually bridge the gap between cloning and disease.

QTL fine mapping involves careful analysis of recombinants within an interval previously found to contain the gene, a concept termed genetic chromosome dissection (GCD). Although GCD was first introduced by Drosophila geneticists (109), this experimental approach has been successfully adapted to animal models (110-112). For a compilation of the various experimental designs currently available, the reader is referred to an excellent recent review by Darvasi (113). One of the most attractive strategies exploits the high mapping resolution present in RI strains (recombinant inbred segregation test, RIST). Using the RIST design, a QTL of moderate effect, previously mapped to a 25 cM interval in an F2 interstrain cross, can be mapped to a 1 cM interval with less than 1000 animals and only two stages of two generations each. Once the QTL has been resolved to such a narrow region, an examination of candidate genes within that region can take place. Several thousand cDNA clones have now been partially sequenced and mapped as expressed sequence tags (ESTs), and the pace is certain to accelerate in the future. This effort will create a map of anonymous genes as candidates for disease whenever a region is spotlighted by human or animal linkage studies. This new resource is likely to transform current positional cloning strategy into a positional candidate approach in the future.

Transgenic technology creates a very effective tool for analyzing the physiological roles of specific genes. A transgenic animal contains a segment of exogenous genetic material stably incorporated into its genome, resulting in a new trait that can be transmitted to further generations. Two widely used methods introduce exogenous genetic material into the genome: 1) microinjection of one-cell fertilized embryos and 2) genetic manipulation of embryonic stem (ES) cells. In contrast to traditional "gain-of-function" mutations, typically created by microinjection of the gene of interest into the one-celled zygote, gene-targeting via homologous recombination in pluripotential ES cells allows one to precisely modify the gene of interest (114). Employing ES methodology, investigators have generated site-specific deletions ("knock-outs"), insertions ("knock-ins"), gene duplications, gene rearrangements, and point mutations. In addition to facilitating the study of known candidate genes, molecular complementation (transfer of specific genes) of selected phenotypes is a potentially important tool for gene identification. The recent success of transgenic technologies employing yeast artificial chromosomes (YAC transgenics) holds great promise for studying QTLs that influence a developmentally restricted phenotype which requires the transfer of both the locus and the long-range regulatory element(s) responsible for normal temporal or regional expression of the gene (115). Traditionally, the mouse has been considered the optimal animal model for conducting transgenic and gene-targeting experiments. Although investigators have succeeded in creating transgenic rats (116), the considerable time and expense involved limit the feasibility of widespread use of this animal model. Furthermore, gene-targeting technology to "knock-out" endogenous genes is currently feasible only in the mouse.

Classical transmission genetics can also be used to transfer a gene of interest from a donor strain or mutant onto the genetic background of an inbred strain. Using this approach, one is able to transfer regions containing risk or protective QTLs, or even multiple QTLs, onto appropriate background strains. Such congenic strains are produced by repeated backcrossing to the background inbred strain and genotypic selection of the desired allele at a marker or markers at each backcross generation (78,117,118). After 7 backcross generations, the congenic and background strains can be expected to be about 98% genetically identical except for the transferred (introgressed) chromosomal region (118). The primary advantage of the congenics is that the influence of an individual QTL on any trait can be tested using the congenic vs. background strain comparison at any level from the molecular to the physiological. Any differences found would strongly implicate a QTL in the introgressed chromosomal region as the cause of the differences. When there are several congenic strains for a given QTL, their differing sites of recombination can aid in attaining higher resolution mapping of the QTL with respect to neighboring markers. The near elimination of "genetic noise" due to unlinked loci greatly aids the search for candidate genes associated with each QTL, and for studies of differential gene expression (119). The differential region of congenic strains can be small enough to permit chromosome walking to the target gene but still large enough to contain restriction fragment length polymorphisms. Genetically directed representational difference analysis (GDRDA) is a new technique designed to identify previously uncharacterized differences between two DNA samples that are genetically identical except in the region of interest (119). This subtractive technique is unique in that it targets and reveals polymorphic markers linked to a particular trait without prior knowledge of their biochemical function. The ultimate resolution of this approach should be limited only by the actual density of polymorphisms detectable by GDRDA, estimated to be 1 to 2 per megabase. Ultimately, congenic strains can greatly facilitate positional cloning of a QTL. In addition, congenic strains provide an invaluable resource for further defining specific genes of interest and for in depth studies of the mechanisms by which they affect skeletal phenotype.

Conclusion

Peak bone mass is a major determinant of risk of osteoporotic fracture. However, BMD is a complex trait whose expression is complicated by environmental influences and polygenic inheritance. The number, locations and effects of the individual genes contributing to natural variation in this trait are all unknown. Experimental animal models furnish a means to largely circumvent confounding environmental factors, and the availability of dense genetic maps based on molecular markers now provides the opportunity to resolve quantitative genetic variation into individual regions of the genome (QTLs) influencing a given trait. Animals are easily bred to provide the sample sizes needed. Inbred strains are homozygous at all loci. Therefore all members of any inbred strain are genetically identical, eliminating the problem of genetic heterogeneity. Phenotypes can be carefully measured and laboratory conditions held uniform to reduce phenotypic variation.

The systematic analysis of inbred strain databases is beginning to reveal important aspects of the genetic regulation of bone mass acquisition and maintenance. The recent advances in genetic mapping of complex traits, such as QTL mapping, are especially promising. A major strength of this approach is that it enables the provisional identification of candidate genes in the absence of any prior hypothesis about the mechanism by which the phenotype is expressed. The identification of those chromosomal regions where marker allelic and trait variation significantly covary is now a straight-forward (although large-scale) enterprise. QTL mapping offers an attractive interface between forward and reverse genetics. Molecular cloning has shown that almost all genes in mice have homologues in humans, and vice-versa (120). Thus, identification and mapping of genes in the mouse offers immediate hope for extrapolation to the human genome. For the future, more molecularly based techniques are likely to be on the leading edge of progress. As candidate genes are identified as having important skeletal functions, the tools of molecular biology will allow the genetic diversity underlying their expression and function to be more fully examined. Discoveries made with animal models can often set the stage for skeletal research in human subjects to augment the results from animals and confirm their relevance to our own species. Perhaps the most versatile aspect of animal model systems is in their use as a proving ground for hypotheses regarding the genetic as well as the epigenetic basis of osteoporosis. Old ideas regarding disease mechanisms can now be rigorously tested in vivo, and what is more important, provocative new concepts can emerge.

References

1. Matkovic V 1992 Osteoporosis as a pediatric disease: role of calcium and heredity. J Rheum 33(Suppl):54-9.

2. Hui SL, Slemenda CW, Johnston CCJ 1988 Age and bone mass as predictors of fracture in a prospective study. J Clin Invest 81:1804-1809.

3. Cummings SR, Black DM, Nevitt MC, Browner WS, Cauley JA, Genant HK, Mascioli SR, Scott JC, Seeley P, Steiger P, Vogt TM 1990 Appendicular bone density and age predict hip fracture in women. JAMA 263:665-668.

4. Nguyen T, Sambrook P, Kelly P, Jones G, Lord S, Freund J, Eisman J 1993 Prediction of osteoporotic fractures by postural instability and bone density. Br Med J 307:1111-1115.

5. Econs MJ, Speer MC 1996 Genetic studies of complex diseases: let the reader beware. J Bone Miner Res 11:1835-1840.

6. Lander ES, Schork NJ 1994 Genetic dissection of complex traits. Science 265:2037-2048.

7. Risch N, Merikangas K 1996 The future of genetic studies of complex human disease. Science 272:1516-1517.

8. Lander ES, Botstein D 1989 Mapping mendelian factors underlying quantitative traits using RFLP linkage maps. Genetics 121:185-199.

48

9. Dietrich W, Katz H, Lincoln SE, Shin HS, Friedman J, Dracopoli N, Lander ES 1992 A genetic map of the mouse suitable for typing intraspecific crosses. Genetics 131:423-447.

10. Dietrich WF, Miller JC, Steen RG, Merchant M, Damron D, Nahf R, Gross A, Joyce DC, Wessel M, Dredge RD 1994 A genetic map of the mouse with 4,006 simple sequence length polymorphisms. Nature Genet 7:220-245.

11. Weeks DE, Lathrop GM 1995 Polygenic disease: methods for mapping complex disease traits. Trends Genet 11:513-519.

12. Schork N, Chakravarti A 1996 A nonmathematical overview of modern gene mapping techniques applied to human diseases. In: Mockrin S (ed.) Molecular genetics and gene therapy of cardiovascular disease. Marcel Dekker, New York, pp 79-109.

13. Botstein D, White R, Skolnick M, Davis R 1980 Construction of a genetic linkage map in man using restriction fragment length polymorphisms. Am J Hum Genet 32:314-331.

14. Riordan JR, Rommens JM, Kerem Z-S, Alon N, Rozmahel R, Grzeiczak Z, Zielenski J, Lok S, Plvsic N, Chou J-L, Drumm ML, Iannuzzi MC, Collins FS, Tsui L-C 1989 Identification of the cystic fibrosis gene: cloning and characterization of complementary DNA. Science 245:1066-1073.

15. Wallace M, Marchuk D, Andersen L, Letcher R, Odeh H, Saulino A, Fountain J, Brereton A, Nicholson J, Mitchell A, Brownstein B, Collins F 1990 Type 1 neurofibromatosis gene: Identification of large transcript disrupted in three NF1 patients. Science 249:181-186.

16. Lander ES, Botstein D 1986 Mapping complex genetic traits in humans: New strategies using a complete RFLP linkage map. Cold Spring Harbor Symp Quant Biol 51:46-61.

17. Schork NJ 1997 Genetically complex cardiovascular traits: origins, problems, and potential solutions. Hypertension 29:145-149.

18. Schork NJ 1993 Extended multipoint identity-by-descent analysis of human quantitative traits: Efficiency, power, and modeling considerations. Am J Hum Genet 53:1306-1319.

19. Schork NJ, Xu X 1996 Sibpairs versus pedigrees: What are the advantages? Diabetes Reviews 5:1-7.

20. Schork NJ, Nath SP, Lindpaintner K, Jacob HJ 1996 Extensions of quantitative trait locus mapping in experimental organisms. Hypertension 28:1104-1111.

21. Kruglyak L, Lander ES 1995 High-resolution genetic mapping of complex traits. Am J Hum Genet 56:1212-1223.

22. Flint J, Corley R 1996 Do animal models have a place in the genetic analysis of quantitative human beavioural traits? J Mol Med 74:515-521.

23. Miller SC, Bowman BM, Jee WSS 1995 Available animal models of osteopenia - small and large. Bone 17(Suppl):117S-123S.

24. Kimmel DB 1996 Animal models for in vivo experimentation in osteoporosis research. In: Marcus R (ed.) Osteoporosis. Academic Press, Sna Diego, pp 671-690.

25. Aerssens J, Boonen S, Lowet G, Dequeker J 1998 Interspecies differences in bone composition, density, and quality: Potential implications for in vivo bone research. Endocrinol 139:663-670.

26. Bar-Shira-Maymon B, Coleman R, Cohen A, Steinhagen-Thiessen E, Slibermann M 1989 Age-related loss in lumbar vertebrae of CW-1 female mice: A histomorphometric study. Calcif Tiss Int 44:36-45.

27. Weiss A, Arbell I, Steinhagen-Thiessen E, Silbermann M 1991 Structural changes in aging bone: Osteopenia in the proximal femurs of female mice. Bone 12:165-172.

28. Kimmel DB 1992 Quantitative histologic changes in the proximal tibial epiphyseal growth cartilage of aged female rats. Cells Mater 1(Suppl)(11-18).

29. Schapira D, Laton-Miller R, Barzilai D, Silbermann M 1992 The rat as a model for studies of the aging skeleton. Cells Mater 1(Suppl):181-188.

30. Li XJ, Jee WJS, Ke HZ, Mori S, Akamine T 1992 Age-related changes of cancellous and cortical bone histomorphometry in female Sprague-Dawley rats. Cells Mater 1(Suppl):25-37.

31. Suzuki HK 1958 Effects of estradiol-17-ß-n-valerate on endosteal ossification and linear growth in the mouse femur. Endocrinol 60:743-747.

32. Edwards MW, Bain SD, Bailey MC, lantry MM, Howard GA 1992 17-ß-estradiol stimulation of endosteal bone formation in the ovariectomized mouse: An animal model for the evaluation of bone-targeted estrogens. Bone 13:29-34.

33. Donahue LR, Rosen CJ, Beamer WG 1994 Reduced bone density in hypogonadal mice. J Bone Miner Res 9(Suppl 1):S193.

34. Kalu DN 1991 The ovariectomized rat as a a model of postmenopausal osteopenia. Bone Miner 15:175-191.

35. Wronski TJ 1992 The ovariectomized rat as an animal model for postmenopausal bone loss. Cells Mater 1(Suppl):69-74.

36. Mosekilde L, Danielsen CC, Knudsen UB 1993 The effect of aging and ovariectomy on the vertebral bone mass and biomechanical properties of mature rats. Bone 14:1-6.

37. Matsushita M, Tsuboyama T, Kasai R, Okumura H, Yamamuro T, Higuchi K, Coin A, Yonezu T, Utani A, Umezawa M, Takeda T 1986 Age-related changes in the senescence-accelerated mouse (SAM). Am J Pathol 125:276-283.

38. Tsuboyama T, Takahashi K, Matsushita M, Okumura H, Yamamuro T, Umezawa M, Takeda T 1989 Decreased endosteal formation during cortical bone modeling in SAM-P/6 mice with a low peak bone mass. Bone Miner 7:1-12.

39. Tsuboyama T, Matsushita M, Okumura H, Yamamuro T, Hanada K, Takeda T 1989 Modification of strain-specific femoral bone density by bone marrow chimerism in mice: A study on the spontaneously osteoporotic mouse (SAM-P/6). Bone 10:269-277.

40. Takahashi K, Tsuboyama T, Matsushita M, Kasai R, Okumura H, Yamamuro T, Okamoto Y, Toriyama K, Kitagawa K, Takeda T 1994 Modification of strain-specific femoral bone density by bone marrow-derived factors administered neonatally: A study on the spontaneously osteoporotic mouse (SAM-P/6). Bone Miner 23:57-64.

41. Takahashi K, Tsuboyama T, Matsushita M, Kasai R, Okumura H, Yamamuro T, Okamoto Y, Kitagawa K, Takeda T 1994 Effective intervention of low peak bone mass and modeling in the spontaneous murine model of senile osteoporosis, SAM-P/6, by calcium supplement and hormone treatment. Bone 15:209-215.

42. Tsuboyama T, Takahashi K, Yamamuro T, Hosokawa M, Takeda T 1993 Cross-mating study on bone mass in the spontaneously osteoporotic mouse (SAM-P/6). Bone Miner 23:57-64.

43. Jilka RL, Weinstein RS, Takahashi K, Parfitt MA, Manolagos SC 1996 Linkage of decreased bone mass with impaired osteoblastogenesis in a murine model of accelerated senescence. J Clin Invest 97:1732-1740.

44. Weinstein RS, Jilka RL, Parfitt AM, Manolagos SC 1997 The effects of androgen deficiency on murine bone remodeling and bone mineral density are mediated via cells of the osteoblastic lineage. Endocrinol 138:4013-4021.

45. Schnitzler CM, Ripamonti U, Mesquita JM 1993 Histomorphometry of iliac crest trabecular bone in adult male baboons in captivity. Calcif Tiss Int 52:447-454.

46. Jayo MJ, Jerome CP, Lees CJ, Rankin SE, Weaver DS 1994 Bone mass in female cynomolgus macaques: A cross-sectional and longitudinal study by age. Calcif Tiss Int 54:231-236.

47. Pope NS, Gould KG, Anderson DC, Mann DR 1989 Effects of age and sex on bone density in the rhesus monkey. Bone 10:109-112.

48. Jayo MJ, Rankin SE, Weaver DS, Carlson CS, Clarkson TB 1991 Accuracy and precision of lumbar bone mineral content by DXA in live female monkeys. Calcif Tiss Int 49:438-440.

49. Jerome C, Kimmel DB, McAlister JA, Weaver DS 1986 Effects of ovariectomy on iliac trabecular bone in baboons (Papio anubis). Calcif Tiss Int 39:206-208.

50. Miller C, Weaver D 1986 Bone loss in ovariectomized monkeys. Calcif Tiss Int 38:62-65.

51. Lundon K, Dumitriu M, Grynpas M 1994 The long-term effect of ovariectomy on the quality and quantitiy of cancellous bone in young macaques. Bone Miner 24:135-149.

52. Aufdemorte TB, Fox WC, Miller D, Buffum K, Holt GR, Carey KD 1993 A non-human primate model for the study of osteoporosis and oral bone loss. Bone 14:581-586.

53. Grynpas MD, Huckell CB, Reichs KJ, Derousseau CJ, Greenwood C, Kessler MJ 1993 Effect of age and osteoarthritis on bone mineral in rhesus monkey vertebrae. J Bone Miner Res 8:909-917.

51

54. Carlson CS, Loeser RF, Jayo MJ, Weaver DS, Adams MR, Jerome CP 1994 Osteoarthritis in cynomolgus macaques: A primate model of naturally occuring disease. J Orthop Res 12:331-339.

55. Kimmel DB, Lane NE, Kammerer CM, Stegman MR, Rice KS, Recker RR 1993 Spinal pathology in adult baboons. J Bone Miner Res 8(Suppl 1):S279.

56. Hughes KP, Kimmel DB, Kammerer CM, Stegman MR, Rice KS, Recker RR 1994 Vertebral morphometry in adult female baboons. J Bone Miner Res 9(Suppl 1):S209.

57. Orwoll ES, Oviatt SK, Mann T 1990 The impact of osteophytic and vascular calcifications on vertebral mineral density measurements in men. J Clin Endocrinol Metab 70:1202-1207.

58. Paigen K 1995 A miracle enough: The power of mice. Nature Med 1:215-220.

59. Frankel WN 1995 Taking stock of complex trait genetics in mice. Trends Genet 11:471-477.

60. VandeBerg JL, Williams-Blangero S 1997 Advantages and limitations of nonhuman primates as animal models in genetic research on complex diseases. J Med Primatol 26:113-119.

61. Rogers J, Hixson JE 1997 Insights from model systems: Baboons as an animal model for genetic studies of common human disease. Am J Hum Genet 61:489-493.

62. Kaye M, Kusy RP 1995 Genetic lineage, bone mass, and physical activity. Bone 17:131-135.

63. Beamer WG, Donahue LR, Rosen CJ, Baylink DJ 1996 Genetic variability in adult bone density among inbred strains of mice. Bone 18:397-403.

64. Rosen CJ, Dimai HP, Vereault D, Donahue LR, Beamer WG, Farley J, Linkhart S, Linkhart T, Mohan S, Baylink DJ 1997 Circulating and skeletal insulin-like growth factor-I (IGF-I) concentrations in two inbred strains of mice with different bone mineral densities. Bone 21:217-223.

65. Green MC 1989 Catalogue of mutant genes and polymorphic loci. In: Searle M (ed.) Genetic variants and strains of the laboratory mouse. Oxford University Press, Oxford, U.K., pp 12-403.

66. Green MC 1951 Further morphological effects of the short-ear gene in the house mouse. J Morph 88:1-22.

67. Green MC 1958 Effects of the short-ear gene in the mouse on cartilage formation in healing bone fractures. J Exp Zool 137:75-88.

68. Mikiç B, van der Meulen MC, Kingsley DM, Carter DR 1995 Long bone geometry and strength in adult BMP-5 deficient mice. Bone 16(4):445-54.

69. Kingsley DM, Bland AE, Grubber JM, Marker PC, Russell LB, Copeland NG, Jenkins NA 1992 The mouse short ear skeletal morphogenesis locus is associated with defects in a bone morphogenetic member of the TGF beta superfamily. Cell 71(3):399-410.

70. Lohler J, Timpl R, Jaenisch R 1984 Embryonic lethal mutation in mouse collagen I gene causes rupture of blood vessels and is associated with erythropoietic and mesenchymal cell death. Cell 38:597-607.

71. Bonadio J, Saunders TL, Tsai E, Goldstein SA, Morris-Wiman J, Brinkley L, Dolan DF, Altschuler RA, Hawkins JE, Bateman JF 1990 A transgenic mouse model of osteogenesis imperfecta type I. Proc Natl Acad Sci USA 87:7145-7149.

72. Khillan JS, Olsen AS, Kontsaari S, Sokolov B, Prockop DJ 1991 Transgenic mice that express a mini-gene version of the human gene for type I procollagen (COL1A!) develop a phenotype resembling a lethal form of osteogenesis imperfecta. J Biol Chem 266:23373-23379.

73. Pereira RF, Hume EL, Halford KW, Prockop DJ 1995 Bone fragility in transgenic mice expressing a mutated gene for type I procollagen (COL1A1) parallels the age-dependent phenotype of human osteogenesis imperfecta. J Bone Miner Res 10:1837-1843.

74. Yoshida H, Hayashi S, Kunisada T, Ogawa M, Nishikawa S, Okamura H, Sudo T, Shultz LD, Nishikawa S 1990 The murine mutation osteopetrosis is in the coding region of the macrophage colony stimulating factor gene. nature 345:442-444.

75. Soriano P, Montgomery C, Geske R, Bradley A 1991 Targeted disruption of the c-src proto-oncogene leads to osteopetrosis in mice. Cell 64:693-702.

76. Wang Z, Ovitt C, Grigoriadis AE, Mohle-Steinlein U, Ruther U, Wagner EF 1992 Bone and hematopoietic defects in mice lacking c-fos. Nature 360:741-745.

77. Hodgkinson CA, Moore KJ, Nakayama A, Steingrimsson E, Copeland NG, Jenkins NA, Arnheiter H 1993 Mutations at the mouse microphthalmia locus are associated with defects in a gene encoding a novel basic-helix-loop-helix-zipper protein. Cell 74:395-404.

78. Bailey DW 1981 Recombinant inbred strains and bilineal congenic strains. In: Foster HL, Small JD, Fox JG (eds.) The mouse in biomedical research., vol. I. Academic Press, New York City, pp 223-239.

79. Taylor BA 1978 Recombinant inbred strains: Use in gene mapping. In: Morse HC (ed.) Origins of inbred mice. Academic Press, New York City, pp 423-438.

80. Gora Maslak G, McClearn GE, Crabbe JC, Phillips TJ, Belknap JK, Plomin R 1991 Use of recombinant inbred strains to identify quantitative trait loci in psychopharmacology. Psychopharmacology Berl 104(4):413-24.

81. Plomin R, McClearn GE, Gora Maslak G, Neiderhiser JM 1991 Use of recombinant inbred strains to detect quantitative trait loci associated with behavior. Behav Genet 21(2):99-116.

82. Plomin R, McClearn GE 1993 Quantitative trait loci (QTL) analyses and alcohol-related behaviors. Behav Genet 23(2):197-211.

83. Takeda K, Hosokawa M, Higuchi K 1991 Senescence-accelerated mouse (SAM): A novel murine model of accelerated senescence. J Am Ger Soc 39:911-919.

84. Benes H, Dennis R, Zheng W, Weinstein RS, Shelton R, Jilka RL, Roberson P, Manolagas SC, Shmookler Reis RJ 1997 Genetic mapping of osteopenia-associated loci using crosses between closely related mouse strains with differing bone mineral density. J Bone Miner Res 12(Suppl 1):F598.

85. Klein RF, Mitchell SR, Phillips TJ, Belknap JK, Orwoll ES 1998 Quantitative trait loci affecting peak bone mineral density in mice. J Bone Miner Res (in press).

86. Russell ES 1979 Genetic origins and some research uses of C57BL/6J, DBA/2, and B6D2F1 mice. In: Gibson DC (ed.) Development of the rodent as a model system of aging. USPHS-DHEW, Pub # (NIH) 79-161, Washington, D.C., pp 37-44.

87. Johnson ML, Gong G, Kimberling W, Recker SM, Kimmel DB, Recker RR 1997 Linkage of a gene causing high bone mass to human chromosome 11 (11q12-13). Am J Hum Genet 60:1326-1332.

88. McClearn GE 1997 Prospects for quantitative trait locus methodology in gerontology. Exp Gerontol 32:49-54.

89. Liel Y, Edwards J, Shary J, Spicer KM, Gordon L, Bell NH 1988 The effects of race and body habitus on bone mineral density of the radius, hip, and spine in premenopausal women. J Clin Endocrinol Metab 66:1247-1250.

90. Slemenda CW, Hui SL, Longcope C, Wellman H, Johnson CC 1990 Predictors of bone mass in perimenopausal women. A prospective study of clinical data using photon absorptiometry. Ann Intern Med 112:96-101.

91. Bauer DC, Browner WS, Cauley JA, Orwoll ES, Scott JC, Black DM 1993 Factors associated with appendicular bone mass in older women: The study of osteoporotic fractures Research Group. Ann Intern Med 118:657-665.

92. Orwoll ES, Bauer DC, Vogt TM, Fox KM 1996 Axial bone mass in older women. Ann Intern Med 124:187-196.

93. Glauber HS, Vollmer WM, Nevitt MC, Ensrud KE, Orwoll ES 1995 Body weight versus body fat distribution, adiposity, and frame size as predictors of bone density. J Clin Endocrinol Metab 80:1118-1123.

94. Keightley PD, Hardge T, May L, Bulfield G 1996 A genetic map of quantitative trait loci for body weight in the mouse. Genetics 142:227-235.

95. Belknap JK, Mitchell SR, O'Toole LA, Helms ML, Crabbe JC 1996 Type I and type II error rates for quantitative trait loci (QTL) mapping studies using recombinant inbred mouse strains. Behav Genet 26:149-160.

96. Pomp D 1997 Genetic dissection of obesity in polygenic animal models. Behav Genet 27:285-306.

97. Lyon MF, Searle AG 1989 Genetic variants and strains of the laboratory mouse., 2nd. ed. Oxford Univesity Press, New York.

54

98. Dietrich WF, Miller J, Steen R, Merchant MA, Damronboles D, Husain Z, Dredge R, Daly MJ, Ingalls KA, O'Connor TJ, Evans CA, Deangelis MM, Levinson DM, Kruglyak L, Goodman N, Copeland NG, Jenkins NA, Hawkins TL, Stein L, Page DC, Lander ES 1996 A comprehensive genetic map of the mouse genome. Nature 380:149-152.

99. Andersson L, Archibald A, Ashburner M, Audun S, Barendse W, Bitgood J, Bottema C, Broad T, Brown S, Burt D, Charlier C, Copeland N, Davis S, Davison M, Edwards J, Eggen A, Elgar G, Eppig JT, Franklin I, Grewe P, Gill T, Graves JAM, Hawken R, Hetzel J, Hilyard A, Jacob H, Jaswinska L, Jenkins N, Kunz H, Levan G, Lie O, Lyons l, Maccarone P, Mellersh C, Montgomery G, Moore S, Moran C, Morizot D, Neff J, Nichola F, O'Brien S, Parsons Y, Peters J, Postlethwait J, Raymond M, Rothschild M, Schook L, Sugimoto Y, Szpirer C, Tate M, Taylor J, Vandeberg J, Wakefield m, Wienberg J, Womack J 1996 Comparative geome organization of vertebrates. Mammal Genome 7:717-734.

100. West DB, Goudey Lefevre J, York B, Truett GE 1994 Dietary obesity linked to genetic loci on chromosomes 9 and 15 in a polygenic mouse model. J Clin Invest 94(4):1410-6.

101. Crabbe JC, Belknap JK, Buck KJ 1994 Genetic animal models of alcohol and drug abuse. Science 264:1715-1723.

102. Beamer W, Shultz K, Frankel W, Donahue L, Baylink D, Rosen C 1997 Genetic loci for cortical bone density in inbred mice. J Bone Miner Res 12(Suppl 1):P291.

103. Dutrillaux B, Viegas-Pequignot E, Masse R 1978 Complete or almost complete analogy of chromosome banding between the baboon (Papio papio) and man. Hum Genet 43:37-46.

104. Rogers J, Witte SM, Kammerer CM, Hixson JE, MacCluer JW 1995 Linkage mapping in Papio baboons: Conservation of a syntenic group of six markers on human chromosome 1. Genomics 28:251-254.

105. Kammerer CM, Sparks ML, Rogers J 1995 Effects of age, sex and heredity on measures of bone mass in baboons. J Med Primatol 24:236-242.

106. Mahaney MC, Kammerer CM, Whittam NJ, Hodgson WJ, Dyer T, Lichter JB, Rogers JA 1995 Genetic and environmental correlations between bone mineral densities at six vertebral and long-bone sites in pedigreed baboons. J Bone Miner Res 10:S364.

107. Mahaney MC, Morin P, Rodriguez LA, Newman DE, Rogers JA 1997 A quantitative trait locus on chromosome 11 may influence bone mineral density at several sites: Linkage analyses in pedigreed baboons. J Bone Miner Res 12(Suppl 1):64.

108. Perelygin AA, Kammerer CM, Stowell NC, Rogers J 1996 Conservation of human chromosome 18 in baboons (Papio hamadryas): A linkage map of eight human microsatellites. Cytogenet Cell Genet 75:207-209.

109. Breese EL, Mather K 1957 The organization of polygenic activity within a chromosome in Drosophila: 1. Hair characters. Heredity 11:373-395.

110. Darvasi A 1997 Interval-specific congenic strains (ISCS): An experimental design for mapping a QTL into a 1-centimorgan interval. Mamm Genome 8:163-167.

111. Jacob HJ, Lindpaintner K, Lincoln SE, Kusumi K, Bunker RK, Mao YP, Ganten D, Dzau VJ, Lander ES 1991 Genetic mapping of a gene causing hypertension in the stroke-prone spontaneously hypertensive rat. Cell 67:213-224.

112. Rapp JP, Deng AY 1995 Detection and positional cloning of blood pressure quantitative trait loci: Is it possible? Hypertension 25:1121-1128.

113. Darvasi A 1998 Experimental strategies for the genetic dissection of complex traits in animal models. Nat Genet 18:19-24.

114. Moreadith RW, Radford NB 1997 Gene targeting in embryonic stem cells: The new physiology and metabolism. J Mol Med 75:208-216.

115. Porcu S, Kitamura M, Witkowska E, Zhang Z, Mutero A, Lin C, Chang J, Gaensler KM 1997 The human beta globin locus introduced by YAC transfer exhibits a specific and reproducible pattern of developmental regulation in transgenic mice. Blood 90:4602-4609.

116. Mullins JJ, Peters J, Ganten D 1990 Fulminant hypertension in transgenic rats harbouring the mouse Ren-2 gene. Nature 234:541-544.

117. Dudek BC, Underwood K 1993 Selective breeding, congenic strains, and other classical genetic approaches to the analysis of alcohol-related polygenic pleotropisms. Behav Genet 23:179-190.

118. Flaherty L 1981 Congenic strains. In: Foster HL, Small JD, Fox JG (eds.) The mouse in biomedical research. Volume I: History, genetics, and wild mice. Academic Press, New York, pp 215-222.

119. Lisitsyn NA, Segre JA, Kusumi K, Lisitsyn NM, Nadeau JH, Frankel WN, Wigler MH, Lander ES 1994 Direct isolation of polymorphic markers linked to a trait by genetically directed representational difference analysis. Nature Genet 6:57-63.

120. Silver LM, Nadeau JH, Goodfellow PN 1994 Encyclopedia of the mouse genome. IV. Mammal Genome 6:S1-S295.

5 Interdependence of Genetic and Epigenetic Factors in Determining Bone Strength

Janet Rubin, M.D.

Clinton T. Rubin, Ph.D.

Natural selection can only eliminate the unfit... something else must create the fit.

S.J. Gould 1982

Bone: The Ultimate Smart Material

Bone is an elegant biologic structure that succeeds at withstanding extremes of functional loading while simultaneously serving as the organism's principal reservoir of mineral. The strength of the skeleton is realized via a sophisticated structural and ultrastructural organization that has evolved to meet specific functional demands. Bone's success as a structure cannot be quantified simply by density (**Figure 1**). Trabecular girth, orientation and connectivity, cell responsiveness to anabolic and catabolic agents, the distribution, organization and competence of the organic constituents, and even the neuromuscular (postural stability, falling reflex) and cardiovascular systems (metabolite distribution) are all critical to the structural success of the skeleton. The multifold functional demands on the skeleton and the need to continually sense and adjust to those demands suggest that a simple genetic template cannot be the sole determinant of skeletal morphology.

When considering the extent to which genetics influences bone strength, it is essential to consider how the genome influences not only the *amount* of bone, but the *quality* of bone. The nature of bone allows for variations in many interdependent parameters to achieve the optimal morphology for a specific function. The goal of this chapter is to identify those parameters that can influence and can be modified to "optimize" the diverse structural responsibility held by bone. This goal will be approached by emphasizing that the genome provides more than a template for bone length and girth – it allows bone to be a tissue which responds to the metabolic and functional needs of the organism. The responsive nature of bone, or its adaptability, is further influenced by epigenetic factors. Epigenetic factors determine the portion of the phenotype that develops out of environmental influences or constraints. Even the best of the smart materials engineered by man are poor cousins to the material attributes of the skeleton. Imagine a bridge that could repair corrosive or fatigue damage without shutdown or an airplane that modulated the span and stiffness of its wings in relation to its cargo load or to wind turbulence. By emphasizing the biologic aspects of bone tissue, it becomes clear that the genome has contributed immensely, but not exclusively, to bone becoming the ideal "smart material" that can perceive, respond, and even adapt to changes in its functional, nutritional and hormonal environment.

To appreciate how the skeleton survives a lifetime of compressive, torsional and distortional forces, it is necessary to view bone as a complex composite material 'engineered' for strength without undue weight, and as a cellular tissue capable of continual remodeling, adapting to the changing needs of the organism. The criteria that define the engineering limits of a structure can be considered at three levels: the gross structural properties (size and shape), the ultrastructural properties (material), and the physical demands (functional loading) to which the structure is subject. These goals are achieved by a sophisticated interaction between the criterion of genomic success, defined by evolutionary selection pressure, and the ability of the individual (via the genome) to adapt to a changing functional environment. We will consider each of these subjects in terms of properties and genetic/epigenetic influences on the strength of the skeleton.

Gross Structural Components of Bone Strength

Gross structural properties are those aspects that define the overall shape and mass of the structure. In the case of bone, size, density, and architecture effectively describe these gross structural properties. During growth, size and density are strongly influenced by inherited factors. Other, more subtle properties ultimately contribute to the structural efficacy of bone. These include morphologic contributions such as the long bone curvature, the girth and geometry of the cross-sectional area, and the trabecular organization (e.g., connectivity). These properties are highly influenced by epigenetic factors such as functional load bearing.

A major component of bone strength is derived from the size of the bone as defined by both the length and girth. The most commonly used *clinical* predictor of bone strength, dual energy x-ray absorptiometry (DEXA), measuring grams of mineral per unit area, provides only a unidimensional indication of these critical descriptors. For example, a real bone density (g/cm^2) from DEXA suggests that white women have less dense cortical bone than either white men or black women. As pointed out by Seeman (1), this is a misinterpretation of the bone density data which arises because the bones of white women are smaller, both lengthwise and crosswise. The DEXA scan across the bone fails to normalize for these size scaling issues, and in reality the actual mineral content per volume is strikingly similar between white women, white men and black women. It should not be surprising that the bone mineral making up the femoral neck of a petite woman is far less than that measured in a male or female twice her size. A more powerful use of DEXA, at least in terms of estimating strength, would be to normalize not only to age and sex, as well to a criteria of individual size.

Height is a size trait commonly accepted to be inheritable. Although stature is normally distributed in populations, stature of groups (e.g., Scandinavians versus Pygmies) varies greatly. Racial phenotype influences bone size and possibly cortical thickness (2). There is also a strong parent-child polygenic heritability. However, despite years of interest in promoting height, the genes designating height remain unknown. In one study using sibling-pair linkage analysis of more than 500 Pima Indians, Thompson (3) showed that a genetic determinant governing stature was located on chromosome 20. Although BMP-2 is located in this region of the genome and was considered as a possible candidate gene for governing stature, this association was not supported by the data. The study of embryological growth of endochondral bones has suggested other genetic targets that contribute to the final length of bones. Vortkamp et al (4) have shown that the longitudinal growth of a bone can be controlled at the transition of proliferating to hypertrophic chondrocytes. When this occurs, osteoblasts are recruited and ossification begins, limiting further longitudinal growth. The molecular controls over chondrocytic maturation may in the future be revealed to be important determinants of stature.

Although genes may be the principal determinant of height, there are also environmental influences on final height. In many studies of the heritability of height, measurements have been performed between two generations - therefore nutritional and environmental contributions to height over several generations are often overlooked. In America, increased nutrition has resulted in increased height as well as growth rate (5). In Japan, the same response has been noted: the average height at maturity increased 10 cm for both genders in citizens born after 1960 compared with those born before 1920 (6). In the genetically similar Japanese population, the increase in height must be strongly influenced by improved dietary factors. While the degree to which nutrition influences peak height has not yet been determined, the role of only a single ion in the diet, calcium, has been shown to be a critical rate determining step in achieving the template designated by the genome: increased milk consumption in young Japanese women living in Hawaii was associated with longer leg length and even greater sitting height (7).

What about the influences of genetics on appendicular bone girth? Studies of black and white children of ages 6 to 20 years showed that bone width after adjusting for height (and with it the bone mineral content, BMC, as g/cm^2) was increased in males but there was no difference between the racial groups (8). It is worth noting that the BMC normalized for bone width was similar between sexes, again inviting concern regarding the widespread use of DEXA, or a real bone density, to estimate bone strength and relative risk of fracture. After adjusting for height, the bone mass of black girls was not increased before puberty. Eventually black women attain higher bone size than white women, with about a 15% larger cortical area (Garn 75). The regulation of ethnic differences in bone size and microarchitecture is unknown.

Our understanding of the effect of genes on bone and body size has been enhanced by paleoanthropological studies of the 2 million year evolution of the genus *Homo*. A recent study emphasizes that caution should be used when evaluating partial skeletons to assess final size. Body mass estimates for Pleistocene *Homo* have varied by as much as 50% for the same individuals (Ruff 97). Paleoanthropologists have previously used lower limb long bone diaphyseal and articular breadths to estimate body size. Early *Homo* groups appear to have had larger diaphyseal breadths than modern humans, an attribute used to hypothesize that the culture of our predecessors resulted in a greater degree of mechanical loading of the skeleton. Since it previously had been determined that articulations were less environmentally sensitive predictors of body size, Ruff and colleagues used two independent articular measurements for body-mass estimation: the femoral head size and the pelvic breadth, neither which depend on mechanical relationships (i.e., support of body weight). These skeletal dimensions for Pleistocene *Homo* specimens dated at 150,000 to 600,000 years old suggested that the average body size was actually greater than that of modern day man. The authors suggest that the recent increases in stature achieved through better nutrition (noted above) are a result of rebounding to early Pleistocene heights. This again raises the point that the size and shape of the skeleton arise from a genomic template, but are subject to modification by epigenetic factors.

Bone strength is affected by geometry as well as by size. Several studies have shown that the geometry of the femoral neck contributes to its susceptibility to fracture (Gluer 94, Slemenda 96). The longer the hip axis, or distance from the inner pelvic brim to the outer edge of the trochanter, the more strain will arise in the tissue of the neck for a given load. Hip axis length (HAL) is a measure of femoral geometry and has predictive value for hip fracture in older women: each standard deviation of increase in HAL was associated with nearly a 2 fold increase in fracture risk in one 2 year study (Faulkner 93). Furthermore, this risk was independent of BMD, as well as of other fracture locations, suggesting that a particular geometry may predispose the femur to fracture. Flicker (96) then studied the genetic component of the HAL in older white women. Adjusting for weight, height was found to be responsible for 25% of the variation in HAL, which was fixed by age 15. Genetic factors were responsible for 95% of the final height (within one generation). The only major independent determinant of HAL was body stature. These authors suggest, however, that even the combination of HAL and BMD explain less than half of the increased risk associated with maternal hip fracture, leaving the bone *quality* issue unexplicated.

Slemenda et al (96), in their studies of the distribution of bone mineral in twin pairs, also considered femoral neck geometry and found it to be an independent predictor of fracture risk. The study revealed significant familial influences on distribution of femoral bone mass and on the calculated structural strength of the proximal femur, but insignificant influences on the femoral neck length.

Finally, it is clear that the most widely studied of the structural components - bone mineral density - is strongly influenced by the genome. In 1973 Smith et al examined monozygotic and dizygotic twins with regard to their midshaft radial bone mass. Their data showed an intraclass correlation that was significantly larger in monozygotic pairs at age 44-55. Analysis indicated that major genetic influences on the adult male midshaft bone mass were due to inherited variation in bone size, i.e., that genetic causes of variation in male bone mass were primarily due to genes influencing skeletal size. This conclusion was similarly reached by Seeman (A J Physiol 1996) who showed that a genetic factor accounted for about 66% of individual variance in femoral neck bone mineral density as well as lean mass. This study suggested again that a greater muscle mass predicted bone mineral density and contributed to the final skeletal form, often indirectly.

A decrease in mineral density accompanies normal aging; the loss of bone density has been estimated to account for as much as 80% of the decrease in strength associated with aging (Singer 95). Christian et al (89) restudied Smith's (73) (see above) twin subjects 16 years later. As these subjects lost bone at a rate of 0.49% BMD per year, they exhibited decreasing genetic correlation for bone density. The familial variations in the *loss* of radial mass and density, and subsequent decrease in bone strength with aging, predicted an epigenetic cause of bone mineral loss, not a genetic one. Therefore, although the peak bone mass (or size) may be largely genetically determined, this peak number does not predict the rate of bone loss. That the loss of bone mass with aging or menopause is not necessarily controlled by the genome is also supported by the recent histomorphometric data of Han, et al (97). These authors showed that bone loss at menopause was equivalent in black and white women, as well as in white men, despite differences in genetically determined bone size.

The monozygotic twin studies of Pocock (87) suggest that genes may variably influence bone density at different sites in the skeleton. The 38 monozygotic, and 27 dizygotic, mostly female, subjects had bone mineral densities which were more highly correlated in the spine than in the appendicular sites (proximal femur and distal forearm). Therefore, epigenetic factors appear to have more dominant influences in the proximal femur and distal forearm than in the spine. This suggests that the density of the spine is largely determined by genetic controls of body size whereas physical demand may be more important in the appendicular skeleton. This may also help to explain why some pharmacologic interventions influence the hip more so than the spine (or vice versa). In fact, Pocock noted that the correlation of VO_2 max between the twin pairs was stronger than the correlation of bone density, implicating physical fitness in certain local areas of bone density. Along these lines, Kanders et al (88) showed that while calcium nutrition affected the bone mass of young women, its incorporation into the skeleton was dependent on the presence of adequate physical strain.

In the laboratory, Beamer and colleagues, studying 11 inbred strains of mice, demonstrated a large variability in volumetric bone mass: they measured significant and even striking differences in the pQCT derived bone density of femur, proximal phalanges and L5-6 vertebrae in the different strains (Beamer 96). Differences in the femoral and phalangeal bones with respect to total and cortical density, mineral and volume were apparent by 2 months despite continued lengthening of femurs for up to 8 months thereafter. These results not only agree that intrastrain bone mass is largely genetically derived, but that the genes which regulate length and density appear to be different. It will be fascinating to explore possible changes in microstructure in these mouse strains that may compensate for, or cause, the gross differences in the cortical bone densities when solving for loading requirements. Since these mice essentially are exposed to a similar environment, genetic influences may predominate at the age the mice were examined, although epigenetic influences on these intrastrain differences might also influence the final phenotype. For instance, Kaye and Kusy (95) also found that C57BL/6J mice had higher bone densities than A/J inbred mice at both femoral and tibial sites. Since the increased bone mass was, as well, associated with larger quadriceps muscles in the C57BL/6J animals, the authors asked if muscle mass was also increased and associated with BMD. Interestingly they found that the C57BL/6J animals were more active. Muscle mass is certainly more malleable than BMD.

Weight training of twins can increase muscle strength by 25% while BMD is changed hardly at all (Seeman 96). This study, while again revealing the strong genetic prediction of BMD, showed an independent association between lean mass and BMD. There were no associations between BMD and the increased muscle strength. These murine models promise to be interesting models for studying genetic and epigenetic contributions of structure, ultrastructure and function to bone morphology in the future. Extreme genetic cases are less clear in studies of the human skeleton, where a long life marries countless epigenetic factors into the final morphology.

Finally, ethnicity has been shown to have a significant influence on fracture rate. The possibility that microarchitecture rather than bone density underlies the variable fracture rate has only lately been considered. Although blacks have a higher a real bone density than whites (grams of density per surface area), as discussed above, they have a similar amount of mineral per volume. As shown in the elegant work of Han et al (96, 97), the amount of a real density rises as a result of increased bone size in black women. Certainly an increased bone size influences the fracture rate as discussed above. As well, black women appear to have a greater cortical thickness, which might contribute to the reduced fracture incidence (Garn and Clark 75, Seeman 97). By performing histomorphometric studies, Han et al (97) have shown that trabeculae in black women, although present in the same numbers compared with white women, are thicker, leaving a decreased surface area with regard to the total bone. Because these differences are present by young adulthood, these are thought to be largely genetically determined (Han 96). It appears, from both the Han studies (96, 97) and those of Weinstein and Bell (88), that black adults have lower bone turnover, in the latter study only 35% that seen in white adults. The lower bone turnover may contribute, as well to the lower fracture rate measured in blacks.

Structural components are therefore regulated by both genetic and epigenetic factors. The relative contribution, and thus importance, of these components may change as the skeleton grows, matures, and ultimately, ages.

Ultrastructural Components of Bone Strength

What *ultrastructural* components might be used to build a support structure that must be strong yet light enough to allow locomotion? For an inanimate structure, an intelligent engineer would select a composite with a fundamental component of ceramic to allow it to withstand compression, and then mix in rope-like components to provide the capacity to resist tension, bending and twisting. Composite materials have been recognized by engineers for centuries, but only relatively recently, at the turn of this century, has the advent of reinforced concrete (adding steel bars as rope-like resistors of tension) allowed for bigger and taller buildings. This is also the strategy bone has used, reflected in the complex interaction of the inorganic phase of the tissue (the ceramic), and the principal component of the protein matrix, the collagen. Importantly, these interactions, including even the interrelationship of the hydroxyapatite crystals to the organic constituents of bone, are determined by a combination of genetic and epigenetic factors. For instance, the makeup of the apatite crystal is influenced predominantly by genetic factors, but the organization of the crystal, and its relationship to constituents such as collagen, is influenced by external factors such as hormones, cytokines and functional stimuli. Considering the large degree of bending to which bone is subject, the ability to resist tension is critical. The design need for elements supplying high tensile strength in bone is fulfilled by collagen fibrils. The ultrastructural characteristics of these chains contribute not only to the strength, but also to the toughness of the material. The collagen triple helical molecules are further organized into plate like structures called lamellae, which, when mineralized, add to the tensile strength of the bone, much like the added strength that layering contributes to plywood. Lamellae vary in thickness, and the collagen orientation between adjacent plates can rotate by as much as ninety degrees permitting the tissue to resist forces and moments acting from several different directions (Alexander 94). While this organization is, in part, defined by the genome, the functional environment contributes to the distribution of lamellae as well the osteons that house them (Skedros et al, 1996).

With much of bone strain arising from bending, some areas of the same cross-section are subject to tensile strain and others to compressive deformation. To withstand compression the composite material must have a ceramic component; in the case of bone, this compression-resistant material is calcium hydroxyapatite. Individual calcium phosphate crystals of an exceedingly wide range of sizes are imbedded in and around the fibrils of the collagen type I lattice (Weiner 92). The number of crystals, which is the substance measured by bone mineral density, clearly contributes to compression resistant strength - but it is not everything. Fluoroapetite, for instance, arising in fluoride poisoning, is denser than hydroxyapatite, but shatters easily (Kroger 94).

Not only are the collagen's tensile strength and the mineral's compressive strength important, their relative proportions largely define the function of the tissue. Currey has demonstrated that bone structure can be defined by the *interaction* of the organic and inorganic constituents by comparing the material properties of antler, tibia and tympanic bulla (Currey 1979). Proportionately, an antler has much more collagen than the other two, allowing the structure to absorb impact during battle. Conversely, the tympanic bulla, which must be highly efficient at transmitting acoustic waves in the ear, is essentially 100% mineral, a non-elastic structure which really doesn't need to bend. The material properties of the tibia, which must bend and resist compression, lie somewhere between the extremes of a tough-bendable and a brittle resistant material. Thus, the density in and of itself does not define the strength of the bone, nor do the ingredients per se. Rather it is the interaction, proportion and organization of these components that ultimately grant strength. What these examples also emphasize is that bone has responsibilities other than locomotion, and that the ultrastructure of bone has evolved to "idealize" the composite to the functional needs. There is truly an intelligent engineer at work here, somewhere.

Alterations in either the organic (e.g., collagen) or inorganic (e.g., hydroxyapatite) matrix components, will bring about changes in the bone strength, some of which are indirect, and some of which can be catastrophic. An entire spectrum of bone diseases is caused by mutations in collagen gene, a principal symptom of which is a skeleton more prone to fracture. In osteogenesis imperfecta (OI), mutations in primary structure of type I procollagen lead to brittle and easily fractured bones (Prockop 84). The origin of the fracturability of OI bone is not completely understood, but points to microarchitectural changes. Recently this disease has been studied using several mouse models, including the osteogenesis imperfecta mouse model (*oim*) which produces only collagen a1. The bone crystals in the absence of collagen a2 appear to be thinner and possibly disoriented (Misof 97). When this collagen, using the tail tendon, is strained beyond 5%, the oim mouse shows reduced tensile strength. Misof and colleagues suggest that mineral crystals within the collagen fibrils disallow further extension of the coiled tri-helix at high tensile strengths.

Another disorder of collagen resulting in excessively fragile bone is fibrogenesis imperfecta ossium (Carr 95), a rare disorder where the skeleton is replaced by disorganized collagen-deficient tissue. The natural history of this disorder reveals a progressive replacement of bone by abnormal collagen with randomly orientated fibrils of varying thickness. Calcification of the collagen is greatly delayed, implying that the highly organized morphology of the collagen substrate is important not only for strength, but for biomineralization.

As severe as these ultrastructural mutations may be, the ability of the skeleton to compensate for them at the structural level must not be overlooked. This compensatory strategy is highlighted in the studies of Bonadio and his colleagues (96), who "knocked out" the collagen I gene in mice. The homozygous mice lacking any type I collagen died at mid-gestation, but the heterozygotes survived to adulthood, while producing 50% less type I collagen. In this case, the bone was completely changed, with a reduced collagen component predicted to increase the brittleness of the ceramic component. Changes of this type in the collagen of human bone leads to increased fracture susceptibility for patients with osteogenesis imperfecta. In the collagen I-deficient mouse, however, the load to failure values in heterozygotes were not significantly different from normal. At 15 weeks, the load to structural failure even increased. This adaptational response involved the enhanced activity of osteogenic cells that generated new bone along periosteal surfaces, resulting in increased cross-sectional geometry and increased long bone bending strength. Interestingly, the natural history of human osteogenesis imperfecta suggests that the fracture frequency of affected individuals often decreases dramatically at puberty. Perhaps in humans the epigenetic influences begin to compensate for the genetically poor substrate. Microarchitectural changes may underlie these changes; clues to what these might be should be forthcoming in ongoing studies of the collagen I-deficient mouse.

The possibility that interactions between ligands and receptors critical to the mineral homeostatic axis might also contribute to bone strength led to investigations into the association of the vitamin D receptor (VDR) with osteoporosis. An Australian cohort of white women found to have certain allelic variants of the VDR appeared to have lower bone densities as measured by absorptiometry (Morrison 95). This area has generated great controversy, beginning with another group's failure to confirm this relationship (Hustmyer 94). Another study of VDR polymorphisms in 189 dizygotic American twins showed no association with bone density (Arden 96). In a recent paper by Sainz, et al (97), three allelic variants of VDR were examined in normal prepubertal girls of Mexican descent. In this study, VDR gene alleles predicted the density of femoral and vertebral volumetric bone density.

The relationship of the VDR alleles may have to do with calcium intake and availability. In a study of rates of skeletal calcium deposition and resorption, Murray et al (93) demonstrated intrastrain differences in 2 strains of mice (C57Bl/6 and the large SENCAR strains). Although this study did not examine bone strengths, it might contribute to understanding the complex relationship with allelic variations in the VDR. There is now some evidence that different genetic groups might handle calcium differently, as did the two mice strains. In fact, the effects of vitamin D supplementation on BMD were recently shown to be associated with the particular VDR genotype: the bb genotype had a decreased response over 2 years to vitamin D administration compared to that of the BB and Bb phenotypes (Graafmans 97). These results suggest that VDR gene variants might have their final effects on bone density through regulating calcium availability. Again, the interdependence of genetic and epigenetic factors conspire to define the ultimate structural success of the skeleton.

The hormonal status of the individual also contributes, at least to the cellular ability to effectively respond to loading requirements. There is a well known increase in the rate of bone loss following the menopause (Han 97), an association with decreased bone density with hyperthyroidism, and an increase in bone density in growth hormone excess. As well, high corticosteroid levels, as seen in Cushing's disease, cause loss of bone mass despite continued physiologic demand (Adachi 97). The degree and perhaps even the type of response of the skeleton to the changing hormonal milieu thus appear to be influenced by epigenetic events under genetic control.

Bone Strain: A Regulatory Signal of Skeletal Success

A "smart material" should sense and adapt to the functional demands placed on it. A signal ideally placed to influence the bone morphology (gross structure and ultrastructure) is the deformation that arises during loading. While the functional demands made upon the skeleton of a goose are certainly distinct from those of a sloth, at the level of the cell the mechanical signals that arise from distinct loads all resolve into strain of the matrix. If the skeletal structure adapted to provide the greatest strength for a minimal mass, load would be applied axially, generating little bending or torsion. Axial loading results in very little strain for a given load: imagine how strong a pencil is when you press straight down on the long axis of the shaft, yet how easily the pencil is snapped when it is subject to bending. Bending and torsion are the nemesis of any man-made structure. Imagine, now, the neck of the femur while climbing a flight of stairs, or the humorous of a baseball pitcher delivering a fastball – the functional demands on bones, as opposed to pencils, are very complex. Considering the diversity of the functional environment, it is clear that a strategy of minimal skeletal mass will not be successful. Indeed, over 90% of the deformation measured in bone arises from bending (Rubin & Lanyon, 1984), suggesting that bone has evolved to ensure that some critical level of deformation is achieved in the tissue, rather than a situation where deformation is minimized. The degree to which bone has evolved away from being the ideal structure (i.e., one that provokes minimal strain) implies that the biologic benefit provided by induced strain outweighs the structural consequences.

The subtle but successful adjustments bone tissue makes to ensure structural suitability are made possible by genetic mechanisms. It must be emphasized, however, that each bone's structure is ultimately determined by its functional requirements, which are not encoded in the genome. What, then, is the signal to which the bone responds? An ideal candidate for such a regulatory signal is strain, the material deformation resulting from the mechanical load. Regardless of the design or function of a vertebrate, strain is a ubiquitous product of a functionally loaded skeleton. This dimensionless unit derived from dividing the change in length of a structure from its original length, is an efficient means of translating the intensity, duration and manner of functional loading into a site-specific, generic epigenetic signal relevant to osteoregulatory cells.

One obvious goal of this strain mediated form/function formula is to avoid fracture. Since compromising the locomotor apparatus of the organism would have obvious consequences to the perpetuation of the genome, bone loading and architecture must be coordinated to avoid a level of strain where irreversible damage might occur. Peak strain magnitudes measured in diverse vertebrates are remarkably similar, ranging in amplitude from 2000 to 3500 microstrain (Rubin & Lanyon 84). That strains of this magnitude are a factor of two below the failure point (yield strain of bone is 0.7%, or 7000 microstrain) emphasizes that a safety factor reigns, and that the skeleton can survive a misstep or two. Competing pressures between natural selection and the genome have undoubtedly defined this goal. In comparison, the 2000 microstrain (0.2% deformation) experienced by bone represents an exceedingly small change in length from a material's original length when compared with strain in other tissues. Cartilage is subject to 25% compressive deformations, tendons experience functional tensile strain of 20%, and ligaments can stretch 4-5% during functional loading (Woo 94). The bone cell mechanosensory system must therefore be exceedingly sensitive if deformations of this order are to affect cell metabolism.

Many laboratories are currently working to understand how cells sense and respond to their mechanical environment. We have, for example, shown that marrow cultures respond to subtle elevations of pressure by decreasing the numbers of osteoclasts formed in response to vitamin D (Rubin 97). Others have shown that osteoblasts respond to dynamic strain by increasing production of matrix molecules (Toma 97). Osteoblasts can also sense fluid shear stress, created as bone is loaded, responding with changes in cyclic adenosine monophosphate levels (Reich 90). The study of cellular response to mechanical factors should help us to better understand the response of the entire skeleton to dynamic loading during growth and adult life, and perhaps provide some insight into novel approaches to treat skeletal injury and disease.

Understanding and Manipulating Bone Strength in the Future

In conclusion, we might ask what determines the increased risk of hip fracture in a 70-year-old in relation to a 15-year-old, who has essentially the same bone density? The answer will arise out of studies that consider the entire bone structure, rather than the bone mineral density alone. We must consider the fact that the 70-year-old's decreased agility in response to falling must predispose him/her to hip fracture. As importantly, we must consider that aged bone might not respond to the loading environment appropriately, and can not adapt to prevent fractures arising out of this changed environment. The ultrastructure of an "old" bone may not be suited for changing moment of inertia, or decreased muscle mass. Aged bone may have a decreased cellular ability to repair damage, or respond to pharmaceutical treatments developed in young animals. We will need to understand how the cellular component of bone adjusts to changing functional demands, remodeling to maintain structure while still remaining sensitive to mineral needs of the organism. Finally we will need to understand what mechanical factors are important to regulating the adaptive response. The factors that define bone quality, and therefore ultimately bone strength, are both genetic and epigenetic, and the rate at which the bone inevitably degenerates reflects a combination of these influences as well.

In the coming years we will need to design diagnostic devices which can evaluate not only bone mass, but bone morphology. These devices must be sensitive to the quality of the organic as well as inorganic constituents, and determine the viability of the cell population. Pharmaceutical interventions must be developed which augment the complex interactions of the remodeling cycle, not ones that disrupt specific aspects of it. And as for tissue engineering, scientists who focus on construction of biomaterials must appreciate the complex biology of the osteoblast, osteoclast and osteocyte, and scientists concentrating on bone biology must consider the diverse structural responsibilities to which these tissues are subject.

68

As bone biologists, bioengineers and clinicians, we typically view bone in the context of its failures: femoral neck fractures, vascular necrosis, pseudoarthroses and metabolic bone disease, to name a few. Perhaps we should turn towards the remarkable successes of bone if we are to learn how to best optimize bone quality and quantity. The next time severe turbulence jostles your plane flight, imagine how much more comfortable you would feel if the "quality" of the fuselage, rather than simply the mass of the material, were appropriate for the changing environment. Perhaps the aeronautical industry will someday invent a structural material "smart" enough to accommodate its functional challenges. At least take comfort in the fact that nature, through millions of years, has achieved this goal – in the skeleton.

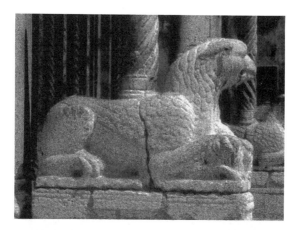

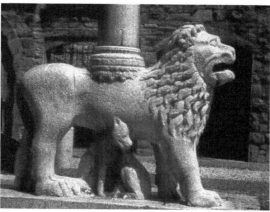

Figure 1. It is clear from the crack in the base of the foundation statue shown at the top (taken from the portico of San Zeno Maggiore, in Verona) that strength of a structure is not derived simply by mass. The less massive statue shown at the bottom (taken from the portico of the church of Santa Maria Maggiore, in Bergamo) shows the strategic placement of the cub has provided structural strength without the need for excess material. Photos courtesy of cub photographer Professor John Currey.

References

1. Seeman E 1997 From density to structure: growing up and growing old on the surfaces of bone. J Bone Miner Res 12:509-521.

2. Garn SN, Clark DC 1975 Nutrition, growth, development, and maturation: findings from the ten state nutrition survey of 1968-1979. Pediatrics 56:306-319.

3. Thompson DB, Ossowski V, Janssen RC, Knowler WC, Bogardus C 1995 Linkage between stature and a region on chromosome 20 and analysis of a candidate gene, BMP-2. Am J Medical Gene 59:495-500.

4. Vortkamp A, Lee K, Lanske B, Segre GV, Kronenberg H, Tabin CJ 1996 Regulation of rate of cartilage differentiation by Indian Hedgehog and PTH-related protein. Science 27:613-663.

5. Willit WC 1990 Nutritional Epidemiology New York: Oxford University Press 217-244.

6. Health Services Bureau, Health Promotion and Nutrition Division 1988 The National Nutrition Survey in Japan. Daiichi Shuppan, Tokyo.

7. Novotny R, Davis JW, Ross PD, Wasnich RD 1996 Adolescent milk consumption, menarche, birth weight, and ethnicity influence height of women in Hawaii. J Am Diet Assoc 96:802-804.

8. Patel DN, Pettifor JM, Becker PJ, Grieve C, Leschner K 1992 The effect of ethnic group on appendicular bone mass in cildren. J Bone Miner Res 7:263-272.

9. Alexander M 1994 Bones: The unity of form and function.

10. Arden NK, Keen RW, Lanchbury JS, Spector TD 1996 Polymorphisms of the VDR gene do not predict quantitative ultrasound of the calcaneus of hip axis length. Osteoporosis Int 6:334-337.

11. Beamer WB, Donahue LR, Rosen CJ, Baylink DJ 1996 Genetic variability in adult bone density among inbred strains of mice. Bone 18(5):397-403.

12. Bonadio J, Jepsen KJ, Mansoura MK, Jaenisch R, Kuhn JL, Goldstein SA 1993 A murine skeletal adaptation that significantly increases cortical bone mechanical properties. J Clin Inv 92(4):1697-1705.

13. Burr DB, Forwood MR, Fyhrie DP, Martin RB, Schaffler MB, Turner CH 1997 Bone microdamage and skeletal fragility in osteoporotic and stress fractures. J Bone Miner Res 12:6-15.

14. Carr AJ, Smith R, Athanasou N, Woods CG 1995 Fibrogenesis imperfecta ossium. J Bone Jt Surgery Br J 77:B:820-829.

15. Christian JC, Yu P, Slemenda CW, Johnston CC 1989 Heritability of bone mass. Am J Hum Genet 44:429-433.

16. Currey, J. 1979 Mechanical properties of bone with greatly differing functions. J. Biomech. 12:313-319

17. Ducy P, Desbois C, Boyce B, Pinero G, Story B, Dunstan C, Smith E, Bonadio J, Goldstein S, Gundberg C, Bradley A, Karsenty G 1996 Increased bone formation in osteocalcin-deficient mice. Nature 382:448-452.

18. Faulkner KG, Cummings SR, Black D, Palermo L, Gluer C, Genant HK 1993 Simple measurement of femoral geometry predicts hip fracture. J Bone Miner Res 8:1211-1217.

19. Flicker L, Faulkner KG, Hopper JL, Green RM, Kaymakci B, Nowson CA, Young D, Wark JD 1996 Determinants of hip axis length in women aged 10-89 years: a twin study. Bone 18(1):41-45.

20. Gluer C, Cummings SR, Pressman A, Li J, Gluer K, Faulkner KG, Gramp S, Genant HK 1994 Prediction of hip fractures from elvic radiographs the study of osteoporotic fractures. J Bone Miner Res 9:671-679.

21. Graafmans WX, Lips P, Ooms ME, van Leeuwen JPTM, Pols HAP, Uitterlinden AG 1997 The effect of vitamin D supplementation on the bone mineral density of the femoral neck is associated with vitamin D receptor genotype. J Bone Miner Res 12:1241-1245.

22. Han ZH, Palnitkar S, Sudhaker Rao D, Nelson D, Parfitt AM 1996 Effect of ethnicity and age or menopause on the structure and geometry of iliac bone. J Bone Miner Res 11:1967-1975.

23. Han ZH, Palnitkar S, Sudhaker Rao D, Nelson D, Parfitt AM 1997 Effects of ethnicity and age or menopause on the remodeling and turnover of iliac bone: implications for mechanisms of bone loss. J Bone Miner Res 12:498-508.

24. Hustmyer FG, Peacock M, Hui S, Johnston CC, Christian J 1994 Bone mineral density in relation to polymorphism at the VDR gene locus. J Clin Invest 94:2130-2134.

25. Kanders B, Dempster DW, Lindsay R 1988 Interaction of calcium nutrition and physical activity on bone mass in young women. J Bone Miner Res 3:145-149.

26. Kaye M, Kusy RP 1995 Genetic lineage, bone mass and physical activity in mice. Bone 17:131-135.

27. Kroger, H, Alhava, E, Honkanen, R, Tuppurainen, M and Saarikoski, S 1994 The effect of fluoridated drinking water on axial bone mineral density - a population based study Bone & Min 27:33-41

28. Misof K, Landis WJ, Klaushofer K, Frati P 1997 Collagen from the osteogenesis imperfecta mouse model (oim) shows reduced resistance against tensile stress. J Clin Invest 100:40-45.

29. Morrison NA, Qi JI, Tokita A, Kelly PJ, Crofts L, Nguyen TV et al. 1994 Prediction of bone density from vitamin D receptor alleles. Nature 367:284-287.

30. Murray EJ, Song MK, Laird EC, Murray SS 1993 Strain dependent differences in vertebral bone mass, serum osteocalcin and calcitonin in calcium-replete and -deficient mice. Proc Soc Exp Biol Med 203:64-73

31. Pocock NA, Eisman JA, Hopper JL, Yeates MG, Sambrook PN, Eberl S 1987 Genetic determinants of bone mass in adults. J Clin Inv 80:706-710.

32. Prockop DJ, Kivirikko KI 1984 Heritable diseases of collagen. NEJM 311:376-386.

33. Prockop KJ 1990 Mutations that alter the primary structure of type I collagen. J Biol Chem 265:15349-15352.

34. Reich KM, Gay CV, Frangos JA 1990 Fluid shear stress as a mediator of osteoblast cyclic adenosine monophosphate production. J Cell Physio l 143:11-104.

35. Rubin CT and Lanyon L 1984 Dynamic strain similarity in vertebrates: An alternative to allometric limb bone scaling in vertebrates. J. Theor. Biol. 107:321-327

36. Rubin J, Fan X, Biskobing D, Rubin C, McLeod K, Taylor WR 1997 Pressure regulates osteoclast formation and MCSF expression in marrow culture, J Cell Physiology 170:81-87.

37. Ruff CB, Trinkaus E, Holliday TW 1997 Body mass and encephalization in Pleistocene Homo. Nature 387:173-176.

38. Sainz J, Tornout J, Loro L, Sayre J, Roe TF, Gilsanz V 1997 Vitamin D-receptor gene polymorphisms and bone density in prepubertal American girls of Mexican descent. N Engl J Med 337:77-82.

39. Seeman E, Hopper JL, Young NR, Formica C, Goss P, Tsalamandris C 1996 Do genetic factors explain associations between muscle strength, lean mass, and bone density? A twin study. Am J Physiol 270:E320-327.

40. Singer K, Edmonston S, Day R, Breidahl P, Price R 1995 Prediction of thoracic and lumbar vertebral body compressive strength: correlations with bone mineral density and vertebral region. Bone 17:167-174.

41. Skedros JG, Mason, MW, Nelson, MC and Bloebaum, RD 1996 Evidence of structural and material adaptation to specific strain features in cortical bone. Anat. Rec. 246:47-63

42. Slemenda CW, Turner CH, Peacock M, Christian JC, Sorbel J, Hui SL, Johnston CC 1996 The genetics of proximal femur geometry, distribution of bone mass and bone mineral density. Osteoporosis Int 6:178-182.

43. Smith DM, Nance WE, Kang KW, Christian JC, Johnston CC 1973 Genetic factors in determining bone mass. J Clin Invest 52:2800-2808.

44. Weiner S, Traub W 1992 Bone structure: from angstroms to microns. FASEB J 6:879-885.

45. Weinstein RS, Bell NH 1988 Diminished rates of bone formation in normal black adults. N Eng J Med 319:1698-701.

46. Woo, S, An, K Arnoczky, S, Wayne, J, Fitghian, D and Myers, B   1994 Anatomy, biology and biomechanics of tendon, ligament and meniscus. Orth. Basic Science ed: S. Simon, Amer. Acad. Orth Surgs. 2:45-87

II. Diagnosis, Prevention, and Treatment

6 Quantitation of Bone Mineral Density in the Growing Skeleton: Methods and Meaning

Vicente Gilsanz, M.D.

Introduction

With the advent of quantitative techniques to measure bone mineral content a little more than a decade ago, our ability to quantify changes in bone mass and assess osteoporosis has markedly improved. For pediatric purposes, this development has awarded us the facility to diagnose and quantify the loss of bone mineral associated with the various disorders that cause osteopenia in children (1). It has also enhanced our understanding of the childhood antecedents of a condition that happens to manifest in elderly subjects: osteoporosis. Prior to the introduction of quantitative imagery analysis, the evaluation of bone mineral was done by conventional radiography, which provided a relatively insensitive depiction, as bone mass may have already decreased by as much as 40 percent by the time osteoporosis was appreciated (2).

Several modalities for the assessment of bone mineral content have been developed, each with its own method for data acquisition and each with beneficial and disadvantageous properties. Ideally, the technique employed should be 1] easy to perform without any need for sedation of the patient, 2] noninvasive, 3] harmless, 4] accurate, and 5] reproducible. It should be able to assess the size of the bones and the two components of bone mass (bone volume and bone density) in the axial and appendicular skeleton, as well as allow for determination of cancellous and cortical bone separately. The measurements should not be influenced by soft tissues, by the size of the bones, or by body size. Lastly, the ideal technique should be inexpensive.

Unfortunately, none of the techniques currently available fulfill all of the above criteria. Single-photon absorptiometry (SPA) and dual-photon absorptiometry (DPA) were used extensively in the past, but have been superseded. Magnetic resonance imaging is a promising technique for the analysis of cancellous bone, but it is still under investigation. In this chapter, we will describe the three modalities most commonly employed for bone measurements in pediatrics: dual-energy x-ray absorptiometry (DEXA), quantitative computed tomography (QCT) and quantitative ultrasound (QUS). It should be stressed that comparison between these techniques is difficult, and, more often than not, judgment regarding their value has been, at least partially, subjective.

DXA

Currently, DXA is the most widely used technique for bone mass measurements in the world. It has the major advantages of simplicity, availability and cost-effectiveness, coupled with a very low radiation exposure dosage. DXA represents an evolution of other projection methods, SPA and DPA, that used a radionuclide source (gadolinium 153) (3). With DXA, an x-ray tube is the source of photons resulting in a 1,000-fold higher photon flux, better edge detection and, therefore, better precision than its predecessors. Bone mineral measurements by DXA rely on the attenuation (absorption) of energy that occurs as the beam of x-ray photons scan across the region of interest. Two different energy photons are used; low energy photons that penetrate only the soft tissue surrounding the bone, and high energy photons that penetrate both the soft tissue and the bone. A detector measures the photons exiting from the region of interest and a computer subtracts the low energy values from the high energy measurements. The attenuation values are converted into measurements of mass of mineral with the use of calibration materials and the results are expressed as bone mineral content or BMC (in grams). Frequently, BMC values are divided by the projected area of the bone analyzed and the resulting measurements are conventionally referred to as bone mineral density or BMD (g/cm^2). Because these measurements are not representative of the true density of bone they are commonly referred to as area density.

Bone mineral measurements by DXA are routinely obtained at the lumbar spine, the proximal femur and the whole body, but peripheral sites, such as the forearm and the hand, can also be scanned. The examination procedure initially took 6 to 15 minutes, but newly developed devices using enhanced generators or a fan beam instead of a pencil beam source have reduced the time to approximately 2 minutes. Radiation exposure involved in DXA examinations is extremely low. The subject effective dose has been estimated to be about 1 μSv for lumbar spine measurements and about 4 μSv for whole skeleton scans (**Table 1**) (4,5). The in vivo precision of the posteroanterior DXA measurements has been calculated as ranging from 0.8% to 2.3% in children and from 1.55% to 2.5% in infants (6-11).

Table 1. Whole Body Equivalent Doses in Microsieverts (μSv) for Children at Different Ages

Exam		Age (years)		
		5	10	20
Chest X-ray		44	39	32
Lumbar Spine	Anteroposterior	21	20	18
	Lateral	131	121	112
DXA	PA Spine	~1	~1	~1
	Lat Spine	~3	~3	~3
	Proximal Femur	~1	~1	~1
	Whole Body	~4	~4	~4
QCT Spine	Scout View	48	45	41
	Axial Scan	9	9	8
Natural Background (per month)		224	181	107
Transcontinental Flight		37	30	18

Adapted from references 4,5,41.

It should be noted that bone measurements with DXA "densitometers" from different manufacturers display substantial variation in BMD values of the same bone. This variation arises from differences in bone standards, edge detection algorithms and regions of interest that are incorporated into the different devices. Recently, leading manufacturers of DXA equipment have proposed a standardization of BMD for measurements in the lumbar spine (**Figure 1**) (12). To provide similar standardization at other sites, such as the femoral neck, changes of the analysis software may be required because of substantial differences in the regions of interest that the various manufacturers have incorporated into the design of their devices. Lastly, the standard software from most DXA manufacturers was designed for adults. Although several manufacturers have developed special software to be used in pediatrics, this software requires longer scanning time.

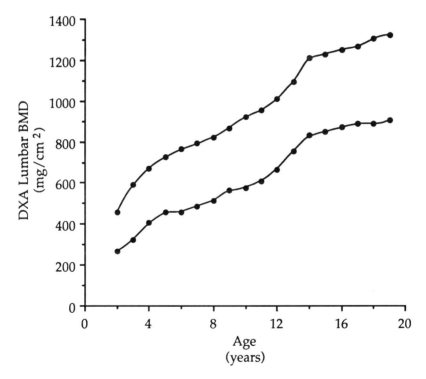

Figure 1. DXA values for the lumbar spine in relation to age in healthy, Caucasian girls (**Figure 1a**) and boys (**Figure 1b**). Measurements were obtained with a Lunar DPX-L absorptiometer (Lunar Corp., Madison, USA) (6), and have been standardized according to the method of Genant (12). Values represent 95% confidence limits and are expressed as mg/cm².

While bone measurements by DXA in the adult skeleton are accurate and reproducible, the major changes in body composition, body size and skeletal mass that occur during growth limit the utility of this technique in children. DXA is a projectional technique based on the two-dimensional projection of a three-dimensional structure. Its measurements are a function of the size of the bone being examined, the amount of bone and its mineral density (13). These values are frequently expressed as measurements of the bone content per surface area (gm/cm^2), as determined by scan radiographs. However, scan radiographs only provide an approximation of the size of the bone and any correction based on these radiographs is only a very rough estimate of the "density". Attempts to overcome this disadvantage with the use of correction factors; i.e., the squared root of the projected area, the height of the subject, the width of the bone, assuming the cross-sectional area of the vertebrae is a square, a circle or an ellipse, or that the femur can be modeled as a cylinder, etc., (7,14-17), are subject to error, as there is no closed formula that defines the size of the vertebrae or the femur. While the inability of DXA to account for bone size is not of great concern when studying the mature skeleton, in growing children, longitudinal DXA values are subject to considerable error, as they reflect both the changes in skeletal size and in bone mass.

DXA values are also influenced by the composition of soft tissues in the beam path of the region of interest. Because corrections for the soft tissues are based on a homogenous distribution of fat around the bone, changes in DXA measurements are observed if fat is distributed inhomogeneously around the bone measured. It has been determined that inhomogeneous fat distribution in soft tissues, resulting in a difference of 2 cm fat layer between soft tissue area and bone area, will influence DXA measurements by 10% (18). While this is not a limitation when studying subjects whose weight and body size remain constant, longitudinal DXA values in children are subject to considerable error, as the measurements may reflect the changes in body size and composition. This disadvantage especially limits studies in children with eating disorders, such as obesity or anorexia nervosa.

Other limitations of DXA studies in very young children include their lack of cooperation, resulting in motion and the presence of artifacts in the scan. Correct positioning is also of the utmost importance in studies of children. Lumbar studies may be inaccurate with even the mildest bending of the trunk, and exact positioning of the foot is required for proper assessment of the proximal femur. Recent studies have shown that motion artifacts may increase the values of the projected bone area by 9%, of BMC by 13% and of BMD by 4% (17). In an attempt to overcome these errors, children have been restrained (6,10), sedated (9,20), or studied while asleep (21).

Although normative data for DXA values of children exists in the literature and is included in most DXA software packages (**Table 2**), caution is advised before using this data for clinical use. Significant differences have been described in normal DXA values, mainly attributable to variations between devices, scanning protocols and body size of the subjects studied, and institutional and device-specific norms are preferable to published references.

Table 2. DXA Measurements of Healthy, Caucasian Children

Age (yrs)	Boys Femoral Neck	Boys Trochanter	Boys Total Body	Girls Femoral Neck	Girls Trochanter	Girls Total Body
2	0.22-0.82	0.29-0.61	0.59-0.78	0.42-0.50	0.28-0.48	0.66-0.81
3	0.34-0.74	0.16-0.80	0.62-0.87	0.38-0.62	0.20-0.64	0.60-0.90
4	0.41-0.73	0.26-0.74	0.64-0.94	0.27-0.79	0.22-0.70	0.65-0.84
5	0.41-0.89	0.28-0.84	0.71-0.90	0.18-0.98	0.13-0.85	0.63-0.94
6	0.4-1.0	0.29-0.85	0.62-0.98	0.28-0.96	0.25-0.77	0.70-0.85
7	0.41-1.01	0.33-0.89	0.72-0.91	0.35-0.91	0.29-0.77	0.70-0.89
8	0.43-1.03	0.30-0.98	0.74-0.91	0.32-0.96	0.20-0.88	0.68-0.90
9	0.41-1.09	0.32-0.92	0.72-0.94	0.37-0.93	0.23-0.87	0.70-0.91
10	0.45-1.09	0.26-1.02	0.70-0.10	0.53-0.85	0.39-0.75	0.68-0.90
11	0.44-1.12	0.32-0.96	0.83-0.87	0.38-1.06	0.45-0.77	0.70-0.91
12	0.48-1.12	0.35-0.99	0.74-1.01	0.35-1.19	0.51-0.83	0.65-1.01
13	0.42-1.30	0.54-1.02	0.91-0.96	0.43-1.31	0.55-0.91	0.74-0.96
14	1.42-1.38	0.33-1.29	0.93-1.01	0.46-1.46	0.56-0.96	0.68-1.05
15	0.57-1.45	0.48-1.32	0.83-1.16	0.41-1.45	0.52-1.00	0.76-1.17
16	0.55-1.63	0.42-1.50	0.94-1.26	0.40-1.48	0.56-0.96	0.82-1.19
17	0.47-1.83	0.46-1.46	0.93-1.34	0.46-1.38	0.38-1.14	0.85-1.24
18-20	0.46-1.86	0.32-1.56	0.95-1.38	0.29-1.61	0.26-1.26	0.92-1.23

Values represent the 95% confidence intervals for BMD measurements, are expressed as g/cm2 and were obtained from Zanchetta, et al with a Norland XR-26 absorptiometer (Norland Corp., Fort Atkinson, USA) (8).

Bone measurements with DXA have been done in children of all ages, (9-11,20-22) and, generally, values measured at all skeletal sites increase from infancy to adulthood (6,8,14,16,23-30). The relationship between age and bone mineral content in the lumbar spine, the femur and the entire skeleton appears to be represented by a segmented polynomial curve (6,8,24,26,27); a rapid increase during childhood is followed by an even greater increase during puberty that ends in the third decade of life (6-8,15,16,23-27,31). Interestingly, radial DXA values in children have not been found to be influenced by puberty (8).

Studies assessing racial and gender differences in DXA measurements of bone mass in children have yielded variable results. The majority of the studies indicate that by the age of 12 or 13 years girls have greater BMD than boys in the lumbar spine (6,14,23,26,28), while most (8,14,23,24), but not all (17,27), of the studies in the femoral neck have found greater BMC in boys than in girls 14 to 16 years of age. In the radius, one study found no gender differences (8), while boys had greater values than girls in another study (28). Similarly, some investigators found no racial differences in bone measurements by DXA between African-American girls and Caucasian girls (16,29), while others report higher values for African-American girls at all ages (32). A recent study found that Asian-American children have lower spine, femur and whole body DXA values when compared to Caucasian children and suggested the difference to be size related (33).

In summary, the relatively low cost, availability and ease of use are the main advantages of DXA. The main disadvantage is the inability of DXA to account for the large changes in body and skeletal size that occur during growth limits its use in longitudinal studies in children.

QCT

Computed tomography (CT) introduced the technique of digital imaging to diagnostic radiology. The transverse anatomic sections afforded by this digital technique provide a three-dimensional image unobscured by overlying structures. However, the pictorial display has overshadowed the very basis of that image - the digital data representing the attenuation values or CT numbers of the object scanned. These numerical values are stored in digital form and are accessible for future study, as needed. The use of this digital data for quantitative information has been labeled quantitative computed tomography (QCT).

Using a standard clinical CT scanner, with an external bone mineral reference phantom and specially developed software, QCT bone measurements can be obtained at any skeletal site. In the past, QCT was principally utilized for measurements of cancellous bone density (mg/cm^3) in the vertebrae. Cancellous bone is made up of a three dimensional lattice of plates and columns (trabeculae), that divide the area within the bone into interlinking pores filled with red and yellow marrow (34). Because of the relatively small size of the trabeculae when compared to the pixel (the CT unit of measurement), QCT values for cancellous bone reflect the amount of bone, as well as the amount of marrow per pixel (35).

A similar limitation applies to the vitro study of the volumetric density of cancellous bone, which is determined by washing the marrow from the pores, weighing it, and dividing the weight by the volume of the specimen, including the pores (34). Thus, QCT and in vitro bone density values for cancellous bone are directly proportional to the bone volume fraction and inversely proportional to the porosity of the bone. The rather large coefficient of variation for values of cancellous bone density reflect the considerable variations in the dimensions of the pores throughout the vertebra. It should be noted that the precision and accuracy of QCT cancellous bone density values are based on the percentage of fat in the marrow of the bone. In children, vertebral bone marrow contains very little fat, thereby increasing the precision and accuracy of the QCT values by 1% - 2% over those obtained in adults (36).

Vertebral dimensions can also be obtained from the same CT scan images taken for measurements of cancellous bone density. The coefficient of variation for determinations of vertebral body height has been calculated to be 1.3% and that for vertebral cross-sectional area to be 0.8% (37).

Recently, QCT has been applied to assess the bones in the appendicular skeleton, markedly improving our ability to measure cortical bone. Three bone parameters can be measured by QCT in the appendicular skeleton, the cross-sectional area (cm^2) of the bone, the cortical bone area (cm^2) and the cortical bone density (1,38). To this effect, the outer and inner boundaries of the cortex are identified by specially developed software at the place of the maximum slope of the profile through the bone. The area within the outer cortical shell represents the cross-sectional area, while the area between the outer and inner shells represents the cortical bone area. The mean CT numbers of the pixels within the inner and outer cortical shells provide the average density of bone. The coefficients of variation for repeated QCT measurements of cortical bone density, cortical bone area and cross-sectional area of the femur range between 0.6 and 1.5% (39).

The relative lack of porosity of cortical bone allows the material density of the bone (the amount of collagen and mineral in a given volume of bone) to be reflected in QCT values if the cortex is sufficiently thick to circumvent volume averaging errors (38). The minimum thickness necessary for an accurate density evaluation of cortical bone by QCT is 2-2.5 mm; below this threshold QCT values fall in a linear way relative to width. Above this thickness, the measured pixel represents the combination of the attenuation coefficients defined by the densities and concentrations of osteoid and mineral. While the nonmineral fraction may contribute to minor fluctuations in measurements of cortical bone density, QCT numbers are primarily based on the high attenuation coefficient of the calcified bone fraction (38). These measurements are analogous to in vitro determinations of the intrinsic mineral density of bone, which are commonly expressed as the ash weight per unit volume of bone (40). In children, the material density of cortical bone in the appendicular skeleton when measured by QCT remains fairly constant; 2.00 ± 0.065 gm/cm^3 (**Figure 2**), and is not influenced by age, body mass, race or gender (38).

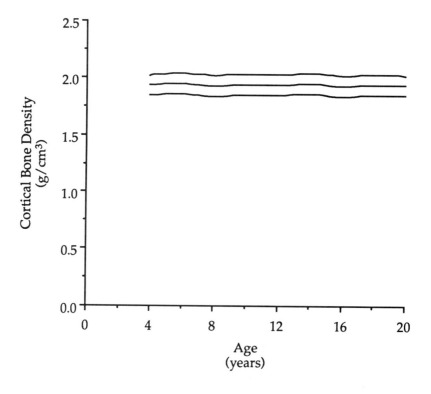

Figure 2. QCT values for cortical bone density at the midshaft of the femur in healthy children. Values represent the mean ± 1 SD, are expressed as g/cm3 and were obtained from reference 38.

While quantitative CT values provide precise, reproducible and accurate measurements of bone in children, this technique presents with various limitations that need to be addressed. In the past, with the exception of lack of availability, radiation exposure was the primary drawback of utilizing CT scans for bone measurements in pediatric research. Recent data, however, indicates that exposure from QCT measurements can be as low as 150 mrem (1.5 mSv), is related to the technique employed, and is far lower than that associated with other CT procedures. The total body equivalent dose of radiation is approximately 4 to 9 mrems (40 to 90 μSv), and this figure includes the radiation associated with screening digital radiographs used to localize the site of measurement (4,41). Radiation from QCT is also less than many other commonly used radiographic diagnostic tests. (**Table 1**) (4,41). Other limitations include the expense and costly maintenance of the equipment, the considerable technological expertise necessary for proper function, and the location of the scanner, which is usually in the radiology department of a facility and under constant demand for clinical purposes. These disadvantages have been partially overcome by the development of smaller, mobile, less expensive peripheral QCT scanners designed exclusively for bone measurements. Peripheral scanners, however, can only assess the bones of the appendicular skeleton.

Studies in healthy children using QCT have shown that events during puberty have a major influence on increases in cancellous bone density during growth (44), and that peak values are achieved around the time of cessation of longitudinal growth and epiphyseal closure (38,43). QCT studies have also shown a greater increase in vertebral cancellous bone density in African-American girls than in Caucasian girls during the later stages of puberty (44,45). Studies analyzing the influence of gender on QCT bone measurements during childhood indicate that the lower vertebral bone mass of women, when compared to men, results from early gender differences in the size of the bones rather than differences in cancellous bone density (37,46). Even after accounting for differences in body size, the cross-sectional area of the vertebral body is approximately 15%-20% smaller in girls than in boys (37). In contrast, QCT measurements of the cross-sectional area at the midshaft of the femur do not differ between boys and girls matched for age and anthropometric parameters (39). The size and the amount of bone in the femur does, however, correlate strongly with all anthropometric indices, suggesting that weight bearing and mechanical stresses are the major determinants of the increases in the size and the volume of cortical bone during growth (42).

In summary, QCT is able to assess the volume and the density of the bones in both the axial and appendicular skeletons. Its capability of providing accurate, precise measurements without influence from soft tissues or skeletal size is the major advantage for using this modality in children. Unfortunately, the cost and inaccessibility of CT scanners has markedly limited its use for bone measurements.

Ultrasound

Ultrasound has recently been utilized for quantitative bone measurements in the calcaneus, the patella, the tibia and the phalanges. Values are obtained by placing two transducers, a transmitter and a receiver, on opposite sides of the bone and measuring the changes that occur in the velocity and the energy of the ultrasound waves as they go through the bone. The ultrasound transmission velocity (UTV, also known as speed of sound, or SOS) is expressed in meters per second (m/s) and is procured by dividing the width of the region of interest by the transit time. When the ultrasound wave is absorbed and/or scattered by the medium through which it is being propagated, acoustic energy is lost and results in a reduction of wave amplitude, specifically referred to as broadband ultrasound attenuation (BUA). Between 200-600 kHz there is a linear relation between ultrasound attenuation and ultrasound frequency in most biological tissues. BUA is defined as the slope of attenuation versus the frequency in this range and is expressed in decibels per megahertz (dB/MHz).

The low cost, portability, simplicity and lack of ionizing radiation make ultrasound very appealing for pediatric use. Several limitations for measurements of bone in children, however, need to be addressed. First, it is believed that both BUA and UTV values are determined by the number, the thickness, the mineral content, and the three-dimensional arrangement of the trabeculae, and BUA values have been known to vary by as much as 50% depending upon the principle orientation of the trabeculae (35). These values are further influenced by the amount and composition of marrow in the bone and by other soft tissues in the path of the ultrasound waves (35). Second, all currently available ultrasound equipment for bone measurements is designed for adult use and employ relatively large transducers. When studying children, smaller transducers are needed to allow closer contact with the region of interest to be scanned without interference from air. On average, the diameter of the specially designed transducers for pediatric studies has been 1 cm (47-50). In addition, specially developed foot pads or calipers for small feet are necessary when studying children to maintain the correct position of the transducer near the bone. QUS measurements in children have been obtained at the calcaneus, the patella and the phalanges of the thumb, although no device has been used to measure more than one skeletal site.

In studies of children, UTV and BUA values increased with age but exhibited considerable variability (47,50). The influence of puberty on these values has been investigated with the findings that UTV values increase substantially between early and mid-puberty in girls, while the increase is constant throughout puberty in boys (49). Reported intra-observer coefficients of variation in children range from 0.5% to 1.2% for UTV (47,48,50) and from 3% to 5% for BUA (47,49).

Ultrasound is able to adequately predict fracture risk independent of bone mass determinations in elderly patients with osteoporosis, and, therefore, these measurements must be related to some aspect of bone strength (51). However, ultrasound values vary markedly and are dependent on so many structural parameters, that it is difficult to use this information in a meaningful way in children. Because these values seem to correlate more with bone size than with changes in the amount, the density, or the geometry of bone, increases seen during childhood may be related to changes in skeletal size (52). Multiple studies have failed to find strong correlations between QUS measurements and values from other bone measurement techniques, suggesting that ultrasound should not be utilized as a substitute for other modalities (35).

1. **References**

2. Kovanlikaya A, Loro ML, Hangartner TN, Reynolds RA, Roe TF, Gilsanz V 1996 Osteopenia in children: CT assessment. Radiology 98:781-784.

3. Lachman E 1985 Osteoporosis: the potentialities and limitations of its radiologic diagnosis. AJR 4:712-717.

4. Sartoris DJ, Resnick D 1989 Dual-energy radiographic absorptiometry for bone densitometry: current status and perspective. Am J Roentgenol 152:241-246.

5. Kalender WA 1992 Effective dose values in bone mineral measurements by photon absorptiometry and computed tomography. Osteoporosis Int 2:82-87.

6. Lewis MK, Blake GM, Fogelman I 1994 Patient dose in dual x-ray absorptiometry. Osteoporosis Int 4:11-15.

7. Del Rio L, Carrascosa A, Pons F, Gusinyé M, Yeste D, Domenech FM 1994 Bone mineral density of the lumbar spine in white mediterranean spanish children and adolescents: changes related to age, sex, and puberty. Pediatr Res 35:362-366.

8. Kröger H, Kotaniemi A, Kröger L, Alhava E 1993 Development of bone mass and bone density of the spine and femoral neck - a prospective study of 65 children and adolescents. J Bone Miner Res 23:171-182.

9. Zanchetta JR, Plotkin H, Alvarez Filgueira ML 1995 Bone mass in children: normative values for the 2-20-year-old population. Bone 14:3S-399S.

10. Braillon PM, Salle BL, Brunet J, Glorieux FH, Delmas PD, Meunier PJ 1992 Dual energy x-ray absorptiometry measurement of bone mineral content in newborns: validation of the technique. Pediatr Res 32:77-80.

11. Koo WWK, Massom LR, Walters J 1995 Validation of accuracy and precision of dual energy x-ray absorptiometry for infants. J Bone Miner Res 10:1111-1115

12. Venkataraman P, Ahluwalia BW 1992 Total bone mineral content and body composition by x-ray densitometry in newborns. Pediatrics 90:767-770.

13. Genant HK 1995 Letter to the Editor: Universal standardization for dual x-ray absorptiometry: patient and phantom cross-calibration results. J Bone Miner Res 10:997-998.

14. Carter DR, Bouxsein ML, Marcus R 1992 New approaches for interpreting projected bone densitometry data. J Bone Miner Res 7:137-145.

15. Kröger H, Kotaniemi A, Vainio P, Alhava E 1992 Bone densitometry of the spine and femur in children by dual-energy x-ray absorptiometry. J Bone Miner Res 17:75-85.

16. Katzman DK, Bachrach LK, Carter DR, Marcus R 1991 Clinical and anthropometric correlates of bone mineral acquisition in healthy adolescent girls. J Clin Endocrinol Metab 73:1332-1339.

17. Plotkin H, Núñez M, M.L. AF, Zanchetta JR 1996 Lumbar spine bone density in Argentine children. Calcif Tissue Int 58:144-149.

18. Moro M, van der Meulen MCH, Kiratli BJ, Marcus R, Bachrach LK, Carter DR 1996 Body mass is the primary determinant of midfemoral bone acquisition during adolescent growth. J Bone Miner Res 19:519-526.

19. Hangartner T 1990 Influence of fat on bone measurements with dual-energy absorptiometry. J Bone Miner Res 9:71-78.

20. Koo WW, Walters J, Bush AJ 1995 Technical considerations of dual-energy x-ray absorptiometry-based bone mineral measurements for pediatric subjects. J Bone Miner Res 10:1998-2004.

21. Lapillonne AA, Glorieux FH, Salle BL, Braillon PM, Chambon M, Rigo J, Putet G, Senterre J 1994 Mineral balance and whole body bone mineral content in very low-birth-weight infants. Acta Paediatr Suppl 405:117-122.

22. Chan GM 1992 Performance of dual-energy x-ray absorptiometry in evaluating bone, lean body mass, and fat in pediatric subjects. J Bone Miner Res 7:369-374.

23. Rupich RC, Specker BL, Lieuw-A-Fa M, Ho M 1996 Gender and race differences in bone mass during infancy. Calcif Tissue Int 58:395-397.

24. Bonjour J-P, Theintz G, Buchs B, Slosman D, Rizzoli R 1991 Critical years and stages of puberty for spinal and femoral bone mass accumulation during adolescence. J Clin Endocrinol Metab 73:555-563.

25. Faulkner RA, Bailey DA, Drinkwater DT, McKay HA, Arnold C, Wilkinson AA 1996 Bone densitometry in canadian children 8-17 years of age. Calcif Tissue Int 59:344-351.

26. Faulkner RA, Bailey DA, Drinkwater DT, Wilkinson AA, Houston CS, McKay HA 1993 Regional and total body bone mineral content, bone mineral density, and total body tissue composition in children 8-16 years of age. Calcif Tissue Int 53:7-12.

27. Glastre C, Braillon P, David L, Cochat P, Meunier PJ, Delmas PD 1990 Measurement of bone mineral content of the lumbar spine by dual energy x-ray absorptiometry in normal children: correlations with growth parameters. J Clin Endocrinol Metab 70:1330-1333.

28. Lu PW, Briody JN, Ogle GD, Morley K, Humphries IRJ, Allen J, Howman-Giles R, Sillence D, Cowell CT 1994 Bone mineral density of total body, spine, and femoral neck in children and young adults: a cross-sectional and longitudinal study. J Bone Miner Res 9:1451-1458.

29. Moreira-Andrés MN, Cañizo FJ, Papapietro K, Rejas J, Hawkins FG 1995 Comparison between spinal and radial bone mineral density in children measured by x-ray absorptiometry. J Pediatr Endocrinol Metab 8:35-41.

30. Southard RN, Morris JD, Mahan JD, Hayes JR, Torch MA, Sommer A, Zipf WB 1991 Bone mass in healthy children: measurement with quantitative DXA. Radiology 179:735-738

31. Tsukahara H, Sudo M, Umezaki M, Hiraoka M, Yamamoto K, Ishii Y, Haruki S 1992 Dual-energy x-ray absorptiometry in the lumbar spine, proximal femur and distal radius in children. Pediatr Radiol 22:560-562.

32. Theintz G, Buchs B, Rizzoli R, Slosman D, Clavien H, Sizonenko PC, Bonjour JP 1992 Longitudinal monitoring of bone mass accumulation in healthy adolescents: evidence for a marked reduction after 16 years of age at the levels of lumbar spine and femoral neck in female subjects. J Clin Endocrinol Metab 75:1060-1065.

33. Bell NH, Shary J, Stevens J, Garza M, Gordon L, Edwards J 1991 Demonstration that bone mass is greater in black than in white children. J Bone Miner Res 6:719-723.

34. Bhudhikanok GS, Wang M-C, Eckert K, Matkin C, Marcus R, Bachrach L 1996 Differences in bone mineral in young Asian and Caucasian Americans may reflect differences in bone size. J Bone Miner Res 11:1545-1556.

35. Dyson ED, Jackson CK, Whitehouse WJ 1970 Scanning electron microscope studies of human trabecular bone. Nature 225:957-959.

36. Genant HK, Engelke K, Fuerst T 1996 Noninvasive assessment of bone mineral and structure: state of the art. J Bone Miner Res 11:707-730.

37. Gilsanz V 1988 Quantitative computed tomography. Siegel M, (ed) Pediatric Body CT. 349-369.

38. Gilsanz V, Boechat MI, Roe TF, Loro ML, Sayre JW, Goodman WG 1994 Gender differences in vertebral body sizes in children and adolescents. Radiology 190:673-677.

39. Hangartner T, Gilsanz V 1996 Evaluation of cortical bone by computed tomography. J Bone Miner Res 11:1518-1525.

40. Gilsanz V, Kovanlikaya A, Costin G, Roe TF, Sayre J, Kaufman F 1997 Differential effect of gender on the size of the bones in the axial and appendicular skeletons. J Clin Endocrinol Metab 82:1603-1607.

41. Gong JK, Arnold JS, Cohn SH 1964 Composition of trabecular and cortical bone. Anat Rec 149:325-331.

42. Cann CE 1991 Why, when and how to measure bone mass: a guide for the beginning user. In: Frey GD, Yester MV (eds) Expanding the role of medical physics in nuclear medicine. American Physics Institute Washington, DC 250-279

43. Mora S, Goodman WG, Loro ML, Roe TF, Sayre J, Gilsanz V 1994 Age-related changes in cortical and cancellous vertebral bone density in girls: assessment with quantitative CT. AJR 162:405-409.

44. Gilsanz V, Gibbens DT, Carlson M, Boechat MI, Cann CE, Schulz EE 1988 Peak trabecular vertebral density: a comparison of adolescent and adult females. Calcif Tissue Int 43:260-262.

45. Gilsanz V, Gibbens DT, Roe TF, Carlson M, Senac MO, Boechat MI, Huang HK, Schulz EE, Libanati CR, Cann CC 1988 Vertebral bone density in children: effect of puberty. Radiology 166:847-850.

46. Gilsanz V, Roe TF, Mora S, Costin G, Goodman WG 1991 Changes in vertebral bone density in black girls and white girls during childhood and puberty. N Engl J Med 325:1597-1600.

47. Gilsanz V, Boechat MI, Gilsanz R, Loro ML, Roe TF, Goodman WG 1994 Gender differences in vertebral sizes in adults: biomechanical implications. Radiology 190:678-682.

48. Jaworski M, Lebiedowski M, Lorenc RS, Trempe J 1995 Ultrasound bone measurement in pediatric subjects. Calcif Tissue Int 56:368-371.

49. Lappe JM, Recker RR, Malleck MK, Stegmane MR, Packard PP, Heaney RP 1995 Patellar ultrasound transmission velocity in healthy children and adolescents. Bone 16:251S-256S.

50. Mughal MZ, Langton CM, Utretch G, Morrison J, Specker BL 1996 Comparison between broad-band ultrasound attenuation of the calcaneum and total body bone mineral density in children. Acta Paediatr 85:663-665.

51. Schönau E, Radermacher A, Wentzlik U, Klein K, Michalk D 1994 The determination of ultrasound velocity in the os calcis, thumb and patella during childhood. Eur J Pediatr 153:252-256.

52. Gluer CC, Cummings SR, Bauer DC, Stone K, Pressman A, Mathur A, Genant HK 1996 Osteoporosis: association of recent fractures with quantitative US findings. Radiology 199:725-732.

53. Serpe L, Rho J 1996 Broadband ultrasound attenuation value dependence on bone width in vitro. Phys Med Biol 41:197-202.

7 Prevention of Osteoporosis: Strategies for Optimizing Peak Bone Mass

Susan H. Allen, M.D., Ph.D.

Introduction

An important determinant of osteoporotic fracture risk is peak bone mass, defined as the amount of bony tissue present at the end of skeletal maturation (1). Heredity plays a major role in influencing bone mass and is estimated to contribute 75-80% of the variance in bone mass (2). Environmental factors including nutritional and endocrine factors, mechanical forces and exposure to risk factors account for the remaining 20-25% as summarized in **Table 1**.

TABLE 1. DETERMINANTS OF BONE MASS ACCUMULATION

INTRINSIC FACTORS

Heredity
Gender
Endocrine Factors
    Sex Steroids
    Calcitriol
    Insulin-Like Growth Factor

EXTRINSIC FACTORS

Nutritional Factors
    Calcium
    Energy
    Proteins
Mechanical Factors
    Physical Activity
    Body Weight

EXPOSURE TO RISK FACTORS

Hypothalamic Amenorrhea
Cigarette Smoking, Alcohol, Caffeine
Chronic Illnesses
Rheumatoid Arthritis
Cushing's Syndrome
Malabsorption Syndromes
    Cystic Fibrosis
Medications
    Glucocorticoids
    Thyroid Hormone
    Anti-Convulsants

Skeletal and Sexual Maturation

After infancy in which there is rapid skeletal accretion, the growth pattern in childhood is gradual for both boys and girls (**Figure 1**) (3). In contrast adolescence is characterized by accelerated skeletal growth and accretion. Both bone mineral content (BMC), a measure of bone size, and a real bone mineral density (BMD), a measurement partially correcting for bone size calculated as BMC per unit area, increase as a function of age. Approximately 37% of the total skeletal mass of adults accumulates during puberty (4). **Figure 1** illustrates the divergence in skeletal and sexual maturation between genders during puberty. Girls begin puberty at a mean chronological age of 11 years, reaching a mean peak height velocity of 9 cm/year at age 12 years (3,5). Menarche usually occurs just after the growth spurt and estradiol levels peak at a mean age 14 years (6). Epiphyseal closure occurs at age 15 to 16 when total body BMD also plateaus (7). Puberty in boys begins 2 years later and lasts at least a year longer than in girls (8). Mean peak height velocity is 10.3 cm per year and occurs at a mean age 14 (3). Testosterone levels continue to increase in Tanner stage 5 (6). Total body BMD also continues to increase after epiphyses close at age 17 to 18 (7).

The linear growth and accrual of mass of the appendicular skeleton are completed prior to the axial skeleton. Peak growth velocity precedes peak mass in both the leg and spine by 0.5-1.0 years, with completion of growth of the leg occurring about 0.7 year prior to the spine (9).

No gender differences in bone mass or density measurements are demonstrable until puberty when gender differences in skeletal maturation become apparent. Bone size, cortical shell, trabecular bone and cortical bone densities are greater in boys compared with girls (10). Differences may be due to a more prolonged duration of pubertal maturation experienced by boys (1). However, no difference is observed in the volumetric or true trabecular density of boys and girls as measured by quantitative computed tomography (11). Most studies have reported either BMC or a real BMD, but not volumetric bone mass. Because a real BMD attempts to partially correct for size differences, BMD will be reported in this chapter, unless BMC is the only reported measurement of bone mass. Bone mineral apparent density (BMAD), a measure of volumetric density derived from BMD adjusting for width, will be reported when available.

The consensus is that peak bone mass is achieved by late adolescence or the early twenties in industrialized countries: North America (12,13), western Europe (7,14), Australia (15) or Japan (16). The timing of peak bone mass acquisition depends upon gender and skeletal site and is summarized below.

Total Body. Gender differences in total body BMD emerge in late adolescence when boys have greater TBBMD compared with girls and TBBMD peaks later (7,12,15) as illustrated in **Figure 1** (7).

91

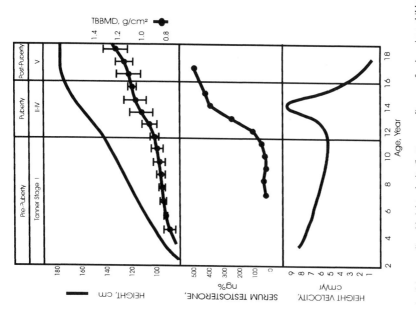

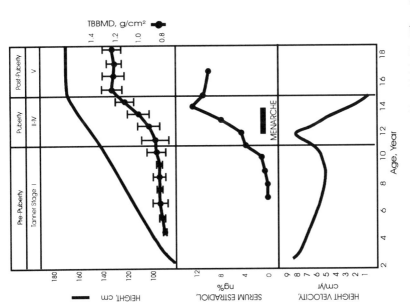

Figure 1 Skeletal and sexual maturation of girls (left) and boys (right). The 50th centile height attained (top panel) and height velocity (bottom panel) curves for American children of average growth tempo (ref. 3). The middle panels show the mean trends by age for serum estradiol derived from the longitudinal study of 58 female subjects (ref. 6) and for serum testosterone from the longitudinal study of 56 male subjects (ref. 6). The relationship between age and mean total body bone mineral density (TBBMD) and SDs is plotted in the top panel (from data published in ref. 7). Used with permission.

Lumbar Spine. Most studies of the lumbar spine density show that peak BMD occurs by the end of the second decade of life. Bonjour and coworkers (14) compared lumbar BMD of the adolescents grouped by age with a young adult cohort, 20 to 35 years of age. Peak bone mass of the lumbar spine was achieved in girls at age 14 or 15 years and in boys at age 17 or 18 years. These results have been corroborated in Canadian (12) and Australian (15) studies. In the North American cross-sectional study of Caucasian females, BMD of the lumbar spine reached peak values by 18.5 years of age (13). Slemenda and coworkers (17) reported that 17-year-old girls who had reached Tanner stage 5 by the age of 14 years had 97% of lumbar spine BMD compared with 30 year old women. In the Young Finns Study Group, lumbar BMD was not significantly different in males or females between the ages of 20 to 29 years, suggesting that peak bone mass had been achieved by the age 20 (18). In contrast, a longitudinal study of college coeds suggested that during the third decade of life, lumbar spine BMD increased 0.7% per year (19).

In a longitudinal study of both boys and girls, aged 9 to 19 years, Theintz et al., (20) reported the rate of change in the lumbar BMD was greatest from age 11 to 14 years in girls and 13 to 17 years in boys. In girls significant changes in rates were complete by age 16 years or by the second year after menarche. BMD in boys continued to increase from age 17 to 20 years for the lumbar spine. Rubin and co-investigators (21) showed similar results: the greatest change in girls for the lumbar BMD was age 10 to 15 years and in boys 13 to 17 years.

The BMAD of the lumbar spine in boys was less than girls in all age groups (7), but in Japanese children, lumbar BMD was higher in girls after the age of 13 years (16). BMAD reached a plateau by 15 to 16 years in girls compared with late adolescence in boys.

Skeletal age, rather than chronological age, is now appreciated as a better predictor of bone mass in children (22,23). Sabetier and coworkers measured lateral and anterior-posterior (AP) lumbar spine BMD in 574 females between skeletal ages 10 and 24 years (23). AP lumbar spine BMD increased dramatically between skeletal ages of 10 to 14, or until the first year after menarche (mean age at menarche was 13.1 ± 1.0 years) and increased moderately between ages 14 to 17 years. No further increase was observed beyond the fourth year after menarche. Lateral BMD showed no change after skeletal age of 14 years.

Femur. Bonjour and co-investigators (14) also compared the BMD of the femoral neck and shaft in adolescents with a young adult cohort, aged 20 to 35 years. In girls, peak bone mass was achieved in the femoral neck by age 14 to 15 years, but the femoral shaft did not reach peak values until age 17 to 18 years. In males, bone mass of the femoral shaft and neck continued to increase between ages 15 and 18 years. The femoral neck reached peak bone density at age 14.1 years and 17.5 years for Australian girls and boys, respectively (15). Slemenda and coworkers (17) showed that 17-year-old girls had 100% of the femoral neck BMD of 30 year old women. In the Finnish cohort study, a decreasing trend for femoral neck BMD was observed for both men and women from the ages of 20 to 29 years (18).

The rate of greatest change of BMD of the femoral neck and shaft occurred at the same ages as reported for the lumbar spine (20).

BMD of the femoral neck, trochanter, intertrochanter, and total hip was greater in boys but estimated volumetric BMD of the femoral neck showed no significant change in either boys or girls with age (12). In Japanese children BMAD appears to have no correlation with age in females, but a negative correlation with age was observed for males after ages 17 to 19 years (16). Because shape changes occur in the proximal hip during puberty, interpretation of these results is limited.

Radius. The radial BMD increases gradually and linearly in both girls and boys until the age of 15 years, when the change in BMD for boys accelerates (21). A large cross-sectional study of Caucasian females, aged 8-50 years, suggested that most of the radial BMD is accumulated by age 22 years but that BMD gradually increases until the age of 50 years (13). Similarly, in a large cross-sectional study of Finnish females, aged 7 to 47 years, most of the BMD of the distal one-third radius was achieved by 18.8 years and gradually increased thereafter (24). However, the BMAD of the distal radius slightly decreased (slope of the linear equation was -0.0001 g/cm3 per year). Girls in Tanner stage 5 at the beginning of a three-year observational study and age 17 years at the study's conclusion had 91% of the BMD of 30 year old adult women (17). The BMD of the radius of 18 year old daughters had 95% of their premenopausal mothers (25). In a prospective study of women, aged 21.4 ± 1.68 years at entry and studied for 1 to 5 years, median BMD of the distal one-third radius measured by single-photon absorptiometry increased 4.8% in the third decade or 0.5% per year (19).

Summary. The timing of peak bone mass is dependent upon bone site and type of bone. Lumbar spine and proximal hip BMD peak several years later in boys compared to girls. Girls acquire the majority of bone mass by the age of 14 to 15 years or by the first year after menarche. Boys attain peak bone mass at 16 to 17 years of age. BMD of the femoral neck peaks approximately one to two years earlier compared to the lumbar spine in girls (12,13,15,16,24,26) and boys (12,24,26). However, BMD of total body, lumbar spine and femoral neck peak in Japanese boys at age 17.5 years (16).

Determinants of Peak Bone Mass

Excluding genetic factors, the four most important primary determinants of skeletal mineralization include sexual maturation, calcium intake, body weight, and physical activity. Each will be considered separately, and then inter-relationships will be summarized. The complexities of these interactions will be illustrated by considering three specific groups of adolescents who are at great risk of compromising bone health.

Sexual maturation

The influence of sexual maturation is an important independent determinant of bone mass acquisition (7,17,26-28). The timings of the onset of puberty and maturation vary widely for both boys and girls. In boys, the first sign of puberty occurs between the chronological ages of 9.5 and 13.5 years (8). In girls the first evidence of pubertal change occurs between the chronological ages of 8.5 and 13.5 years (5). Boys reach sexual maturity between the ages of 13 and 17 years (8) and girls between ages 12 and 19 years (5). Sexual maturation or Tanner stage is a better predictor of bone density compared with chronological age.

Lumbar Spine. BMD of the lumbar spine increases approximately 33-70% between Tanner stage 1 and 5 in both sexes (7, 14, 21, 26). No gender differences in BMD of the lumbar spine have been demonstrated when BMD is compared for the same pubertal maturation stage (14, 26) except in the study of Rubin et al., (21) who found that girls had a significantly greater BMD in mid-puberty (stage 3). By using quantitative computed tomography (QCT), Gilsanz and coworkers showed that cortical bone density of lumbar vertebrae increased steadily from Tanner stage 1 to 5, but trabecular bone did not significantly increase until Tanner stage 4 and 5 in Caucasian females (29). Age at menarche also influences lumbar peak bone mass. Rice and coworkers (30) determined that the age at first menses accounted for 8% variance in lumbar spine BMC. A Japanese study of 519 women, aged 21 to 74 years, found that women who experienced earlier menarche had greater spinal BMD as determined by both dual-energy x-ray absorptiometry and QCT (31). In another Japanese study of 18 to 19 year old females, those who experienced menarche before the age of 12 years had 7% greater lumbar spinal BMD compared with those girls who experienced menarche after the age of 14 years (16). In addition, girls with central precocious puberty had lumbar BMD values 17% greater than age-matched girls. In contrast hypogonadal girls between the ages of 16 to 20 years, had lumbar BMD significantly lower than aged-matched controls and BMAD levels at the prepubertal level. Similarly, the spinal BMD of men with a history of delayed puberty was 9.7% lower than normal men when measured in the third decade of life (32).

Femur. BMD of the femoral neck (14, 26) and femoral shaft (14) increases about 33-38% and 40-50%, respectively, comparing Tanner stages 1 and 5 (14, 26). Boys had higher BMD in the femoral neck and femoral shaft compared with girls in the same Tanner stage of development, reaching significance in Tanner 1 (14, 26) and Tanner 5 (14) for the femoral neck and in Tanner stages 2, 4 and 5 for the femoral shaft (14).

Radius. One study showed distal radial BMD had no correlation with Tanner stage in Finnish girls, aged 8 to 20 years (28). In contrast, pubertal stage was an important determinant in the distal third of the radial BMD of children (21). Tylavsky and coworkers found that 18 to 22 year old females who were 10 to 12 years post-menarcheal had 10-12% greater mid- and distal radial BMD and BMC compared with those females of the same chronological age but 3 to 6 years after menarche (33). The distal radial BMD of men with a history of delayed puberty was 9.6% lower than normal men when measured in the third decade of life (32).

Mechanism. Hormones play an important independent role in increasing BMD during puberty. Growth hormone and insulin-like growth factor or IGF-1 act in synergy (34). Growth hormone and IGF-I peak at Tanner breast stage 3 to 4 in girls and Tanner genital stage 4 in boys. Indeed, Sabetier and coworkers observed IGF-I levels peaked at a skeletal age of 13 to 14 years in girls, corresponding to pubertal stage 4 or the first year after menarche (23).

Summary. During puberty, the rate of change of BMD in the lumbar spine is greater than in the proximal hip. The greatest increases of BMD occur at sites with more trabecular bone (lumbar spine and trochanter) compared with the distal radius which contains more cortical bone.

Calcium intake

The conclusion of a meta-analysis of 33 studies performed by Welten and coworkers (35) was that calcium intake has a positive effect on bone mass in young and premenopausal women. Several studies suggest that women whose intake of calcium was below the RDA during childhood or adolescence have clinically significantly lower BMD. Only a few studies have been published in children, but most indicate that calcium intake is an important determinant in obtaining peak bone mass. The effect of calcium intake varies according to skeletal site and age group. The results of each skeletal site are summarized below with prepubertal, pubertal and young adults age groups considered separately. Cross-sectional studies are summarized before the interventional and longitudinal cohort studies.

Lumbar Spine. The cross-sectional study of 299 children, aged 6 to 18 years, reported by Rubin et al., (21) showed no effect of calcium intake on the lumbar spine BMD after adjusting for pubertal stage, height, weight and age. The mean daily intake of calcium for male subjects less than 11 years and greater or equal to 11 years was 1090 mg and 1220 mg, respectively. In females, the mean daily calcium intake was 932 mg in subjects less than 11 years and 947 mg in subjects 11 years and older. No standard deviations were reported.

In a cross-sectional study of Finnish girls, aged 8 to 20 years, no significant effect of calcium was observed at the lumbar spine of the girls in the prepubertal cohort (age 9.2 ± 1.1year, N=40), Tanner stage 2-3 (N=54) or Tanner 4-5 (N=81) (28). Average daily spontaneous calcium intake for the three groups was relatively high (Tanner 1: 1018 ± 361mg, Tanner 2-3: 1059 mg ± 460 mg and Tanner 4-5: 1231 ± 565 mg).

Boot et al., (7) in a large cross-sectionally designed study examined the influence of calcium intake on the lumbar BMD of boys and girls, aged 4 to 20 years and found that calcium intake (1180 ± 516 mg/day) was not significantly associated with BMD of the lumbar spine in either gender.

Ruiz and coworkers measured BMD in French boys and girls, ages 7 to 15.3 years, stratified by Tanner stage (26). In contrast to the Finnish study (28), the mean calcium intake of girls (N =16) and boys (N=33) was lower in Tanner stage 1, amounting to 800 ± 425 mg and 862 ± 321 mg, respectively. Thirty-four of the prepubertal children had a calcium intake less than the RDA, with two children having a calcium intake less than 400 mg/day. Calcium intake was an independent determinant of lumbar BMD in multiple regression analysis. Although Z scores were not reported for the prepubertal group alone, 26% of the 101 children and adolescents with a calcium intake less than 1000 mg/day had Z scores < -1 compared to 4% of the 50 children with a calcium intake greater than 1000 mg/day. No significant association of calcium intake was observed in pubertal children (N=102). When comparing the entire male cohort with the female cohort, the calcium intake was significantly associated with the lumbar BMD.

In a three-year double-blind placebo-controlled study of 22 male and female prepubertal twins (mean age 6.9 ± 1.4 years), the effect of supplementation with 700 mg of calcium citrate malate (total calcium intake of 1612 mg/day) was compared with a baseline intake of 908 mg/day (36). The supplemented twin gained 2.8% more bone mass in the lumbar spine compared to the twin receiving the baseline calcium dose. No difference was observed in the lumbar spine of the pubertal subjects. A limitation of this study was that both boys and girls were included in the analysis of pubertal twins, a sexual maturation period in which there are marked gender differences.

Two randomized double-blind placebo-controlled studies of premenarcheal girls have been reported by Lloyd and coworkers. In the first study girls, aged 11.9 ± 0.5 years with a baseline calcium intake of 960 mg were compared to a group supplemented with an additional 354 mg calcium citrate malate for 18 months (37). The net gain of the supplemented group was 2.9% greater in the lumbar spine. Approximately 65% had reached menarche by the end of the study. In a two-year intervention study comparing a baseline daily calcium intake of 983 mg with a similar group supplemented with an additional 500 mg of calcium citrate malate in girls, aged 11.9 ± 0.5 years, Lloyd and coworkers demonstrated a net gain of 2.9% in lumbar spine BMD (and 2.8% in pelvis BMD) in the supplemented girls (27). Three-fourths of the girls had reached menarche at the conclusion of the study. Only those subjects with above-median Tanner scores were affected by calcium supplementation.

In a twelve-month randomized study of girls staged as Tanner 2 with a mean age of 11 ± 1 years, Chan et al., (38) observed a 9.9% greater gain in the lumbar BMD in girls supplemented with dairy products (daily calcium intake 728 ± 321 mg in controls versus 1437 ± 366 mg in the supplemented group). It should be noted that the supplemented group also had significantly higher intake of protein, phosphorus, and vitamin D, but not fat or total calories compared with the control group.

The Finish prospective cohort study of 9 to 18 year old females demonstrated no significant association of vertebral BMD adjusted for weight obtained between the ages of 20 to 29 years with daily calcium intake ranging from 996 ± 262 mg to 1083 ± 256 mg women (18). The effect of age of menarche was not considered in the statistical analysis.

Finally, a Dutch study of 98 females showed no significant effect of calcium on the BMD of the lumbar spine obtained at the age of 27 years in a multiple regression model after adjusting for body weight and weight-bearing activity (35). Daily calcium intake of 941 to 1204 mg since the age of 12 years was documented.

Femur. The BMD of the femoral neck in the 49 prepubertal and 102 pubertal French subjects (26) was not significantly associated with calcium intake. Many of these subjects had a calcium intake less than 1000 mg/day. In the Finnish cross-sectional study summarized above, the femoral neck BMD showed no significant association with calcium (mean calcium intake greater than 1000 mg/day) in either the prepubertal or pubertal subjects (28).

Three calcium intervention studies have shown none to small gains in BMD of supplemented subjects. In the three-year longitudinal twin study reported by Johnston et al., (36), the net gains observed in the Ward's triangle and trochanter, were 2.9% and 3.5% greater, respectively, in the supplemented prepubertal twin. In contrast to the gain observed in lumbar BMD of the Tanner 2 girls supplemented with dairy products, no differences were observed in the femoral BMD after one year of supplementation (38). In the Swiss study (39), the femoral diaphysis, neck and trochanter of the prepubertal girls supplemented with 850 mg of calcium demonstrated BMD gains of 1.1, 1.4, and 1.9%, respectively, compared with the girls receiving the placebo.

In the Finnish prospective cohort study (20), femoral BMD, adjusted for age, weight, and exercise, was 4.7% higher in those women who consumed more than 800 mg calcium during adolescence compared with the group consuming less than 800 mg.

Radius. In the cross-sectional study of American subjects reported by Rubin and coworkers (21), daily calcium intake was positively associated with radial BMD. In a cross-sectional study of 495 Norwegian children (8-11 years) and adolescents (11-17 years), adolescents with a daily average calcium intake of 1443 ± 351 mg had 4.3% greater BMD of the ultradistal radius compared to those with a calcium intake of 677 ± 226 mg/day (40). The distal radial BMD was not associated with calcium intake in adolescents. BMD of both radial sites was not associated with calcium intake in children. The Finnish cross-sectional study (28) revealed no significant association between calcium intake and radial BMD for prepubertal or pubertal children.

Lee and coworkers reported (41) an 18-month randomized double-blind placebo-controlled trial of prepubertal male and female Chinese children (mean age 7.2 ± 0.2 years). Subjects with a baseline intake of calcium of 280 mg were compared with subjects supplemented with an additional 300 mg of calcium carbonate. In spite of the calcium intake below the RDA, a 3.14% gain was observed in the radial diaphysis of the supplemented subjects.

The longitudinal study conducted by Johnston et al., (36), the supplemented prepubertal twin gained 5.1% more bone mass in the mid-radius and 3.8% in the distal radius compared to the twin receiving the baseline calcium dose during the three-year study. Unlike the prepubertal twins, the pubertal twins, aged 10.6 ± 2.0 years, supplemented with calcium showed no benefit in bone density of the mid-radial shaft. However, there was a net gain of 2.9% in the ultradistal radius, a site containing more trabecular bone compared with the radial diaphysis.

Swiss prepubertal girls supplemented with calcium-enriched milk extract for 12 months had a net gain in the BMD of the radial diaphysis and metaphysis of 1.4% and 1.5%, respectively, compared with those receiving the placebo (39). No significant differences were noted in BMD of the distal third of the radius in girls staged as Tanner 2 after 12 months supplementation with dairy foods (38).

Tylavsky and coworkers (33) demonstrated a 2.6% higher distal radial BMD in 18 to 22 year old females who had higher long-term milk and cheese consumption (>842 mg/day during high school and > 660 mg/day in college) compared with those with a lower calcium intake (<287 mg/day during high school and <209 mg/day during college). BMD was corrected for body mass-index and age at menarche.

In a cross-sectional study of 181 premenopausal women, aged 20-50, Halioua and Anderson (42) assessed the effect of lifetime calcium intake on radial BMD adjusted for age and lean body mass. The respective gain in BMD of distal and mid-radial BMD was 10-13% and 5.9-8.5% in women who had consumed more than 500 mg calcium per day compared with those consuming less than 500 mg/day.

Summary. These studies are consistent with the concept that calcium is a threshold nutrient for the skeleton. The effect of calcium appears to be greater on the prepubertal appendicular skeleton compared with the axial skeleton. In pubertal subjects interventional studies, but not cross-sectional studies, show a positive effect of calcium intake on the BMD of the axial skeleton. Trabecular bone is affected to a greater extent than cortical bone. By the third decade evidence suggests that adequate lifelong calcium intake results in significantly greater radial bone density compared to sub-optimal intake.

Weight

Body weight is an important independent determinant of BMD and is thought to be due to increased skeletal loading (43).

Lumbar spine. Most studies of either boys or girls have found that weight is positively correlated with the lumbar BMD (7, 6, 17, 28, 30, 35, 44, 45).

Femur. Weight was also positively correlated with the BMD of the proximal femur in several studies: the upper femur (head, neck, trochanter and upper third of the diaphysis) in boys and girls, especially Tanner 1 and 2 (26); the femoral neck in girls (28); and the trochanter in prepubertal children but the femoral neck in pubertal children (17). In the three-year observational study, Slemenda and coworkers observed that weight was positively correlated with the trochanter in prepubertal children, and the femoral neck in pubertal children (17). Lean body mass was a stronger determinant of femoral neck BMD in a study of adolescent children than body mass (46). In contrast, a population-based study of girls (N=39) and boys (N=48), aged 15.2 ± 0.4 years, in whom height and weights were documented by the public health service for the first 6 years of life, demonstrated that weight was a predictor of total body BMC but not total body BMD or femoral neck BMD and BMC (47).

Radius. Only one study has shown that weight is positively correlated with radial BMD (21).

Physical Activity

Several cross-sectional studies have reported a positive association of physical activity with BMD at various sites in both prepubertal and pubertal children as well as young adults. No consistent measure of "physical activity" was used in these studies. This must be kept in mind when evaluating the significance of varying degrees of physical activity on bone density. To my knowledge, no prospective trial of exercise has been reported and only one observational prospective study has been reported in normal children (17). However, BMD of athletes performing high impact activities has been compared with the BMD of children engaged in 'normal' activities (48-50). Several prospective cohort studies of children and adolescents have analyzed the effect of physical activity (20, 51) on BMD. Keeping in mind the limitations of these studies, several conclusions can be made.

Lumbar Spine. Two studies by Slemenda and coworkers evaluated the effect of physical activity on BMD. In a cross-sectional study of 59 pairs of male and female twins, ages 5.3 to 14 years, total weight-bearing activity as determined by a questionnaire was 12.4 ± 8.0 hours/week for boys and 9.8 ± 8.4 hours/week for girls (52). Seventy-seven per cent of the males and 61% of the females were staged as prepubertal. Tanner stage and calcium intake, two potential confounding variables, were not considered. General linear models were constructed for age since the older children were noted to be more active. Weight-bearing activity was not significantly related to vertebral BMD. Forty-five pairs of twins in the same cohort were studied three years later and prepubertal and pubertal children were analyzed as separate groups (17). The effect of activity was significantly associated with lumbar BMD in the prepubertal children, but not the pubertal twins.

Rubin and coworkers evaluated the contribution of physical activity as determined by a daily measure of kilocalorie energy expenditure in children, aged 6 to 18 years, and found a significant association with vertebral BMD after adjusting for weight (21).

The cross-sectional French study of 151 children and adolescents, aged 7 to 15.3 years, including 33 prepubertal boys and 16 prepubertal girls, evaluated the effect of calcium intake and physical activity on BMD (26). Physical activity was determined by hours spent per week in organized sports. The more intense activity profile was defined as 3-12 hours/week whereas the usual activity level was considered to be 1-3 hours/week. For the prepubertal subjects the physical activity was 5.0 ± 2.3 hours/week for girls and 4.9 ± 2.5 hours/week for boys. The mean calcium intake of all of the subjects was 810 mg/day, but 69% of the prepubertal subjects had an intake below 1000 mg/day. Multiple regression analysis showed that sports activity was not significantly associated with lumbar BMD in the prepubertal children. However, it should be noted that non-weight-bearing activities such as swimming were included and accounted for 36% of the time spent in activities. In contrast, sports activity was significantly associated with BMD of the lumbar spine during puberty.

In the Finish cross-sectional study of females, ages 8-20 years, physically active subjects were defined as those who competed and exercised regularly in an athletic club (28). Normally active children participated only in physical educational classes. Absolute values of BMD were reported by Tanner group. Thirteen of the 41 (32%) prepubertal subjects were physically active (the mean calcium intake was 1000 ± 361 mg/day). The vertebral BMD, adjusted by weight, was 4.3% greater in the more active children. The greatest changes in BMD of the lumbar spine occurred in Tanner 2-3 peripubertal children. Thirty of the 54 (56%) children were physically active. Weight-adjusted BMD was 10.3% greater in physically active peripubertal children compared with the normally active children. Only a 1.7% increment was noted in the vertebral BMD of physically active Tanner 4-5 children.

Boot and others evaluated the effect of physical activity on the spinal density in both girls and boys, aged 4 to 20 years (7). Physical activity was measured in terms of minutes per week of activities including organized sports, physical education classes, recreational activities, walking and cycling. Statistical analysis was performed on the entire group, rather than separating the prepubertal children from the pubertal children. The activity level of boys (9.1 ± 5.4 h/week) was significantly greater than that of girls (7.5 ± 4.0 h/week) ($p < 0.001$) and had a positive association with lumbar BMD after adjustment for age. The authors suggested that the physical activity level in girls was not correlated with BMD because of low variance in activity.

Dyson and coworkers (48) studied 16 pre-adolescent Canadian gymnasts, age 7 to 11 years, with 2 years of training involving high impact loading training of at least 15 hours per week. BMD of the spine was 4.5% greater than controls, but was not statistically different from the controls. When normalized for bone size

(BMAD) the lumbar spine density was 8% greater in the gymnasts compared with controls (p<0.05).

Alfredson and others (49) studied the effect of high impact loading in female soccer players, mean age 20.9 ± 2.2 years, who trained 6 hours/week for an average of 5.2 years. The lumbar spine BMD was 10.7% greater compared to age-, weight- and height-matched controls. Twenty Swedish male ice hockey players, aged 15.9 ± 0.3 years, who trained 10 hours a week, showed no significant difference when compared with a control group (50).

In the Finnish ten-year prospective cohort study of lifestyle in men and women, BMD was measured between the ages of 20 to 29 years after 11 years follow up (18). The effect of physical activity, based on a sum parameter of the weekly frequency of activities of greater than 30 minutes for four age cohorts, was significant for men but not women. When adjusted for age and weight, the lumbar BMD of men was 8.2% greater in the group with the greatest activity index compared to the lowest. The BMD was not adjusted for age of menarche. The mean calcium intake was approximately 1000 mg/day for women and 1400 mg/day for males.

Welten and associates (51) studied the effect of weight-bearing activity on vertebral BMD in 27-year old Dutch males and females followed longitudinally starting at age 13 years (Amsterdam Growth and Health Study). Weight-bearing activity, was converted to an activity score based on time spent engaged at three levels of intensity (4-7, 7-10, or >10 times the basal metabolic rate (MET) or resting oxygen uptake) during the three months prior to the interview. Three time periods were examined: 13 to 17, 13 to 21, 13 to 27 years. Weight-bearing activity was a significant independent predictor of spinal BMD in men, but not women in whom weight was the best predictor of BMD.

Femur. The association of physical activity with femoral BMD in the above mentioned studies are summarized briefly. Physical activity in prepubertal and pubertal children reported by Slemenda and others (17) was also significantly associated with BMD of the femoral neck and trochanter. However, in the French study, no significant association of physical activity was found with the femoral BMD in prepubertal or pubertal children (26). In the Finnish study, BMD of the femoral neck was 1% greater in the physically active prepubertal girls compared with the normally active subjects (28). Respective weight-adjusted BMD of the femur in Tanner stages 2-3 and 4-5 was 12.8% and 3.7% greater in the physically active group compared with the normally active group (28). In the Finnish study, both men and women had greater femoral neck BMD, 10.5% and 7.6% respectively, in the group with the highest activity index compared with the lowest (18).

The BMD of the femoral neck and trochanter were 7.8% and 16% greater in the gymnasts compared with controls (48). The young adult female soccer players described above (49) also had significantly elevated BMD in the femoral neck (13.7%), Ward's triangle (19.6%), and distal femur (12.6%) compared with controls (49). The BMD of the proximal femur and total femur were 7.2% and 5.6% greater in the high-activity ice hockey players, respectively (50).

Radius. Variable associations of activity and radial BMD have been observed in prepubertal children. Slemenda and coworkers (17) reported that physical activity was significantly associated with mid-radial BMD. In the Finnish study, a 12.4% greater radial BMD was noted in the more active girls (28). However, data were available for only 5 physically active girls and 12 normally active girls compared with the larger sample sizes used in the analysis of the femur and spine. In a study of 159 children, aged 8 to 11 years, simple regression analysis showed radial BMD was not associated with weight-bearing activity (30). None of the studies showed a significant association of physical activity with radial BMD in pubertal subjects (17, 21, 28).

Anderson and coworkers reported three studies evaluating the effect of moderate exercise and calcium intake in adult females. In the first cross-sectional study (N=181; ages 20 to 50 years), moderate to strenuous lifetime physical activity > 45 minutes four times a week was associated with greater BMD of the mid- and distal radius when adjusted for calcium intake (42). In the second study the effect of calcium intake and physical activity on radial BMD in 38 women, aged 24 to 28 years, was studied to identify factors that might be associated with BMD at a time when peak radial bone mass is achieved (53). In a multiple regression analysis, physical activity was positively associated with distal radial BMD but not mid-radial BMD. A cross-sectional study of 705 college women, aged 18 to 22 years, showed that exercise was an independent determinant of distal radial BMD (33). Distal BMD was 9% greater in the highest activity group compared to the lowest, after adjusting for body mass index and age at menarche.

Summary. Physical activity plays an important role in achieving peak bone mass. The level of activity appears to play a more dominant role in achieving BMD during puberty, especially in Tanner stages 2-3. However, when the skeleton is loaded in high impact activities, prepubertal children can gain up to 4-12% more bone density than children engaged in normal activity. The region of loading (lumbar spine and proximal hip) is most likely to have increased density, although in the longitudinal observational study of prepubertal children, radial BMD was greater in the more active children. BMD of the distal radius, but not the mid-radius, was greater in young adults who had higher activity levels during the second decade of life. The magnitude of change responsive to activity level varies among studies, but may be as great as 10%. Gains in cortical and trabecular BMD are observed when the bone is adequately loaded.

Interplay between sexual maturation, calcium intake, weight, and physical activity.

Many of the summarized studies have used multivariate analysis to identify which determinant plays the most important role in establishing peak bone mass. Some are limited by not including all of the essential independent variables in the research design. When applicable, the excluded variable will be noted in the following summary.

Lee and coworkers evaluated the potential predictors of BMD including weight, height, calcium intake and pubertal status in 84 Chinese children, aged 8.5 years, and 18 months later (54). Dietary intake of calcium was suboptimal (approximately 600 mg per day). Pubertal status was the strongest predictor in the lumbar spine and radius, whereas weight strongly predicted femoral BMD. Physical activity was not evaluated.

Rice and coworkers studied the relationships among whole body and vertebral BMC and BMD and sexual maturation, body mass, and measures of physical activity and fitness in postmenarcheal girls, aged 14 to 19 years, most of whom were staged as Tanner 5 (30). Calcium intake was not considered in the regression model. The major determinant of BMD of the lumbar spine and total body was found to be body mass which explained 34.5% and 30.2% of the variance, respectively. Body mass explained a greater variance in BMC of the lumbar spine (44.7%) and total body (68.2%). Age at first menses explained 4.06 and 8.58% variance in whole- body and lumbar-spine BMC, respectively, but not density.

In a cross-sectional study of boys (N= 205) and girls (N=295) from ages 4 to 20 years, Boot and coworkers evaluated the effect of age, weight, height, Tanner stage, calcium intake (mean intake of 1180 mg per day) and physical activity on BMD in the spine and total body (7). The conclusions from stepwise regression analysis were: (a) In girls, Tanner stage and weight accounted for 80% of the variance for the lumbar spine BMD and 85% of the total body BMD, with Tanner stage being the primary determinant. Calcium intake and physical activity did not have significant associations with BMD in girls. (b) Weight and calcium intake explained 88% of the variance in the total body BMD of boys, with weight being the major independent determinant of BMD (p<0.001). Calcium intake was positively associated with BMD of the total body (p=0.009), but not the lumbar spine BMD or BMAD in boys. Physical activity was significantly associated with lumbar spine BMD and total body BMD (p=0.04).

In the Finish cross-sectional investigation of females, aged 8 to 20 years, body weight seemed to be the most important determinant (28). Exercise positively affected the spine and hip (but not the radius) in the peri- and post-pubertal subjects (28). Calcium intake was adequate. In the Finnish prospective cohort study that focused on lifestyle factors affecting peak bone mass, the independent predictors of femoral neck BMD in females included age, weight and exercise (18). Only weight predicted lumbar spine BMD. In males, weight and exercise were important determinants of both lumbar spine and femoral neck BMD. In addition, age predicted BMD in the femoral neck, but not the lumbar spine in males. Age at menarche or completion of puberty was not included in the research design.

The Amsterdam Growth and Health Study as summarized above (51) concluded that for males, weight-bearing activity was the best determinant of peak bone mass in the spine whereas weight was the best predictor for women. Calcium intake, when adjusted for weight-bearing activity and body weight, was not a significant predictor when highest and lowest quartiles of calcium intake were compared although there was a trend. It should be noted that the mean calcium ranged from 941-1204 mg/day for females and 1100-1435 mg/day for males. Compared with calcium intake, weight-bearing activity has been suggested to be a more important determinant in vertebral BMD in Dutch adolescents and young adults, aged 13 to 27 years (51). Weight accounted for about 17% of the variance in males and 14% in females when the age period from 13 to 27 years was evaluated in this longitudinal observational study. The age of menarche or Tanner stage was not considered in the regression model.

The regression analysis performed by Anderson and coworkers suggested that exercise is a more important determinate of distal radius in college-age women compared with calcium intake (33).

In summary, the greatest changes in BMD of the lumbar spine and hip occur during puberty. Trabecular bone appears to be more sensitive to the hormonal effects associated with puberty, especially in girls. Cortical bone appears to be affected primarily by weight-bearing activity. Body weight has consistently been found to be an important determinant, and may be related to the loading effect on the skeleton. Calcium intake appears to be the least important determinant of peak bone mass, but appears to be important to optimize the effect of physical activity, especially in the prepubertal years.

It is not surprising that individuals at greatest risk for not obtaining peak bone mass are those who enter puberty late and who have sub-optimal nutrition resulting in a negative calcium balance and decreased weight. Obviously, children with growth delay related to chronic diseases are at great risk. Three specific groups of adolescents who potentially compromise their bone health are considered below.

First, individuals with anorexia nervosa have decreased BMD and increased risk for fractures (55). Trabecular bone (spine) is affected to a greater extent than cortical bone (radius and femoral neck) (56). The etiology of osteoporosis is multifactorial and includes low body weight, decreased nutrients including low calcium intake, amenorrhea, reduced physical activity and hypercortisolism (56). A critical amount of fat (22%) is necessary to maintain normal menstrual cycles (57).

Second, it is a well-recognized observation that amenorrheic athletes experience bone loss and are at risk for osteoporotic fractures, in spite of their weight-bearing activities. Rencken and coworkers measured lumbar spine and femoral BMD in 49 amenorrheic athletes, aged 17 to 39 years (58). Seventy-two percent of amenorrheic athletes were osteoporotic or osteopenic by World Health Organization criteria at the spine and femoral neck. When compared with eumenorrheic athletes, the amenorrheic adults had lower BMD especially in sites containing trabecular bone: lumbar spine (88%), proximal hip, including femoral neck, trochanter, Ward's triangle and intertrochanter (ranging from 81 to 89%), compared with sites largely composed of cortical bone: femoral shaft (92%) and tibial shaft (94%). The age at menarche was 14.4 years compared with 13.1 years in the eumenorrheic athletes. Multiple regression analysis indicated that body weight combined with months of amenorrhea and age of menarche predicted vertebral BMD for amenorrheic athletes. Body weight combined with duration of amenorrhea predicted BMD in the tibia and proximal hip. The femoral shaft BMD was predicted by weight alone. Daily calcium intake was 1062 ± 37 mg for the amenorrheic athletes compared to 981 ± 32 mg for eumennorheic athletes. Calcium intake was unrelated to BMD at any site for either group.

Third, excretion of calcium in sweat was significant in African-American collegiate basketball players (59). In the first year of the study, total body BMC decreased 6.1% and BMC of the legs decreased 10.5%. The average dermal loss of calcium was 422 mg per training session. When subjects received calcium supplementation in the following year, BMC of the total body and legs increased 2% and 3%, respectively. The investigators suggested that a calcium intake of at least 2000 mg/d should be considered during intensive athletic training in order to promote mineralization.

Strategies to optimize bone mass- modifiable factors

It is imperative to identify negative lifestyle factors that can potentially limit the acquisition of peak bone mass. The best window of opportunity to maximize bone mineralization is during puberty. Evidence has been presented to support the view that good nutrition and exercise positively affect bone health in children and young adults. Potential risk factors such as anorexia nervosa, athletic amenorrhea, and smoking should be identified and intervention initiated immediately.

Nutrition

Calcium. While it is recognized that a positive calcium balance is imperative during growth to ensure maximal skeletal accretion, several practical issues need to be addressed. First, many children are not consuming an adequate daily amounts of calcium. **Table 2** summarizes results of the United States Department of Agriculture's 1994 and 1995 Continuing Survey of Food Intakes by Individuals (60) for calcium in both males and females for the first three decades of life. A substantial percentage of both males and females are below the RDA for calcium. For example, less than 15% of adolescent girls consume the RDA for calcium. Males have a greater intake of calcium compared to females. Median (50th percentile) intake of calcium for females versus males at ages 6 to 11 years is 729 mg and 838 mg; at ages 12 to 19 years, it is 684 mg versus 1022 mg; and at ages 20 to 29 years it is 498 versus 725 mg, respectively (60). Twenty-five percent of females, aged 12 years or older, consumed less than or equal to 50% of the RDA for calcium (60).

106

AGE, year	0-0.5	0.5-1	1-5	6-11	12-19	20-29
RDA, mg	360	540	800	800	1200	800
PERCENT OF INDIVIDUALS BELOW:						
100% RDA						
Females	28.3		52.1	59.7	86.4	83.8
Males	28.3		52.1	44.4	64.6	59.4
75% RDA						
Females	9.4		29.4	34.0	68.9	66.0
Males	9.4		29.4	22.3	40.0	40.2
50% RDA						
Females	1.9		10.7	10.5	43.3	34.4
Males	1.9		10.7	6.5	19.2	19.3

TABLE 2: Calcium Intake. Percentages of Individuals with Diets Below Selected Levels of the 1989 Recommended Dietary Allowances (RDAs), by Sex and Age, 2-day average, 1994-5, USDA's Continuing Survey of Food Intakes by Individuals (ref.60).

Second, the adequacy of the RDA recommendations has been recently questioned. Peacock (61) suggested that an intake of 1000 mg in boys and 850 mg in girls does not meet the nutritional needs of children. Matkovic and Heaney's review of 34 calcium balance studies indicated that the 1989 RDA for calcium during the life cycle may underestimate the requirement of maximal calcium retention (62). In 1994 the NIH published new guidelines for calcium intake based on age (63). The consensus panel recommended a daily intake of 800-1200 mg for children (compared to the RDA of 800 mg) and 1200-1500 mg for adolescents and young adults (compared to the RDA of 1200 mg).

Only recently has a calcium retention study been performed in which the dose effect of dietary calcium intake has been specifically studied (64). The protocol used four pairs of low and high calcium intake, defined as being above or below the recommended NIH Consensus Conference 1200-1500 mg/day in a crossover design to study adolescent females. Basal dietary calcium of 799 ± 163 mg/day was provided primarily by dairy products. Total calcium intake ranged from 841 to 2173 mg/day and supplemented diets included calcium fortified fruit-flavored beverages containing calcium citrate malate. Potentially confounding variables were minimized by stratifying subjects at baseline according to postmenarcheal age, body-mass index and osteocalcin level. No additional salt intake was permitted during the study. The lower limit of dietary calcium intake for adolescent females to achieve 100% calcium retention in bone was 1300 mg/day. Maximal skeletal calcium retention was 473 ± 114 mg/day (SEM). Maximal calcium retention decreased with postmenarcheal age: the mean ± SEM at 0, 10 and 20 months was 584 ± 165, 510 ± 161, 435 ± 160 mg/day, respectively. Between ages 12 and 15 years, fractional absorption of calcium, net absorption, net bone deposition and calcium balance decrease dramatically in girls (65). Efforts to maximize peak bone mass should occur before the age of 15 years in girls.

In an effort to establish more complete nutritional reference values, the Food and Nutrition Board of the Institute of Medicine, National Academy of Science, is replacing the nutrient requirement estimates previously expressed as Recommended Daily Allowance (RDA) with the development of Dietary Reference Intakes or RDIs (66). In addition to prevention of nutritional deficiencies, the new RDIs are based on evidence pertaining to prevention of disease and developmental disorders. The set of nutrient values of the RDI includes: Estimated Average Requirement (EAR), Recommended Daily Allowance (RDA), Adequate Intake (AI) and the Tolerable Upper Intake Level (UL). The EAR is defined as the intake that meets the estimated nutrient need of 50 percent of the individuals in that group. The RDA is based on the EAR and is the intake that meets the nutrient need of almost all (97 to 98 percent) individuals in that group. When scientific evidence is not available to calculate the EAR, then AIs are utilized. AI is the average observed or experimentally derived intake by a defined population or subgroup (instead of individuals) that appears to sustain a defined nutritional state, such as normal circulating nutrient value, growth, or other functional indicators of health. Finally, the UL is the maximal intake by an individual that is unlikely to pose risks of adverse health effects in almost all (97 to 98 percent) individuals.

The RDIs have been developed for calcium, phosphorus and vitamin D as summarized in **Table 3** for the first three decades of life (66). In the case of calcium, only AIs have been defined for age-specific groups. A gender difference could not be established due to insufficient data in males. During pregnancy and lactation, the AI for calcium is the same as in non-pregnant and non-lactating females. The primary indicator used to define adequacy of calcium intake for children, adolescents, and young adults is maximal calcium retention (calcium balance is the criterion of adequate calcium intake in men and women ages 31 to 50 years and bone mineral mass for pregnancy and lactation). The functional outcome considered to be most important is reduced osteoporotic fracture risk. The UL for calcium has not been determined for infants since they usually do not take calcium supplements, but is 2500 mg/day for all other age groups.

TABLE 3. Reference Dietary Intakes for Calcium, Phosphorus and Vitamin D Based on Age (ref. 66)

Age, years	Calcium AI* mg/d	Phosphorus AI* or EAR** mg/d	 ***RDA mg/d	Vitamin D AI IU/day
0-0.5	210	100*	-	200
0.5-1	270	275*	-	200
1-3	500	380**	460	200
4-5	800	405**	500	200
9-13	1300	1055**	1250	200
14-18	1300	1055**	1250	200
19-30	1000	580**	700	200

*AI = Adequate Intake (average observed intake that appears to sustain a defined nutritional state).

**EAR = Estimated Average Requirement (intake that meets the estimated need of 50% of the individuals).

***RDA = Recommended Daily Allowance (intake that meets the nutrient need of 97-98 % of individuals).

In the United States the mean daily milk consumption of adolescent boys is approximately 1 cup (316 grams) and in girls is less than one cup (207 grams) (60). Furthermore, adolescents drink twice as much carbonated beverages (1 1/3 cups for girls and 2-2/3 cups for boys per day). Clearly, children and adolescents must increase their daily calcium intake, either in dairy products, fortified foods or supplements. Based on a fractional absorption of 32.1%, 96.3 mg of calcium is absorbed per serving of milk. The calcium content in fortified fruit beverages is equivalent to milk but the fractional absorption is approximately 50%. Therefore, about 150 mg of calcium is absorbed per serving of fortified juice (67). The calcium absorption efficiency varies for supplements. Approximately 26% of calcium is absorbed from calcium carbonate and 36% from calcium citrate malate (68). Another consideration is the percent of elemental calcium in different supplements. Calcium carbonate contains 40% elemental calcium, and fewer tablets are required to meet the requirement of calcium. Dairy products are the best source of calcium. Two other at risk groups for consuming inadequate amounts of calcium are the lactose intolerant (69) and strict vegetarians (67). Calcium should be taken on a regular basis since its benefit is lost when calcium is discontinued (54,70).

Vitamin D. In the United States, one cup of milk is fortified with approximately 100 IU of vitamin D (68). Other dietary sources of vitamin D include eggs, fish oils and liver. The AI of vitamin D from birth through age 30 years is 200 IU/day

(60). The UL is 1000 IU/day in the first year of life and 2000 IU/day from the age of 1 year to 30 years (60). Supplementation of vitamin D is not be needed if there is adequate exposure to sunshine.

Vitamin C. Vitamin C is a necessary cofactor for collagen synthesis. Gunnes and Lehmann showed that radial BMD is predicted by vitamin C in adolescents (ages 11 to 17 years), but not in children (ages 8 to 11 years) (40). Results of the USDA 1994-95 survey (60) indicate that 38.0% of girls (aged 12 to 19 years) and 31.1% of boys (aged 12 to 19 years) have a vitamin C intake below 100% of the RDA (50-60 mg). Girls and boys, aged 6 to 11 years, consume 24.2% and 22.8% of the RDA (45 mg) for vitamin C, respectively.

Calcium-Nutrient Interactions. The conclusion of the standing committee on the Scientific Evaluation of Dietary Reference was that no recommendation could be made for adjusting calcium intake based on sodium, protein or caffeine intake (66).

Weight

In developed countries, there is an obsession to be thin, especially by the young. Seventy percent of girls and 30 percent of boys in high school have reported that they are trying to lose weight or not gain weight (70). In the same study, up to 14% of females reported using vomiting and 21% using diet pills to lose weight.

In 1994-5, the USDA reported 50% of females, aged 6 to 19 years, had food energy intake 81-84% of the RDA compared with males who had food energy intake between 91-95% of the RDA (60). At the 25th percentile, food intake of females and males was 63-71% and 71-78% of the RDA, respectively. Between 72-74% of girls, aged 6 to 19 years, had a food energy intake less than the 100% of the RDA compared to 55-62% of boys of the same ages. The mean food energy intake for females aged 6 to 11 years was 1814 kilocalories compared to 2056 kilocalories for boys. For adolescents, aged 12 to 19 years, boys consumed 800 kilocalories more than girls (boys- 2740 kilocalories and girls- 1901 kilocalories).

Growth should be monitored in children and adolescents. Nutrition guidelines need to be reviewed with the child and parents on a periodic basis especially during adolescence. The possibility of under-nutrition or an eating disorder needs to be explored with teenagers and the risks and consequences of such behavior clearly defined.

Physical activity

The cross-sectional studies summarized here suggest that physical activity decreases in girls during adolescence. Rubin et al., reported that the mean kilocalorie energy expenditure score was greater in males than females after age fourteen (21). In the Amsterdam Growth and Health Study (51), light to medium weight-bearing activity was noted to be approximately the same during ages 13 to 17 years, but boys participated more in heavy exercise (boys: 103.5 ± 107 minutes/week, females: 18.06 ± 41.31 minutes/week). Total weight-bearing activity from ages 13 to 17 years was also greater in males (3681 ± 1454 METs) than females (2857 ± 1180 METs). After age 17 years there was no gender difference in these measures of physical activity. On a percentage basis, there was a decline in the number of Finnish girls who participated in athletic club-sponsored activities between Tanner stage 2-3 (56%) and Tanner stage 4 and 5 (42%) (28). In contrast, no difference in physical activity based upon hours per week spent in sports activities was noted when French girls and boys were compared by Tanner stage (26).

What type of activity has the greatest osteogenic effect? Lanyon suggests that activities of high peak strains, high strain rates and strain distributions from different directions are the most osteogenic (72). The number of cycles of repetitions probably does not need to exceed 50 and be performed more than three times a week. A recent study in early post-menopausal women indicated that strengthening (low repetition high-load regimen) exercises rather than endurance (high repetition low-load regimen) resulted in the greater increase in BMD (73).

Power sports and strength sports such as gymnastics or fast ball games such as squash or tennis are the most effective activities (74,75). Running, cross-country skiing and certainly swimming would be less desirable activities for strengthening the bones because they involve large number repetitions of low peak force.

The starting age of physical activity may also be an important determinant in achieving peak bone mass. Kannus and coworkers reported that female tennis and squash players had twice the benefit of exercise on BMC in the dominant arm if they started training at or before menarche instead of after menarche (76). This finding suggests that pubertal subjects should be targeted for high-impact exercise activities. The residual effect of high loading activity on adult bone mass appears to be significant as suggested by a study comparing BMD of former collegiate female gymnasts (mean age, 36.3 ± 1.0 years) with age-matched controls (77). The BMD of the lumbar spine and hip sites were 16% and 18-22% greater in the former gymnasts compared with females who had never engaged in gymnastics.

Limiting Risk Factors

Smoking. A primary risk factor for osteoporosis is smoking. The Finnish prospective cohort study of lifestyle factors during adolescence and young adulthood concluded that men who smoked had a 9.7% lower femoral neck BMD compared to non-smokers when adjusted for weight, age and exercise (18). Smoking did not significantly affect the BMD of women in this study. An earlier report of premenopausal women, aged 20 to 39 years, who had smoked ≥ 2 cigarettes per day for at least one year were found to have a lumbar BMD 4% lower

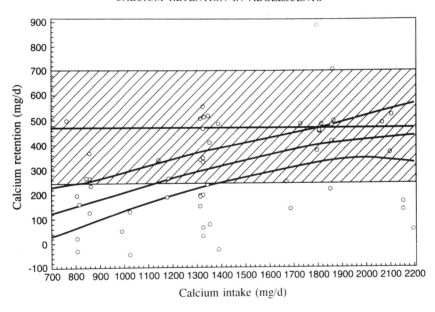

Figure 2 Calcium retention as a function of calcium intake in adolescent females. The three sloped lines represent mean and 95% Confidence Interval resulting from the linear regression model. The slopes of the lines are significantly different from zero (P< 0.05). The horizontal line is the mean maximal calcium retention (473 mg/d). The shaded area indicates the 95% CI for mean maximal retention (ref. 64; used with permission).

112

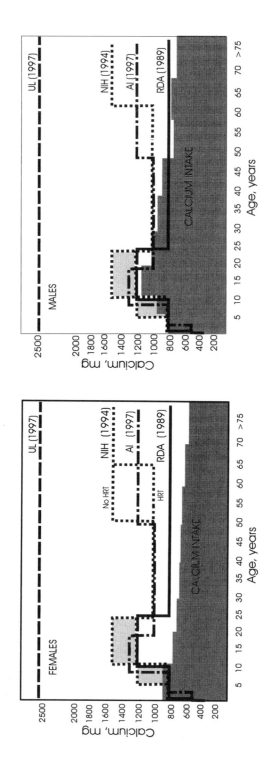

Figure 3 Daily calcium intake of calcium (mg) from the USDA's 1994-95 Continuing Survey of Food Intakes (ref. 60) for females (left) and males (right) compared with the RDA (1989), NIH (1994) and (AI) 1997 recommendations for daily calcium intake. AI is adequate intake and UL is upper limit (see text).

than non-smokers (78). The significance of this risk factor may have a larger impact considering 28.5% of men and 22.9% of women in the United States, aged 18 to 24 years, smoke cigarettes (79).

Amenorrheic athletes. It is imperative to identify patients at risk and to recommend proper nutrition, including adequate intake of calcium and weight gain. Treatment with hormone replacement therapy or oral contraceptives should be considered early. The importance of identifying these individuals is underlined by the recent longitudinal study of former amenorrheic athletes. The vertebral BMD of women, mean age 30.6 years, who had resumed normal menses or been treated with oral contraceptives for 6 to 10 years remained low (80).

Other. Children with chronic diseases such as juvenile rheumatoid arthritis, cystic fibrosis, inflammatory bowel disease, sickle cell disease, and asthma are at risk for osteoporosis. Inadequate nutrition, alcohol use, decreased activity, delayed puberty and therapy with immunosuppressive agents such as glucocorticoids negatively impact the growing skeleton. The treating physician needs to keep in mind the issues relating to optimal peak bone mass when managing medical problems in children with chronic illnesses.

Conclusion

Primary prevention of osteoporosis is fundamental in decreasing fracture risk later in life. An essential prevention strategy is to maximize peak bone mass, especially during adolescence, before peak bone mass is achieved by the second decade of life. Although few longitudinal studies have been reported during childhood, weight-bearing activity and adequate nutrition including calcium intake appear to be important determinants of peak bone mass. The effect of exercise on bone mass is site-specific and load dependent and may play a greater role in reaching peak bone mass compared with calcium intake, at least during adolescence. The calcium intake of children in the United States, especially girls, does not meet the recommended guidelines. Consumption of dairy products or fortified food should be encouraged and supplemented with calcium if necessary to reach optimal calcium intake. High-risk individuals need to be identified and intervention strategies initiated to minimize the deleterious effect of the risk factor on the growth and mineralization of the skeleton.

References

1. Bonjour JP, Theintz G, Law F, Slosman D, Rizzoli R 1994 Peak Bone Mass. Osteoporosis Int 4(Suppl 1):S7-13.

2. Slemenda CW, Christian JC, Williams CJ, Norton JA, Johnston CC Jr 1991 Genetic determinants of bone mass in adult women: a reevaluation of the twin model and the potential importance of gene interaction on heritability estimates. J Bone Miner Res 6:561-567.

3. Tanner JM, Davis PS 1985 Clinical longitudinal standards for height and height velocity for North American children. J Pediatr 107:317-329.

4. Matkovic V 1992 Calcium intake and peak bone mass. N Engl J Med 327:119-120.

5. Marshall WA, Tanner JM 1969 Variations in pattern of pubertal changes in girls Arch Dis Child 44:291-303.

6. Faiman C, Winter JSD 1974 "Gonadotropins and sex hormone patterns in puberty; clinical data." In Grumbach MM, Grave GD, Mayer FE (eds): The Control of the Onset of Puberty. New York, NY: John Wiley & Sons 32-61.

7. Boot AM, DeRidder MAJ, Pols HAP, Krenning EP, DeMuinck Keizer-Schrama SMPF 1997 Bone mineral density in children and adolescents: Relation to puberty, calcium intake, and physical activity. J Clin Endocrinol Metab 82:57-62.

8. Marshall WA, Tanner JM 1970 Variations in the pattern of pubertal changes in boys. Arch Dis Child 45:13-23.

9. Bass S, Pearce G, DeLuca V, Hendrich E, Seeman E 1997 Heterogeneity in the tempo and growth of axial and appendicular bone size and bone mass. J Bone Miner Res 12 (suppl 1):S342.

10. Gilsanz V, Gibbens DT, Carlson M, Boechat MI, Cann CE, Schulz EE 1988 Peak trabecular vertebral density: A comparison of adolescent and adult females. Calcif Tissue Int 43:260-262.

11. Genant HK, Gluer C-C, Lotz JC 1994 Gender differences in bone density, skeletal geometry, and fracture biomechanics. Radiology 190:636-640.

12. Faulkner RA, Bailey DA, Drinkwater DT, McKay HA, Arnold C, Wilkinson AA 1996 Bone densitometry in Canadian children 8-17 years of age. Calcif Tissue Int 9:344-351.

13. Matkovic V, Jelic T, Wardlaw GM, Ilich JZ, Goel PK, Wright JK, Andon MB, Smith KT, Heaney RP. 1994 Timing of peak bone mass in Caucasian females and its implication for the prevention of osteoporosis. J Clin Invest 93:799-808.

14. Bonjour JP, Theintz G, Buchs B, Slosman D, Rizzoli R 1991 Critical years and stages of puberty for spinal and femoral bone mass accumulation during adolescence. J Clin Endocrinol Metab 73:555-563.

15. Lu PW, Briody JN, Ogle GD, Morley K, Humphries IRJ, Allen J, Howman-Giles R, Sillence D, Cowell CT 1994 Bone mineral density of total body, spine, and femoral neck in children and young adults: A cross sectional and longitudinal study. J Bone Miner Res 9(9):1451-1457.

16. Takahashi Y, Minamitani K, Kobayashi Y, Minagawa M, Yasuda T, Niimi H 1996 Spinal and femoral bone mass accumulation during normal adolescence: Comparison with female patients with sexually precocity and with hypogonadism. J Clin Endocrinol Metab 81:1248-1253.

17. Slemenda CW, Reister TK, Hul SL, Miller JZ, Christian JC, Johnston CC Jr 1994 Influences on skeletal mineralization in children and adolescents: evidence for varying effects of sexual maturation and physical activity. J Pediatr 125:201-207.

18. Valimaki MJ, Karkkainen M, Lamberg-Allardt C, Laitinen K, Alhava E, Heikkinen J, Impivaara O, Makela P, Palmgren J, Seppanen R, Vuori I, and the Cardiovascular Risk in Young Finns Study Group 1994 Exercise, smoking, and calcium intake during adolescence and early adulthood as determinants of peak bone mass. BMJ 309:230-235.

19. Recker RR, Davies KM, Hinders SM, Heaney RP, Stegman MR, Kimmel DB1992 Bone gain in young adult women. JAMA 268(17):2403-2408.

20. Theintz G, Buchs B, Rizzoli R, Slosman D, Clavien H, Sizonenko PC, Bonjour JP 1992 Longitudinal monitoring of bone mass accumulation in healthy adolescents: Evidence for a marked reduction after 16 years of age at the levels of lumbar spine and femoral neck in female subjects. J Clin Endocrinol Metab 75:1060-1065.

21. Rubin K, Schirduan V, Gendreau P, Sarfarazi M, Mendola R, Dalsky G 1993 Predictors of axial and peripheral bone mineral density in healthy children and adolescents, with special attention to the role of puberty. J Pediatr 123:863-870.

22. Ilich JZ, Hangartner TN, Skugor M, Roche AF, Goel PK, Matkovic V 1996 Skeletal age as a determinant of bone mass in preadolescent females. Skeletal Radiol 25:431-439.

23. Sabatier J-P, Guaydier-Souquieres G, Laroche D, Benmalek A, Fournier L, Guillon-Metz F, Delavenne J, Denis AY 1996 Bone mineral acquisition during adolescence and early adulthood: A study in 574 healthy females 10-24 years of age. Osteoporosis Int 6:141-148.

24. Haapasalo H, Kannus P, Sievanen H, Pasanen M, Uusi-Rasi K, Heinonen A, Oja P, Vuori I 1996 Development of mass, density, and estimated mechanical characteristics of bones in Caucasian females. J Bone Miner Res 11:1751-1760.

25. Tylavsky FA, Bortz AD, Hancock RL, Anderson JJB 1989 Familial resemblance of radial bone mass between premenopausal mothers and their college-age daughters. Calcif Tissue Int 45:265-272.

26. Ruiz JC, Mandel C, Garabedian M 1995 Influence of spontaneous calcium intake and physical exercise on the vertebral and femoral bone mineral density of children and adolescents. J Bone Miner Res 10:675-682.

27. Lloyd T, Martel JK, Rollings N, Andon MB, Kulin H, Demers LM, Eggli DF, Kieselhorst K, Chinchilli VM 1996 The effect of calcium supplementation and Tanner stage on bone density, content, and area in teenage women. Osteoporosis Int 6:276-283.

28. Uusi-Rasi K. Haapasalo H, Kannus P, Pasanen M. Sievanen H. Oja P, Vuori I 1997 Determinants of bone mineralization in 8 to 20 year old Finnish females. Eur J Clin Nutr 51:54-59.

29. Mora S, Goodman WG, Loro ML, Roe TF, Sayre J, Gilsanz V 1994 Age-related changes in cortical and cancellous vertebral bone density in girls:Assessment with   quantitative   CT. AJR 162:405-409.

30. Rice S, Blimkie CJR, Webber CE, Levy D, Martin J, Parker D, Gordon CL 1993 Correlates and determinants of bone mineral content and density in healthy adolescent girls. Can J Physiol Pharmacol 71:923-930.

31. Ito M, Yamada M, Hayashi K, Ohki M, Uetani M, Nakamura T 1995 Relation of early menarche to high bone mineral density. Calcif Tissue Int 57:11-14.

32. Finkelstein JS, Neer RM, Biller BMK, Crawford JD, Klibanski A 1992 Osteopenia in men with a history of delayed puberty. N Engl J Med 326:600-604.

33. Tylavski FA, Anderson JJB, Talmage RV, Taft TN 1992 Are calcium intakes and physical activity patterns during adolescence related to radial bone mass of white college-age females? Osteoporosis Int 2:232-240.

34. Clark PA, Rogol AD 1996 Growth hormone and sex steroid interactions at puberty. Endocrinol Metab Clin N Am 25:665-681.

35. Welten DC, Kemper HCG, Post GB, Van Staveren WA 1995 A meta-analysis of the effect of calcium intake on bone mass in young and middle aged females and males. J Nutr 125:2802-2813.

36. Johnston CC, Miller JZ, Slemenda CW, Reister TK, Hui S, Christian JC, Peacock M 1992 Calcium supplementation and increases in bone mineral density in children. N Engl J Med 327:82-87.

37. Lloyd T, Andon MB, Rollings N, Martel JK, Landis JR. Demers LM, Eggli DF, Kieselhorst K, Kulin HE 1993 Calcium supplementation and bone mineral density in adolescent girls. JAMA 270: 841-844.

38. Chan GM, Hoffman K, McMurry M 1995 Effects of dairy products on bone and body composition in pubertal girls. J Pediatr 126:551-556.

39. Bonjour JP, Carrie AL, Ferrari S, Clavien H, Slosman D, Theintz G, Rizzoli R 1997 Calcium-enriched foods and bone mass growth in prepubertal girls: A randomized, double-blind, placebo-controlled trial. J Clin Invest 99:1287-1294.

40. Gunnes M, Lehmann, EH 1995 Dietary calcium, saturated fat, fiber and vitamin C as predictors of forearm cortical and trabecular bone mineral density in healthy children and adolescents. Acta Paediatr 84:388-392.

41. Lee, WTK, Leung SSF, Wang S-H, Xu Y-C, Zeng W-P, Lau J, Oppenheimer SJ, Cheng JCY 1994 Double-blind, controlled calcium supplementation and bone mineral accretion in children accustomed to a low-calcium diet. Am J Clin Nutr 60:744-750.

42. Halioua L, Anderson JJB 1989 Lifetime calcium intake and physical activity habits: independent and combined effects on the radial bone of healthy premenopausal Caucasian women. Am J Clin Nutr 49:524-541.

43. Wardlow GM 1996 Putting body weight and osteoporosis into perspective. Am J Clin Nutr 63(suppl):433S-436S.

44. Nordstrom P, Thorsen K, Nordstrom G, Bergstrom E, Lorentzon R 1995 Bone mass, muscle strength, and different body constitutional parameters in adolescent boys with a low or moderate exercise level. Bone 17:351-356.

45. Jones G, Couper D, Riley M, Goff C, Dwyer T 1997 Determinants of bone mass in prepubertal children: Antenatal, neonatal, and current influences. J Bone Min Res 1997;12(suppl 1):S145.

46. van der Meulin MCH, Moro M, Kiratli BJ, Marcus R, Bachrach LK, Carter DR 1997 Determinants of femoral neck structure during adolescents. J Bone Min Res12(suppl 1):S252.

47. Duppe H, Cooper C, Gardsell P, Johnell O 1997 The relationship between childhood growth, bone mass, and muscle strength in male and female adolescents. Calcif Tissue Int 60:405-409.

48. Dyson K, Blimkie CJR, Davison KS, Webber CE, Adachi JD 1997 Gymnastic training and bone density in pre-adolescent females. Med Sci Sports Exerc 29(4):443-450.

49. Alfredson H, Nordstrom P, Lorentzon R 1996 Total and regional bone mass in female soccer players. Calcif Tissue Int 59:438-442.

50. Nordstrom P, Thorsen K, Bergstrom E, Lorentzon R 1996 High bone mass and altered relationships between bone mass, muscle strength, and body constitution in adolescent boys on a high level of physical activity. Bone 19(2):189-195.

51. Welten DC, Kemper HCG, Post GB, Van Mechelen W, Twisk J, Lips P, Teule GJ 1994 Weight-bearing activity during youth is a more important factor for peak bone mass than calcium intake. J Bone Miner Res 9(7):1089-1096.

52. Slemenda CW, Miller JZ, Jui SL, Reister TK, Johnston CC Jr 1991 Role of physical activity in the development of skeletal mass in children J Bone Miner Res 6(11):1227-1233.

53. Metz JA, Anderson JJB, Gallager Jr PN 1993 Intakes of calcium, phosphorus, and protein, physical-activity level are related to radial bone mass in young adult women. Am J Clin Nutr 58:537-542.

54. Lee WTK, Leung SSF, Leung DMY, Cheng JCY 1996 A follow-up study on the effects of calcium-supplement withdrawal and puberty on bone acquisition of children. Am J Clin Nutr 64:71-77.

55. Maugars Y, Berthelot J-M, Lalande S, Charlier C, Prost A 1996 Osteoporotic fractures revealing anorexia nervosa in five females. Rev Rhum 63:201-206.

118

56. Salisbury JJ, Mitchell JE. 1991 Bone mineral density and anorexia nervosa in women. Am J Psychiatry 148;768-774.

57. Van der Spuy ZM 1985 Nutrition and reproduction. Clin Obstet Gynecol 12:579-604.

58. Rencken ML, Chesnut CH, Drinkwater BL 1996 Bone density at multiple skeletal sites in amenorrheic athletes. JAMA 276(3):238-240.

59. Klesges RC, Ward KD, Shelton ML, Applegate WB, Cantler ED, Palmieri GMA, Harmon K, Davis J 1996 Changes in bone mineral content in male athletes. JAMA 276:226-230.

60. Wilson JW, Enns CW, Goldman JD, Tippett KS, Mickle SJ, Cleveland LE, Chahil PS 1997 Data tables: Combined results from USDA's 1994 and 1995 Continuing Survey of Food Intakes by Individuals and 1994 and 1995 Diet Health Knowledge Survey, [Online]. ARS Food Surveys Research Group. Available (under "Releases"): <http://www.barc.usda.gov/bhnrc/foodsurvey/home.htm>[1997,9].

61. Peacock M 1991 Calcium absorption efficiency and calcium requirements in children and adolescents. Am J Nutr 54:261S-265S.

62. Matkovic V, Heaney RP 1992 Calcium balance during human growth: evidence for threshold behavior. Am J Clin Nutr 55:992-996.

63. National Institutes of Health Consensus Coference 1994 Optimal calcium intake. JAMA 272:1942-1948.

64. Jackman LA, Millane SS, Martin BR, Wood BW, McCabe GP, Peacock M, Weaver CM 1997 Calcium retention in relation to calcium intake and postmenarcheal age in adolescent females. Am J Clin Nutr 66:327-333.

65. Martin BR, Wastney ME, Ng J, Smith D, Peacock M, Weaver CM 1997 Changes in calcium kinetics with post pubertal age. J Bone Miner Res 12(suppl 1):S486.

66. Standing Committee on the Scientific Evaluation of Dietary Reference Intakes 1997 Dietary Reference Intakes: Calcium, Phosphorus, Magnesium, Vitamin D, and Fluoride. Washington DC, National Academy Press, (Prepublication Copy).

67. Miller GD, Jarvis JK, McBean LD 1995 Bone Health and the Vegetarian In: Handbook of Dairy Foods and Nutrition 135-169.

68. Miller GD, Jarvis JK, McBean LD 1995 Dairy foods and Osteoporosis.In: Handbook of Dairy Foods and Nutrition 93-134 .

69. Honkanen R, Pulkkinen P, Jarvinen R, Kroger H, Lindstedt K, Tuppurainen M, Uusitupa M 1996 Does lactose intolerance predispose to low bone density? A population-based study of perimenopausal Finnish women. Bone 19:23-28.

70. Slemenda CW, Reister TK, Peacock M, Johnston CC 1993 Bone growth in children following the cessation of calcium supplementation. J Bone Miner Res 8(suppl 1):S154.

71. Serdula MK, Collins ME, Williamson DF, Anda RF, Pamuk E, Byers TE 1993 Weight control practices of U.S. adolescents and adults. Ann Intern Med 119(7 pt2):667-671.

72. Lanyon LE 1996 Using functional loading to influence bone mass and architecture: Objectives, mechanisms, and relationship with estrogen of the mechanically adaptive process of bone. Bone 18(suppl) 1:37S-43S.

73. Kerr D, Morton A, Dick I, Prince R 1996 Exercise effects on bone mass in postmenopausal women are site specific and load-dependent. J Bone Miner Res 11:218-225.

74. Vuori I 1996 Peak bone mass and physical activity: A short review. Nutr Rev 54(4 Pt 2):S11-S14.

75. Heinonen A, Oja P, Kannus P, Sievanen H, Manttari A, Vuori I 1993 Bone density of female athletes in different sports. J Bone Miner Res 23:1-14.

76. Kannus P, Haapasalo H, Sankelo M, Sievanen H, Pasanen M, Heinonen A, Pja P, Vuori I 1995 Effect of starting age of physical activity on bone mass in the dominant arm of tennis and squash players. Ann Intern Med 123:27-31.

77. Kirchner EM, Lewis RD, O'Cooner PJ 1996 Effect of past gymnastics participation on adult bone mass. J Appl Physiol 80:226-232.

78. Mazess RB, Bardern HS 1991 Bone density in premenopausal women: effects of age, dietary intake, physical activity, smoking, and birth-control pills. Am J Clin Nutr 53:132-142.

79. National Center for Health Statistics 1996 Health, United States, 1995 Hyattsville, Maryland: Public Health Service, p.173.

80. Keen AD, Drinkwater BL 1997 Irreversible bone loss in former amenorrheic athletes. Osteoporosis Int 7:311-315.

8 Skeletal Consequences Of Physical Activity

Robert Marcus, M.D.

Introduction

The beneficial effects of physical activity on the skeleton are widely touted, and optimism abounds that increased activity in the form of recreational exercise will promote peak bone mass, maintain bone density throughout adult life, restore established deficits in bone density, and prevent osteoporotic fracture. This chapter reviews current evidence that addresses these issues. The notion that physical activity may influence the skeleton dates back more than a century to the German scientist, Julius Wolff (1), who crystallized the concept, known subsequently as Wolff's law, that bone responds to the habitual loading environment that is placed on it by modifying its amount and distribution. Thus, if a person increases the customary loads on his femur by gaining weight, femoral mass and trabecular density will also increase until the load experience per unit of bone has been restored to initial values; if he loses weight, bone mass will decrease in a commensurate fashion. The role of this adaptive response appears to be the optimization of load experienced at any point in the skeleton, so that mass and trabecular density are maintained at the minimum level to accommodate demand.

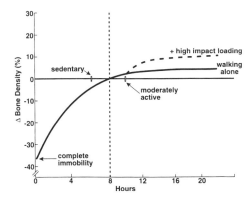

Figure 1. The curvilinear nature of skeletal response. The effect on bone mass of immobility is far greater than that of adding additional walking to an already ambulatory subject. It is more effective to provide a higher intensity stimulus than simply to extend the duration of ordinary loading activity. Ordinary activity, as shown by the region between "sedentary" and "moderately active" defines most individuals, and is characterized by a relatively modest dose-response slope (Copyright Robert Marcus, 1996).

As shown in **Figure 1,** the relationship of bone mass to load experience is non-linear. The slope of response is much steeper when going from complete immobilization to sedentary existence, and attenuates markedly when going from sedentary to very active life. Accordingly, the most extreme case of skeletal adaptation is the case of complete immobilization. Persons rendered quadriplegic may lose 40% of their original bone mass within the first year. Even short-term bed rest results in bone loss that over a years' time would amount to a 6-9% reduction in bone mass. By contrast, substantial evidence shows that elite athletes have a greater bone mass than do sedentary individuals, almost without regard for their particular athletic endeavor (2). It has been tempting to interpret such reports as showing a favorable skeletal response to athletic training itself. However, in considering such evidence, it is very difficult to exclude the problem of ascertainment bias. That is, elite athletes may have been more likely to achieve success in their chosen sports because of some physical characteristic that was present even before serious training began, and therefore they were more likely to qualify in the future to be in a study of athletes. For example, it is not difficult to imagine that a higher genetically determined bone mass might permit an individual to withstand the rigors of football training with few injuries and greater success.

Another area of interpretive difficulty is a technical problem related to bone geometry. The conventional bone mineral density measurement, BMD (g/cm^2), is based on the projected *area* of the bone, and does not take into account differences in bone thickness. Since all bones possess geometric proportionality, longer and wider bones are also thicker, so tall people will have an artifactually higher areal BMD than short people, even if true volumetric mineral density is the same (3). Depending on the sport, athletes may have a body habitus that is either substantially larger (e.g. football player) or smaller (e.g. jockey) than average, permitting a size confound to cloud BMD interpretation.

As will be shown, a reasonable case can be made that exercise training can promote increases in bone density, but the magnitude of changes that follow a training program do not approach the bone mass differences that are observed between athletes and non-athletes. Thus, a substantial portion of these differences is likely related to factors other than exercise training itself.

Relationship of Habitual Physical Activity to Bone Mass of Ordinary People.

Although the number of studies is small, it appears that the skeletons of children are highly susceptible to the effects of physical activity. As pointed out by Dr. Allen in the previous chapter, activity levels of children are directly related to bone mineral density and to changes in bone mineral density over time (4-7). Initiation of exercise training during childhood confers changes not only in bone *density* but also in bone *geometry* that eventuate in a permanent mechanical advantage (8, 9). Habitual childhood activity appears to be an independent determinant of adult bone mass (10). Thus, childhood is probably the most important time to encourage vigorous physical activity. Such a recommendation must be made in recognition of the fact that an immature skeleton may be more susceptible to injury if mechanical loads are inappropriately applied. Most people have heard of serious injuries that occurred with excessive training of Olympic calibre gymnasts or young baseball players whose arms were not sufficiently mature to withstand the repetitive strains associated with various "finesse" pitches.

It has been more difficult to show with consistency that habitual physical activity is related to bone mass in adults. Although many studies show a positive relationship between current or previous habitual activity and bone density (11-17), others fail to confirm this relationship (18-20). Moreover, some of the "positive" reports have not observed significant relationships at all skeletal regions (12, 17). The results of Kanders et al. (13), relating bone mass to total daily energy output, are confounded by failure to account for the effect of body mass. Similarly, the results of Krall et al. (16), which are frequently cited to show a beneficial effect of walking exercise, primarily demonstrate the negative impact of *inactivity*, and offer little evidence for a dose effect of progressive increases in walking.

Several potential explanations may account for this inconsistency. First, of course, there may actually be no consistent relationship between habitual physical activity and bone mass within normal, moderately active populations, or at least any relationship that exists has such a shallow dose-response (as predicted from **Figure 1**), that extraordinarily large study samples would be necessary for an effect to emerge. Alternatively, there may be problems in quantifying a person's habitual skeletal loads. Questionnaires and other validated instruments used in the exercise field have tended to emphasize high metabolic, endurance activities. These instruments may be insensitive to the sorts of loads that stimulate bone. For example, if a man participates in no recreational activity, but his job requires that he open a very heavy door three times each day, his skeletal load history may actually be substantial, but the measurement tool is completely inadequate. In one carefully executed study, Mazess and Bardin (19) assessed the bone densities of a large group of healthy young women, whose physical activities were recorded by an instrument that measured each step taken during a 24-hour period. In this case, the instrumentation may have reliably measured the *number* of cycles for each woman, but was not responsive to cycle *intensity* . Thus, it will be necessary to develop better methods to record ground reaction forces or other indices of load intensity before the relationship of activity to bone mass can be definitively understood.

The Skeletal Effects of Exercise as Determined by Intervention Trials

The most effective defense against ascertainment bias is the randomized intervention trial. Recently published exercise trials have remedied the inadequacies of earlier studies: problems of design, randomization, selection of bones to measure, and standardization of loading regimen have been corrected; duration of exercise training has extended to one and even to two years. As summarized below, most recent studies do generally support the conclusion that exercise promotes bone mass. However, the increases in bone density achieved in these studies have been considerably lower than what might be predicted from the cross-sectional literature. There are several possible explanations for this. First, it is possible that the true maximal effect of imposed exercise on a moderately to very active person is minimal. Second, the weight training protocols that have been employed, using Nautilus and Universal equipment which safely permits training of individual muscle groups in isolation, may not provide adequate skeletal loading even though muscular training is robust. Only one study has documented whether changes in other forms of habitual activity occurred when exercise training was inititated. The importance of this issue can be seen in the example of a woman who ran three miles each day prior to starting weight training. If she elected to decrease her running mileage, walked less, or otherwise modified her daily loading after starting a vigorous weight training program, she might actually have experienced a reduction in total daily loading, at least until her weight training work increased to the point that it equalled her previous equilibrium level.

Exercise trials in young adults.

Several trials have explored the impact of exercise on bone mass at the time that peak bone mass is reached. In one of very few studies in young men, Leichter and colleagues (21) reported positive changes in tibial BMD following short-duration (14 weeks), very high intensity (eight hours per day) physical training. A high incidence of fatigue fractures in that study makes that particular training regimen unsuitable for general application. Studies in young women have not given consistent results. Gleeson et al. (22) found that one year of weight training marginally increased lumbar spine density. Although a significant difference in spine mineral was found between weight trainers and controls, the observed increase of 0.8 % in bone mass over baseline values did not achieve significance. Rockwell et al. (23) reported that women completing one year of weight training *lost* approximately 4% of lumbar spine mineral, and questioned the safety of weight training. Snow-Harter et al. (24) conducted an 8 month exercise trial for healthy college women who were randomly assigned to a control group or to progressive training in either jogging or weightlifting. Lumbar spine BMD increased significantly in both the runners and weight trainers by about 1.3%, whereas bone mineral did not change in control subjects. No measure of bone mineral at the proximal femur changed significantly in any group. Of particular interest in this study was the documentation of a wide variety of non-training physical activities during the course of the protocol. Such activities included hours per day of standing, walking, sitting, and non- protocol recreational exercise. No significant change in other habitual activities was observed in any group. Thus, the observed changes in bone mineral appear to reflect increased mechanical loading specifically due to the exercise program.

A weakness of these studies is their relatively short duration. It is certainly possible that the tempo of skeletal adaptation is slower than that of the cardiovascular or muscular systems. This issue has been addressed by two additional studies which incorporated training regimens similar to those of Snow-Harter et al. (24), but continued to 1.5 and 2 years, respectively. Lohman et al. (25) observed increases in lumbar spine BMD of about 1.3% after a year of training, but no further increase in

BMD by 1.5 years; in fact, some loss of effect was observed at 18 months. Friedlander et al. (26) carried out a mixed endurance/resistance activity training schedule for 2 years. BMD increases in the lumbar spine were about 1.3%, reaching statistical significance by the end of year 2. Thus, it appears that the maximum effect on lumbar spine BMD that can be realistically anticipated from an extended period of intense exercise training, using exercises that are reasonably prescribed for a healthy, non-athlete population, is about 1.3%.

These studies almost uniformly share a failure to observe any effect of exercise on hip BMD. The single exception, Friedlander et al. (26), observed significant gains at the hip at two years, ranging from 0.5-2.5%, depending on the specific hip site (i.e. femoral neck, trochanter, Ward's triangle). This is a surprising result, since the strength training exercises in some of these studies specifically loaded the hip. It is possible that the greater abundance of cortical bone at this site may require more prolonged training for a detectable response. It may also be that habitual loading of the hip during such daily activities as standing and walking is so great that increments in daily loading produced by the intervention were ineffective.

Two recent papers indicate that the hip does respond to increased activity, but requires greater loading impact than is achieved by running or conventional resistance exercise machinery. Bassey and Ramsdale (27) employed a jumping protocol in young women, and demonstrated a 3.4% increase in hip BMD after 6 months. Heinonnen et al. (28) described a "high impact exercise" regimen that led to several percent increase in hip BMD. In this regard, it may be instructive to examine the case of elite gymnasts. These athletes show substantial increases in BMD at virtually all skeletal sites, despite having a high prevalence of amenorrhea, which would ordinarily be associated with deficits in bone mass (29). Moreover, when follow-up examinations were made on gymnasts after a season of training and competition (30), they had gained several percent in BMD, whereas no similar gains had been achieved by a group of elite runners. The magnitude of skeletal loading experienced by gymnasts far exceeds that achieved by the types of exercise we have been considering to this point. Walking imparts loads to the spine of about 1 body weight. Jogging and running may load the spine with 2-4 body weights. The "high impact" schedule of Heinnonen et al. (28) was calculated to provide loads of ~5 body weights. By contrast, when gymnasts dismount from the parallel bars, loads of 11 body weights or more have been estimated. Naturally, if such loads are required for substantial increases (i.e. equivalent to a standard deviation in the population distribution of BMD) in bone mass, it seems most unlikely that the average person could ever safely accomplish this level of activity.

From consideration of the published literature in this area, it seems reasonable to conclude that ordinary endurance and resistance training schedules can achieve modest improvement in lumbar spine BMD, but that achieving significant improvement at the hip has been inconsistent at best, probably because the loads actually imparted to that area of the skeleton are not adequate.

Exercise studies in mid-life.

As exemplified by the woman athlete with amenorrhea, loss of normal reproductive hormone secretion leads to bone loss and increased fracture risk even when exercise levels are high (31, 32). It is of obvious interest, therefore, to know whether an exercise program for recently menopausal women can offer skeletal protection, yet it is remarkable how few studies have actually examined this issue. Pruitt et al. (33) assigned women within 7 years of menopause to a 9-month program of weight-training or a control group. No subject had taken estrogen replacement therapy. Training involved muscle groups in the upper and lower extremeties and in the trunk, and was sufficiently intense to increase strength in all muscle groups. Whereas the control subjects lost 3.6% of bone density at the lumbar spine, no loss was observed in the training group. No significant changes were seen in either group at the femoral neck or distal radius. Thus, resistance activity can offer some skeletal protection to early menopausal women at the spine, but appears to be of no benefit at other sites.

The possibility that estrogen repletion enhances the skeletal response to exercise has been raised by the work of Notelovitz et al. (34), who assigned a group of women who had undergone a surgical menopause to estrogen replacement alone or to estrogen replacement plus weight-training for one year. Whereas BMD at the lumbar spine was maintained in the estrogen-alone group, the weight training group experienced an increase of 8.3%. At the radial shaft, exercisers increased BMD by 4.1% in comparison to no significant change in the hormone only group. It is of particular interest to note that in an earlier unpublished study, these same investigators found no effect of the resistance training program on a group of menopausal women who were not taking estrogen replacement (Notelovitz M, personal communication).

Thus, exercise as a single modality may help to conserve bone at some skeletal regions in recently menopausal women, but for overall skeletal protection, or for meaningful increases in bone mass to occur, it may be necessary to carry out exercise in a state of estrogen repletion.

Exercise studies in older subjects.

Earlier trials in postmenopausal women employed calisthenics and light aerobic activity for 8 to 48 months. Results were generally inconsistent and unimpressive, reflecting a host of inadequacies. For example, low magnitude of exercise stimulus, poor or imprecise measurement techniques, use of exercises that did not load the skeletal site of interest, lack of randomization, permitting subjects to exercise at home without supervision, and short protocol duration are just a few representative deficiencies that abound.

The first adequate trials to demonstrate an exercise-dependent improvement in BMD of older women were reported by Chow et al. in 1987 (35) and Dalsky et al. (35) in 1988. Chow et al. (35) observed an 8% increase in spine bone density with a mixed aerobic/resistance program. Dalsky et al. (36) showed gains of 5.2% in spine bone mineral after a nine month program of mixed weight-bearing and non-weight-bearing resistance exercise. This value increased to 6.1% after an additional 13 months of exercise. A nonrandomized simultaneous group of sedentary controls exhibited no change. These authors were also the first to consider whether gains in bone density are maintained when exercise has been terminated. Following a 13-month detraining period, bone mass was only 1.1% above baseline. This return toward baseline exemplifies the dynamic nature of the skeletal system and reinforces the view that long-term maintenance of activity is essential to achieving sustained benefit.

Subsequently, a number of studies have described the effects of supervised exercise programs on bone mass of older women (37-41). Results have varied, although most support a conclusion that exercise increases bone mass to a modest degree. The least encouraging results have been observed in studies of weight-bearing activity (37, 38). For example, Cavanaugh and Cann (37) examined the effect of walking exercise on spinal trabecular mineral in postmenopausal women. The walkers actually lost trabecular bone (5.6%) while a control group lost 4% over the same interval. These results directly contradict those of Dalsky et al. (36), and may be related to differences in experimental protocol. In addition to walking, Dalsky's exercise group jogged and performed exercises that specifically loaded the vertebrae.

Several reports of resistance exercise have appeared since those of Chow (35) and Dalsky (36). Pruitt et al. (39) trained healthy older women for a full year using either high-intensity/low-repetition or high-repetition/low intensity exercise, in which the total volume of work (loads x repetitions) was the same for the two groups. No change in BMD at any site was observed in either group, nor with a sedentary group randomized to control status. By contrast, Kohrt et al. (40) conducted a trial of similar length, in which women undertook exercise alone, estrogen replacement therapy alone, or exercise plus estrogen. Exercise led to increases in spine and hip BMD of 2-3%. As one might predict from the study of Notelovitz et al. (34), the response to estrogen alone was higher than that observed with exercise alone, but the greatest increase, 3-5%, was observed in women undergoing both modalities in combination.

A novel paper from Kerr et al. (41) established the site-specificity and load-dependence of exercise response in older women. Using a protocol involving unilateral bicycle exercise, in which one leg served as a control for each woman, the authors trained women for a full year with progressive resistance (high intensity) or endurance (high repetitions) schedules. An increase in hip BMD relative to control was seen in the strength-trained group (~2-4%), but no increase was observed in the endurance group. The authors concluded that peak loads were a more important stimulus to bone mass than were the number of loading cycles.

In summary, most evidence indicates that resistance training promotes small increases in BMD for older women. It is interesting to note that the magnitude of increase in these studies, while small, exceeds those observed in younger women. Since habitual physical activity decreases with age, one presumes the older women in various studies were generally less active than their healthy young counterparts. Given the curvilinear nature of skeletal response (**Figure 1**), one would therefore predict a greater effect of imposed activity in a group whose initial level was low.

Exercise for Patients with Established Osteoporosis.

Among the several goals of an exercise program for osteoporotic patients, increased bone mineral density, while desirable, should be considered a secondary outcome. Most importantly, exercise should not be harmful; it should increase a patient's functional capacities; and it should minimize the risk for falls and subsequent fracture. Health professionals who work with osteoporotic patients recognize that back strengthening exercise constitutes a powerful intervention for reducing pain and increasing functional capacity. Many physicians express reluctance to prescribe exercise for osteoporotic patients out of concern for injury and additional fracture. This view may be counterproductive in the long run, since avoidance of activity will certainly aggravate bone loss and place the skeleton at even greater jeopardy. In fact, rehabilitation programs for patients with osteoporosis that are aimed at improving functional capacity and providing social interactions in addition to improving strength and flexibility can safely yield significant improvements in aerobic capacity and bone mass, with high patient adherence. Little information is available concerning the effect of exercise on bone mass of osteoporotic patients. Krølner et al. (42) evaluated the effect of exercise on bone mineral density of women who had previously experienced a Colles' fracture. The results showed a 3.5% increase in lumbar spine BMD in the exercise group compared to a 2.7% loss for the controls. In another controlled trial, Simkin et al. (43) administered a 5 month program of thrice weekly dynamic loading exercise to the distal forearm to older osteoporotic women. Bone mineral content of the distal radius increased by 3.8% in the training group, whereas bone density declined by 1.9% in the controls.

In one of the few exercise studies in patients with vertebral compression, Sinaki and Mikkelsen (44) found that resistance exercise to strengthen the back *extensor* muscles reduced new vertebral fractures compared to a control group, whereas a substantial increase in vertebral deformities was observed in subjects assigned to a program that included *flexion* activity. For patients with vertebral osteoporosis, therefore, it appears that activities that place an anterior load on vertebral bodies, as with back flexion, are particularly harmful, and patient education must emphasize their danger. Even modest weights may be deleterious to the spine because their effect is amplified by leverage. For example, if one lifts a 5 kg weight from a shopping cart using arms that are 50 cm in length, the load is balanced by paraspinous muscles that may be no more than 1 cm long. Thus the load on the vertebral body may be magnified 50-fold to a value of 250 kg:

(Weight x Length = Weight" x Length", or 5 x 50 = 250 x 1).

For severely osteopenic patients, one may appropriately ask what the real benefits could be from the limited improvement documented by these studies. Although the skeletal changes were modest, one should not overlook the possibility that exercise may have produced benefits that were not directly reflected in BMD. Hayes et al. (45) presented evidence that many older individuals have insufficient bone strength at the proximal femur to withstand the impact of a fall. Since more than 90% of hip fractures result directly from a fall, strategies aimed at reducing falls may be more effective at reducing the incidence of hip fracture than those aimed specifically at increasing bone mineral. Muscle weakness is an important antecedent of falls (46), and decreased muscle mass and strength are consequences of normal human aging. It has now been established that progressive resistance exercise can increase muscle strength and promote muscle fiber hypertrophy in older men and women (47-50), even in the 10th decade (51).

Preliminary evidence suggests that increased lower extremity strength may reduce the risk of falls by improving postural stability. Hoy and Marcus (unpublished data) evaluated the act of rising from a chair by healthy elderly and young women. Kinematic and reaction force data were obtained using a video-based motion analysis system and force plates fixed into the chair seat and floor. The elderly women then participated in a 12 week strength training program that emphasized hip and knee musculature, after which the chair tests were repeated. Initial muscle strength was very low in these women, ranging from 37% to 70% of values observed in young women. Instability during the rise from a chair was maximum at the moment of loss of chair contact. The center of body mass was located at its most posterior point at this time, sometimes lying behind the feet. With strength training, muscle strength increased significantly. Stability improved and the center of mass was located more anteriorly. Results of this pilot study indicate that strength training alters movement strategy in a way that favors increased static and dynamic stability. Many falls in the elderly occur at times of "transfer," that is, changing from one position to another. Thus, a widely disseminated program of leg strengthening exercise could lower the risk of falling and reduce hip fracture incidence even if no changes in bone mineral were achieved. The importance of proper attention to safety cannot be overemphasized in this discussion. Although experimental data indicates the danger of loading the spine in flexion, there is very little scientific support for other recommendations. Nonetheless, a few reasonable principles can be offered (**Table 1**).

Table 1. Principles of strength training for patients with osteoporosis

1. Strengthen back extensors

2. Avoid back flexion and trunk torque

3. Use small weights

4. Increase very slowly to reasonable maximal loads (4-6 kg)

5. Exercise all body regions

6. Emphasize proper technique for routine daily activities.

Practical considerations.

Although we still do not fully understand the optimal components for an exercise prescription, it is possible from the foregoing discussion to reach a few general conclusions. The changes in skeletal integrity associated with immmobilization greatly exceed those brought about by increasing the activity of an already mobile person. In adults, exercise-related gains in bone mass appear to be modest. For increases in bone mass to be sustained, exercise needs to be continued. The skeleton adapts to the loads which are imposed on it, and a reduction in loading, even after many years of activity, will predictably lead to a decrease in bone mass. The material reviewed in this chapter has dealt primarily with the skeleton. Exercise directed at other aspects of health, such as flexibility or aerobic fitness, may require different types or intensities of exercise to achieve optimal results. However, exercise is not a way of life for most adults. Men and women commonly state that regular exercise is not necessary at their age; they frequently have unrealistic expectations regarding the health benefits of their usual daily activities, and they seriously exaggerate the risks of vigorous exercise. It is very unlikely, therefore, that very many people will carry out multiple exercise programs to achieve diverse physiological ends. If there is any chance for widespread acceptance of exercise by the population, it will be necessary to define a few sensible and relatively simple exercise strategies that can be carried out by people of average capacity and motivation without major requirements for time or financial investment. Finally, although considerable scientific efforts continue to be directed at the relationship between physical activity and health, for new insights to yield practical benefits it will be necessary to invest a similar effort into motivating a sedentary population to incorporate exercise into daily life.

References:

1. Wolff J, Das Gesetz der Transformation, der Knochen Kirchwald, Berlin, Springer-Verlag, 1892.

2. Snow C, Shaw JM, Matkin CC 1996 Physical activity and risk for osteoporosis. In Marcus R, Feldman D, Kelsey J, Eds, Osteoporosis. Academic Press, San Diego 511-528.

3. Carter DR, Bouxsein ML, Marcus R 1992 New approaches for interpreting projected bone densitometry. J Bone Min Res 7:137-145.

4. Slemenda CW, Miller JZ, Hui SL, Reister TL, Johnston CC Jr 1991 Role of physical activity in the development of skeletal mass in chilren. J Bone Miner Res 6: 1227-1233.

5. Ruiz JC, Mandel C, Garabedian M 1995 Influence of spontaneous calcium intake and physical exercise on the vertebral and femoral bone mineral density of children and adolescents. J Bone Miner Res 10: 675-682.

6. Kröger H, Kotaniemi A, Kröger L, Alhava E 1993 Development of bone mass and bone density of the spine and femoral neck-a prospective study of 65 children and adolescents. J Bone Miner Res 23: 171-182.

7. Cooper C, Cawley M, Bhalla A, Egger P, Ring F, Morton L, Barker D 1995 Childhood growth, physical activity, and peak bone mass in women. J Bone Miner Res 10: 940-9407.

8. Haapasalo H, Sievanen H, Kannus P, Heinonen A, Oja P, Vuori I 1996 Dimensions and estimated mechanical characteristics of the humerus after long-term tennis loading. J Bone Miner Res 11: 864-872.

9.   Morris FL, Naughton GA, Gibbs JL, Carlson JS, Wark JD 1997 Prospective ten-month exercise intervention in premenarcheal girls: positive effects on bone and lean mass. J Bone Miner Res 12: 1453-1462.

10. Teegarden D, Proulx WR, Kern M, Sedlock D, Weaver CM, Johnston CC, Jr, Lyle R 1996 Previous physical activity relates to bone mineral measures in young women. Med Sci Sports Exerc 28: 105-113.

11. Stillman RJ, Lohman TG, Slaughter MH 1986 Physical activity and bone mineral content in women aged 30 to 85 years. Med Sci Sports Exerc 18: 576-580.

12. Aloia JF, Vaswani AN, Yeh JK, Cohn SH 1988 Premenopausal bone mass is related to physical activity. Arch Intern Med 148: 121-123.

13. Kanders B, Dempster DW, Lindsay R 1988 Interaction of calcium nutrition and physical activity on bone mass in young women. J Bone Miner Res 3:145-149.

14. Suominen H, Rahkila P 1991 Bone mineral density of the calcaneus in 70- to 81-yr-old male athletes and a population sample. Med Sci Sports Exerc 23:1227-1233.

15. Snow-Harter C., Whalen R, Myburgh K, Arnaud S, Marcus R 1992 Bone mineral density, muscle strength, and recreational exercise in men. J Bone Miner Res 27: 1291-1296.

16. Krall EA, Dawson-Hughes B 1994 Walking is related to bone density and rates of bone loss. Am J Med 96: 20-26.

17. Greendale GA, Barrett-Connor E, Edelstein S, Ingles S, Haile R 1995 Lifetime leisure exercise and osteoporosis. The Rancho Bernardo Study. Am J Epidemiol 141: 951-959.

18. McCulloch R, Bailey D, Houston C, Dodd BL 1990 Effects of physical activity, dietary calcium intake and selected lifestyle factors on bone density in young women. Can Med Assoc J 142: 221-227.

19. Mazess RB, Barden HS 1991 Bone density in premenopausal women: effects of age, dietary intake, physical activity, smoking, and birth-control pills. Am J Clin Nutr 53: 132-142.

20. White CM, Hergenroeder AC, Klish WJ 1992 Bone mineral density in 15- to 21-year old eumenorrheic and amenorrheic subjects. Am J Dis Child 146: 31-35.

21. Leichter I, Simkin A, Margulies JY 1989 Gain in mass density of bone following strenuous physical activity. J Orthop Res 7:86-90.

22. Gleeson PB, Protas EJ, LeBlanc AD, Schneider VS, Evans HJ 1990 Effects of weight lifting on bone mineral density in premenopausal women. J Bone Miner Res 5:153-158.

23. Rockwell J, Sorensen A, Baker S, Leahey D, Stock J, Michaels J, Baran D 1990 Weight training decreases vertebral bone density in premenopausal women: a prospective study. J Clin Endocrinol Metab 71: 988-93.

24. Snow-Harter C, Bouxsein ML, Lewis BT, Carter DR, Marcus R 1992 Effects of resistance and endurance exercise on bone mineral status of young women: a randomized exercise intervention trial. J Bone Miner Res 7: 761-769.

25. Lohman T, Going S, Pamenter R, Hall M, Boyden T, Houtkooper L, Ritenbaugh C, Bare L, Hill A, Aickin M 1995 Effect of resistance training on regional and total bone mineral density in premenopausal women: a randomized prospective study. J Bone Miner Res 10: 1015-1024.

26. Friedlander AL, Genant HK, Sadowsky S, Byl NN, Glüer CC 1995 A two-year program of aerobics and weight training enhances bone mineral density of young women. J Bone Miner Res 10: 574-585.

27. Bassey EJ, Ramsdale SJ 1994 Increase in femoral bone density in young women following high-impact exercise. Osteoporosis Int 4:72-75.

28. Heinonen A, Kannus P, Sievänen H, Oja P, Pasanen M, Rinne M, Uusi-Rasi K, Vuori I 1996 High-impact exercise and selected risk factors for osteoporotic fractures. An 18-month prospective, randomised trial in premenopausal women. Lancet 348: 1343-1346.

29. Robinson TL, Snow-Harter C, Taaffe DR, Gillis D, Shaw J, Marcus R 1995 Gymnasts exhibit higher bone mass than runners despite similar prevalence of amenorrhea. J Bone Min Res 10: 26-35.

30. Taaffe DR, Robinson TL, Snow CM, Marcus R 1997 High-impact exercise promotes bone gain in well-trained female athletes. J Bone Miner Res 12:255-260.

31. Drinkwater BL, Nilson K, Chesnut CH III, Bremner WJ, Shainholtz S, Southworth MB 1984 Bone mineral content of amenorrheic and eumenorrheic athletes. N Engl J Med 311:277-281.

32. Marcus R, Cann C, Madvig P, Minkoff J, Goddard M, Bayer M, Martin M, Haskell W, Genant H 1985 Menstrual function and bone mass in elite women distance runners: Endocrine metabolic features. Ann Intern Med 102:158-163.

33. Pruitt LA, Jackson RD, Bartels RL, Lehnhard HJ 1992 Weight-training effects on bone mineral density in early postmenopausal women. J Bone Miner Res 7:179-185.

34. Notelovitz M, Martin D, Tesar R, Khan FY, Probart C, Fields C, McKenzie L 1991 Estrogen therapy and variable-resistance weight training increase bone mineral in surgically menopausal women. J Bone Miner Res 6: 583-590.

35. Chow R, Harrison JE, Notarius C 1987 Effect of two randomized exercise programmes on bone mass of healthy post-menopausl women. Br Med J 295:1441-1444.

36. Dalsky G, Stocke KS, Ehsani A 1988 Weight-bearing exercise training and lumbar bone mineral content in postmenopausal women. Ann Int Med 108: 824-828.

37. Cavanaugh DJ, Cann CE 1988 Brisk walking does not stop bone loss in postmenopausal women. Bone 9:201-204.

38. Nelson ME, Fisher EC, Dilmanian FA, Dallal GE, Evans WJ 1991 A 1-y walking program and increased dietary calcium in postmenopausal women: effects on bone. Am J Clin Nutr 53:1304-1311.

39. Pruitt LA, Taaffe DR, Marcus R 1995 Effects of a one-year high- versus low intensity resistance training program on bone mineral density in older women. J Bone Min Res 10:1788-1795.

40. Kohrt WM, Snead DB, Slatopolsky E, Birge SJ Jr 1995 Additive effects of weight-bearing exercise and estrogen on bone mineral density in older women. J Bone Miner Res 10: 1303-1311.

41. Kerr D, Morton A, Dick I, Prince R 1996 Exercise effects on bone mass in postmenopausal women are site-specific and load-dependent. J Bone Miner Ress 11:218-225.

42. Krølner B, Toft B, Pors Nielsen S, Tondevold E 1983 Physical exercise as prophylaxis against involutional vertebral bone loss: a controlled trial. Clin Sci 64: 541-546.

43. Simkin A, Ayalon J, Leichter I 1987 Increased trabecular bone density due to bone-loading exercises in postmenopausal osteoporotic women. Calcif Tiss Intl 40:59-63.

44. Sinaki M, Mikkelsen BA 1984 Postmenopausal spinal osteoporosis: flexion versus extension exercises. Arch Phys Med Rehab 65: 593-596.

45. Hayes WC, Piazza SJ, Zysset PK 1991 Biomechanics of fracture risk prediction of the hip and spine by quantitative computed tomography. Radiol Clin N Amer 29:1-18.

46. Whipple RH, Wolfson LI, Amerman PM 1987 The relationship of knee and ankle weakness to falls in nursing home residents. J Am Geriatr Soc 35:13-20.

47. Frontera WR, Meredith CN, O'Reilly KP, Knuttgen HG, Evans WJ 1988 Strength conditioning in older men: skeletal muscle hypertrophy and improved function. J Appl Physiol 64: 1038-1044.

48. Charette SL, McEvoy L, Pyka G, Snow-Harter C, Guido D, Wiswell RA, Marcus R 1991 Muscle hypertrophy response to resistance training in older women. J Appl Physiol 1991 70:1912-1916.

49. Nichols JF, Omizo DK, Peterson KK, Nelson KP 1993 Efficacy of heavy-resistance training for active women over sixty: muscular strength, body composition, and program adherence. J Am Geriatr Soc 41: 205-210.

50. Pyka G, Lindenberger E, Charette S, Marcus R 1994 Muscle strength and fiber adaptations to a year-long resistance training program in elderly women. J Gerontol 1:M22-27.

51. Fiatarone MA, Marks EC, Ryan ND, Meredith CN, Lipsitz LA, Evans WJ 1990 High-intensity strength training in nonagenarians. Effects on skeletal muscle. J Am Med Assn 263:3029-3034.

9 Postmenopausal Osteoporosis

Patrick M. Doran, M.D.
Sundeep Khosla, M.D.

Definition and Diagnosis

Postmenopausal osteoporosis consists of a metabolic bone disease characterized by low bone mass and microarchitectural deterioration of the skeleton, leading to enhanced bone fragility and a consequent increase in fracture risk. It is estimated that 1.5 million fractures attributable to osteoporosis occur annually in the United States, incurring a total cost estimated at 13.8 billion dollars in 1995 alone (1). Bone density values in the vertebrae, distal radius and proximal femur are in the osteoporotic range, as defined by the World Health Organization, in 25% of women at age 65 and in 70% of them above age 80 (2). Caucasian women have a lifetime risk of fracture of approximately 40% for hip, spine, distal forearm or a combination thereof. The same lifetime risk for hip fracture alone is 17%, an incidence as great as the risks of breast, endometrial, and ovarian cancers combined. Hip fracture is also significant for being the most costly and catastrophic of the osteoporotic complications; about 25% of these patients have a fatal outcome, half of the survivors are unable to walk unassisted, and a quarter become confined to a long-term care institution. However, the other types of osteoporotic fractures may also cause considerable functional impairment (1). Women born during the post-war population rise have begun to reach menopausal age. This fact magnifies the seriousness of postmenopausal osteoporosis and emphasizes the pressing need for effective and widespread treatment and prevention measures.

The application of such interventions requires accurate diagnosis of this condition, preferably before the occurrence of fractures. This diagnostic process should start at the initial history and physical examination. These should aim to detect any osteoporotic risk factors such as previous fractures, early menopause (natural or induced), family history of osteoporosis or fragility fractures, low intake of calcium and vitamin D, poor nutrition, low body weight, and lifestyle factors such as smoking, heavy alcohol intake (more than 2 drinks per day), and low activity level. Although this chapter focuses on primary postmenopausal osteoporosis, the initial encounter should also include a search for secondary causes of reduced bone density, such as the use of some medications, endocrine, gastrointestinal, hepatic, renal and connective tissue disorders, and malignancies.

Plain spine radiographs are too insensitive to diagnose osteoporosis, since a substantial degree of bone loss may have taken place (up to 30%) before radiologic changes can be appreciated. Therefore, spine x-rays should be reserved for defining the presence and extent of vertebral fractures or deformities. Dual-photon absorptiometry (DPA) uses transmission scanning with an isotope source that emits two energy peaks, thereby providing a bone density measurement that is independent of soft tissue thickness and composition. However, DPA has largely been replaced by dual-energy x-ray absorptiometry (DEXA). DEXA in principle is similar to DPA but uses a x-ray tube rather than an isotope to produce photons of two energies. This technique benefits from excellent reproducibility (1% to 2%), low radiation exposure (< 3 mrem), and a shorter scan time (5 to 10 minutes). Since both DPA and DEXA have fields that contain the entire vertebra and surrounding tissues, they are sensitive to the effects of dystrophic calcification (e.g. osteoarthritis, calcification of spinal ligaments and aorta) and vertebral compressions in the scanning area. In such circumstances, DPA and DEXA may yield spuriously elevated BMD measurements. DEXA also can be used to assess bone density in the proximal femur (3). Although still investigational, measuring density by broadband ultrasonographic attenuation is a promising new technique shown to correlate closely with DEXA, while being less expensive and causing no radiation exposure (4).

All patients suspected of having osteoporosis, with or without fracture, should have a bone mineral density (BMD) measurement. Recent legislation approves reimbursement for bone density measurement for the following: 1) estrogen-deficient women at clinical risk for osteoporosis; 2) individuals with vertebral abnormalities demonstrated on x-ray; 3) individuals receiving or expecting glucocorticoid therapy equivalent to 7.5 mg of prednisone or greater per day for more than 3 months; 4) individuals with primary hyperparathyroidism; 5) and individuals being monitored to assess response to an FDA-approved drug of treatment of osteoporosis.

Generally, BMD is still most reliably obtained using DEXA, and it is preferable to measure both the spine and proximal femur sites. The spine consists of 70% cancellous bone and is consequently often the most sensitive site for assessing early postmenopausal bone loss. However, as mentioned above, confounding spinal factors become more prevalent with advancing age and DEXA may give a misleadingly elevated vertebral BMD. This situation is often suggested by a significantly lower femoral BMD in the same patient, and confirmed either by the appearance of the spine on DEXA or by spinal radiography. In such patients, limiting measurements to the proximal femur during future readings may provide a more accurate determination of the extent of bone loss.

The main purpose of measuring BMD is to predict the risk of fracture and determine which patients would benefit most from treatment. Moreover, women who are aware of their BMD values seem more likely to initiate various fracture prevention measures (5). Based on data from a number of prospective studies, every standard deviation (SD) decrease in bone density approximately doubles the risk of fracture. For this reason and in an effort to more fully define the prevalence and incidence of osteoporosis worldwide, the World Health Organization (WHO) convened an expert panel to define osteoporosis on the basis of bone mass measurements. This classification is based on the number of SD units a given individual is below the young adult reference mean BMD (Table 1). Using these criteria, a diagnosis of osteoporosis can now be made solely on the basis of a low bone density, even in the absence of fragility fractures (9).

Table 1. World Health Organization diagnostic criteria for osteoporosis

Normal	BMD within 1 SD of young adult reference mean
Low bone mass (osteopenia)	BMD between −1.0 and −2.5 SD below young adult reference mean
Osteoporosis	BMD −2.5 SD or more below the young adult reference mean
Severe (established) osteoporosis	Osteoporosis with one or more fragility fractures

Most patients with documented osteoporosis should be screened for secondary and potentially reversible processes, since one or more of these are found in approximately 20% of women who present with vertebral or hip fractures. A cost-effective laboratory approach for the more common secondary causes of osteoporosis includes serum calcium, phosphorus, total alkaline phosphatase, creatinine, liver function tests and sensitive thyroid stimulating hormone level. A complete blood count and serum protein electrophoresis can provide important clues to a heretofore unsuspected multiple myeloma or other hematological malignancy. A 24-hour urine collection for calcium excretion can be helpful since the presence of hypercalcuiria may modify the prescription for calcium supplementation and may itself warrant therapy to avert the development of nephrocalcinosis and nephrolithiasis. Conversely, a very low 24-hour urinary calcium level (i.e., <75 mg or less) may indicate the presence of vitamin D malnutrition or malabsorption. The use of additional studies, such as a 24-hour urinary free cortisol to determine the presence of Cushing's syndrome, should be dictated only by the clinician's index of suspicion for other secondary causes of osteoporosis.

Recently, a number of biochemical markers for bone formation and resorption have become available (**Table 2**). These markers have the potential to provide prognostic information on rates of bone loss (10). BMD remains the method of choice for making the diagnoses of osteopenia or of osteoporosis, but it represents only a *static* measurement and cannot predict the *rate* at which a given individual may lose bone. There is accumulating evidence that elevated levels of resorption and formation markers are predictive of increased rates of bone loss when groups of individuals are studied; however, the ability of these markers to accurately predict the rate of bone loss for the individual patient has not yet been established. Several studies now also indicate that elevated bone turnover rates may predict an increased fracture risk, independently of the BMD (11, 12). At present, however, the most practical application of these markers is to monitor the response to treatment. For instance, changes in marker levels after only 3 months of bisphosphonate therapy have been shown to correlate with the changes in BMD eventually observed after 2 years of that treatment (13). In addition, while the changes in bone turnover markers can be appreciated within weeks or a few months after starting therapy, any changes in bone density may not be discernible for 1 to 2 years after initiating treatment.

Table 2. Biochemical markers of bone remodeling.

Bone Formation (serum)
 Osteocalcin
 Bone specific alkaline phosphatase
 Carboxy-terminal extension peptide of type I procollagen

Bone Resorption (urine)
 Pyridinoline
 Deoxypyridinoline
 N-telopeptide of the cross-links of collagen
 C-telopeptide of the cross-links of collagen

Treatment of Postmenopausal Osteoporosis: General Principles

Bone is limited in the ways it can respond to illness, and bone loss is the common denominator to many disease processes. Consequently, what we refer to as "osteoporosis" is actually a syndrome, with many causes and multiple clinical forms. This section concentrates on primary postmenopausal osteoporosis and will not discuss the secondary forms of osteoporosis which are discussed in the final section of this volume.

Maximal bone mass is reached at about age 25 to 30, and as covered in earlier chapters 2, 5, & 7 is probably determined by multiple environmental and genetic factors. After a short period of bone mass stability, bone loss begins and continues throughout the remainder of life. The smaller the total bone mass accumulated during skeletal growth and consolidation, the greater is the risk of fractures later in life as bone loss ensues. Thus, women have an increased predisposition to osteoporosis, not only because of age and menopause-related bone losses, but also because of a lower initial bone mass.

As will be discussed further under the relevant treatment interventions, two distinct phases of bone loss can be recognized in postmenopausal women (14). One is the aforementioned protracted slow phase, age-related and seen in both sexes, which results in similar losses of both cortical and trabecular bone. The other is a transient accelerated phase immediately following menopause and tapering asymptotically with the slow phase over the following 5 to 10 years. This rapid phase results in a disproportionately greater loss of trabecular bone. Cortical bone predominates in the shafts of the long bones, whereas trabecular bone is concentrated in the vertebrae, pelvis and other flat bones, and the ends of long bones. Trabecular bone has greater surface area than cortical bone and is consequently metabolically more active. There is still some uncertainty about how much bone is lost over life with each of these phases, but the following is a reasonable estimate. The slow phase produces a loss of about 25% from the cortical compartment and about 35% from the trabecular compartment, and the accelerated phase an additional 10% from the cortical and 25% from the trabecular compartments (15).

Nonpharmacologic Treatment

Nonpharmacologic measures are clearly essential both as preventive and therapeutic strategies. Although nutrition is discussed elsewhere in this volume, it is important to remind postmenopausal women to avoid high intakes of sodium and caffeine, because of their deleterious effects on calcium balance. The diet should contain sufficient protein, vitamins and calcium (see below), and patients should be advised to discontinue bone toxins such as smoking and excessive alcohol consumption (over two drinks per day).

Several cross-sectional and longitudinal studies have shown a direct relation between weight-bearing exercises and bone mass (16, 17), and postmenopausal women should be encouraged to regularly participate in activities such as walking, jogging or aerobics. Such bone loading has at least modest beneficial effects, both by directly enhancing osteoblast function, and indirectly by increasing muscle mass and improving its protective effects on bone. Also, muscle mass and bone mass are directly correlated. It appears that exercise may have its greatest benefits when accompanied by sufficientl calcium intake (over 1 gam per day) (18).

As much as they should remain reasonably active, women with established osteoporosis should avoid potentially harmful activities such as heavy lifting and sports with significant risk of bony trauma, and should be instructed in the use of optimal body mechanics to reduce unnecessary vertebral stress. Household falls are also an important contributor to osteoporotic fractures. Even though approximately only 1% of all falls result in hip fractures, at least one third of community-dwelling elderly persons experience one or more falls annually, with even higher rates among the institutionalized (19, 20). The elderly are also particularly prone to injury from falls because of 1] decreased strength, 2] delayed reaction time impair their ability to break the impact of a fall, 3] reduced soft tissue mass over the proximal femurs. Attention should be paid to minimizing the risk of falling, such as wearing supportive shoes with an adequate sole, eliminating household hazards such as loose throw rugs and carpets with raised edges, using night lights to facilitate nocturnal trips to the bathroom, and exercising particular care when walking on snow and ice. A home assessment by an occupational therapist is an effective way of optimizing these conditions.

Acute back pain from vertebral collapse can be treated with analgesics, heat, and gentle massage to alleviate muscle spasm. Sometimes, a brief period of rest may be required. Chronic back pain may be secondary to spinal deformity and is often difficult to relieve completely. Measures should be prescribed by a physical therapist trained in this disorder and include instruction in posture and gait, and institution of regular back extension exercises to strengthen paravertebral muscles and improve spine stability. Occasionally, a patient may require a back brace and benefit from an orthopedic consultation.

Pharmacologic Treatment

Theoretical Principles. Bone is continuously being remodeled at discrete skeletal foci known as bone-remodeling units. At each of these sites, bone resorption is initiated by osteoclasts, which are subsequently replaced by osteoblasts, which in turn replenish the space excavated by the osteoclasts. When the bone resorption component of remodeling exceeds bone formation, bone loss ensues. Drugs used in the treatment of osteoporosis can be classified according to which component of remodeling they influence: those that decrease bone resorption and those that increase bone formation. **Figure 1** summarizes the differences in BMD responses between antiresorptive and formation-stimulating drugs. Antiresorptive drugs may act by decreasing the imbalance between bone resorption and formation, by decreasing the overall rate of bone turnover, or by both mechanisms. They are most effective when bone turnover is increased, have a greater influence on cancellous bone than on cortical bone, and can be expected to maintain bone mass or transiently increase it. Antiresorptive agents used clinically include calcium, estrogen, bisphosphonates, and calcitonin. Formation-stimulating agents generally increase both the rate at which new bone-remodeling units are activated and the activity of individual osteoblasts. Thus far, no formation-stimulating drug has been approved by the United States Food and Drug Administration (FDA), although sodium fluoride is currently under review.

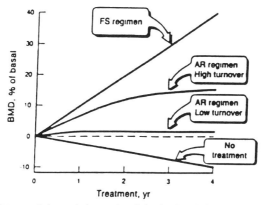

Figure 1. Patterns of change in bone mineral density (BMD) in the lumbar spine of women with osteoporosis during various treatment regimens. When an antiresorptive (AR) drug is given, the response varies directly with the rate of bone turnover at baseline. When the turnover rate is high, gains of 8% to 29% may be achieved but plateau after 2 to 3 years. The mechanism for the waning of therapeutic effect is unknown; the magnitude and duration of the initial increase in bone density seem to be too great to be explained entirely by refilling of increased numbers of resorption cavities present when the bone turnover rate is high. When the turnover rate is normal or low, bone mass is stabilized but does not increase. With no treatment, bone loss continues, although its rate varies among individual patients. When a formation-stimulating (FS) drug, such as fluoride is given, BMD increases linearly up to 10% annually for at least 4 years. Dashed line represents no change in BMD. (From Riggs BL, Melton LJ III. The prevention and treatment of osteoporosis. N Engl J Med 1992; 327: 620-627, with permission.)

Calcium. The first line of intervention in the pharmacologic treatment of osteoporosis consists of ensuring that the patient has an optimal calcium and vitamin D status. Obligatory fecal and urinary losses are in the order of 150 to 250 milligrams daily and account for considerable dietary calcium requirements, even in healthy individuals. These requirements are further increased by an age-related decline in intestinal absorption and renal tubular reabsorption of calcium (21), as well as by changes in vitamin D metabolism (see below). If oral intake is insufficient, the required calcium is withdrawn from bone, which contains 99% of total body stores (22), by way of a compensatory increase in parathyroid hormone (PTH) secretion (23, 24, 25). Evidence for this age-related secondary hyperparathyroidism includes an elevation of parathyroid concentration and increased parathyroid gland size with age (26) as well as functional hyperplasia detected by dynamic studies in the elderly (27). The increased bone resorption caused by secondary hyperparathyroidism combined with an intrinsic defect in compensatory osteoblastic activity with increasing age result in the significant bone loss seen in postmenopausal women (28).

The abnormal PTH secretion and increased bone resorption and bone loss are reversible with sufficient calcium intake (29). These beneficial effects are especially marked in patients with low baseline calcium intake, in older women, and in women with established osteoporosis (30). Also, a recent prospective randomized trial demonstrated that supplemental calcium and vitamin D increased BMD at all sites and decreased the incidence of nonvertebral fractures in elderly men and women (31). Based on the available evidence, a NIH consensus panel developed the following recommendations for total daily intake of elemental calcium: 1000 mg for postmenopausal women on estrogen replacement therapy, and 1500 mg for postmenopausal women not on estrogens and for all women over the age of 65, regardless of estrogen use (32). Of course, these guidelines assume the absence of contraindications to calcium supplementation, such as some forms of nephrolithiasis, etc.

Table 3. Commonly used calcium preparations

Trade Name	Type of salt	Elemental calcium per tablet (mg)	Cost of 1500 mg
Os-Cal* (SmithKline Beecham)	Carbonate	250	$0.54
Os-Cal 500 (SmithKline Beecham)	Carbonate	500	0.30
Generic oyster shell calcium	Carbonate	500	0.15
Tums (SmithKline Beecham)	Carbonate	200	0.29
Posture (Whitehall)	Phosphate	600	0.38
Citracal	Citrate	200	0.70

* Contains 125 IU of cholecalciferol

Table 3 includes some of the currently available calcium supplements. Calcium carbonate is the most widely used, since it is inexpensive and generally well tolerated, except for potential constipation and abdominal discomfort. It should be noted that it is poorly absorbed in the absence of gastric acid. Because a significant percentage of postmenopausal and elderly women have relative achlorhydria and generate free acid only with food, absorption will be optimized if calcium carbonate is taken exclusively with meals. In cases of absolute achlorhydria, calcium citrate is the most favorable alternative, since it is still absorbed, in addition to being less likely to cause constipation. In sum, the choice of calcium supplement should take into account issues such as patient tolerance and underlying conditions, the elemental calcium content of each preparation, as well as medication availability and cost.

Vitamin D. The main regulator of calcium absorption is the biologically active metabolite 1,25-dihydroxyvitamin D (1,25(OH)$_2$D). There is accumulating evidence for a number of age-related abnormalities in vitamin D metabolism. Decreased renal 1a-hydroxylase activity results in reduced synthesis of 1,25 (OH)$_2$D (33), which is compounded by a decreased intestinal responsiveness to this metabolite (34). Other contributing factors include reduced intestinal absorption of dietary vitamin D, and the lessened ability of aging skin to synthesize vitamin D when exposed to ultraviolet light. Thus, vitamin D deficiency in the aging population is not a rare problem; 10-20% of elderly patients with hip fractures were shown to have this condition (35), and in elderly institutionalized women the incidence of hip fractures was significantly reduced with vitamin D and calcium supplementation (36). Vitamin D deficiency should be suspected in the presence of a low 24-hour urinary calcium (<75 mg), and is confirmed by a decreased plasma 25-hydroxyvitamin D concentration.

For the above reasons and in order to increase fractional absorption of calcium, vitamin D is usually given with calcium therapy. For most patients, 400 to 800 International Units (IU) of vitamin D daily (the content of most over the counter multivitamin preparations) are sufficient to ensure adequate vitamin D status. In some patients, however, despite the above doses of calcium and vitamin D, calcium absorption remains low. Thus, for patients with persistently low urinary calcium values of less than 100 mg per day, higher doses of vitamin D (e.g. 50,000 IU every 7 to 10 days) may be required. In addition to tablet form, vitamin D is also available as a liquid preparation (Calciferol ® drops) providing 8,000 IU per ml, or calcidiol (25-hydroxyvitamin D) sold under the name Calderol®. Fifty micrograms of calcidiol is approximately equivalent to 50,000 IU of vitamin D.

Hormone replacement therapy. Estrogen deficiency at menopause is an important cause of bone loss and subsequent fractures, and estrogen replacement therapy (ERT) remains the best current option for prevention and treatment of postmenopausal osteoporosis. Numerous studies have shown a mean vertebral BMD increase of over 5%, and a 50% reduction of hip and vertebral fracture (37). The most effective way to reduce future fracture rates is to initiate ERT at menopause. Nevertheless, recent data indicate that ERT may still reduce bone loss late (>20 years) in the postmenopausal period (38, 39).

The accelerated phase of postmenopausal bone loss is mediated largely by estrogen deficiency and accounts for 1/3 to 1/2 of the total loss. It is characterized by a high bone turnover rate, with radiocalcium kinetic studies showing increased bone accretion with an even greater rate of resorption (40). The primary effect of ERT is to decrease bone resorption. Normal human bone cells contain high-affinity sex steroid receptors and respond directly to estrogens (41). The exact mediators by which estrogen deficiency exerts its effects on the skeleton are still the subjects of intense research. Likely mechanisms include increased local production of bone-resorbing cytokines such as interleukin 1(IL-1), IL-6 and tumor necrosis factor alpha (TNF-a); decreased production of factors such as transforming growth factor beta (TGF-b) which inhibit osteoclastic bone resorption (42, 43); altered skeletal responsiveness to circulating PTH; and osteocyte apoptosis (44). It has also been recognized that estrogen deficiency is associated with extraskeletal abnormalities in calcium metabolism, such as reduced renal tubular calcium reabsorption, decreased intestinal calcium absorption, and possibly a direct disinhibition of PTH secretion, which all contribute to the negative calcium balance of menopause. Other beneficial effects of ERT in postmenopausal women not related to bone include lowering of low-density lipoproteins and elevation of high-density lipoproteins, a decrease in the incidence of coronary artery disease of up to 50% (both directly and via its effects on lipids)(45), and possibly a reduction in clinical Alzheimer's disease.

144

Table 4. Comparable dosages of estrogen preparations

Preparation	Trade name	Dosage (mg/day)
Tablets		
Conjugated estrogen	Premarin (Wyeth-Ayerst)	0.625
Estropipate	Ogen (Abbott)	0.75
Ethinyl estradiol	Estinyl (Schering)	0.02
Estradiol	Estrace (Mead Johnson Labs)	1.0
Dermal patch		
Transdermal estradiol	Estraderm	0.05 (1 patch every 3.5 days)

From Riggs BL, Khosla S. Practical clinical management. In: Riggs BL, Melton LJ III, eds. Osteoporosis: Etiology, Diagnosis, and Management. 2nd ed. New York: Lippincott-Raven Publishers, 1995: 487-502, with permission.

Estrogens can be administered orally or transdermally (**Table 4**). In addition to having the same beneficial effects on bone (46), transdermal estrogens reduce or eliminate the increase in coagulation factors, renin and bile cholesterol, with the resultant thrombosis, hypertension and cholelithiasis, respectively. They also are much less likely than oral estrogens to elevate serum triglycerides. However, they also have less ability to decrease LDL and increase HDL, since they do not undergo first-pass hepatic metabolism. Transdermal estrogens are also considerably more expensive than oral, and previous reservoir-type patches which contain alcohol commonly caused local skin irritation at the site of application, often necessitating discontinuation. More recent matrix patches (Climara®, Vivelle®) do not contain alcohol and reduce the occurrence of cutaneous reactions by as much as 60% (47). In women who have an intact uterus, the additional risk for endometrial cancer incurred by ERT is eliminated by the addition of a progestin, such as medroxyprogesterone acetate 5-10 mg cyclically during the last 12-14 days of each month, or 2.5 mg daily in a continuous fashion. The continuous regimen is proving to be as effective as the cyclical approach in preventing endometrial complications, while eliminating monthly menstrual flow in the majority of women.

Each patient should carefully weigh the advantages cited above with the potential drawbacks of ERT, such as the return of menses, mastodynia, and fluid retention. Undoubtedly the most controversial (and consequently discussed) complication of ERT has been the potential increase in breast carcinoma. A recent metanalysis of the existing literature found that there may be a 30-50% increase in breast cancer risk over baseline after 10 or more years of ERT in current users (48), which translates in a lifetime risk of 13-15%, instead of the 10% in the general population. However, the large numbers of comparable yet conflicting studies prevent us from reaching any firm conclusions at present. It is hoped that the NIH Women's Health Initiative will finally shed some light on this yet unresolved issue. In the meantime, it is reasonable to conclude that for most postmenopausal women, the potential increased risk for breast cancer with ERT is largely outweighed by its beneficial skeletal and cardiovascular effects. Most importantly and as emphasized by Dr. Silverman in the ensuring chapter, is to strive to individualize the treatment regimen according to each patient's underlying conditions and preferences.

Bisphosphonates. These compounds are carbon-substituted analogs of pyrophosphate which act as potent inhibitors of bone resorption. Bisphosphonates have become attractive alternatives for women in whom ERT is either contraindicated or has intolerable side effects. Although it is still not approved by the FDA for this purpose, the first bisphosphonate to be used in the treatment of osteoporosis was etidronate. Initial data indicated that cyclical use of etidronate (400 mg daily for 2 weeks, followed by 11-13 weeks of calcium supplementation alone) decreased the incidence of vertebral fractures after 2 to 3 years (49, 50). However, this was not confirmed by further follow-up, and because of the potential for therapeutic doses of etidronate to impair mineralization, there is concern that etidronate could have adverse long-term effects such as increasing the incidence of fractures.

Second and third generation bisphosphonates such as alendronate, tiludronate and risedronate, are significantly more potent and have a greater therapeutic window between inhibition of bone resorption and inhibition of mineralization than does etidronate. Alendronate is the first second-generation bisphosphonate to be approved for the treatment of osteoporosis. A large scale clinical trial showed a progressive increase of spine and hip BMD continuing to the end of the 3-year treatment period with alendronate 10 mg daily, as well as significant reduction in vertebral fractures compared with placebo (**Figure 2**) (51). Recent data also indicate that this regimen may also lower the incidence of hip fractures (52). Alendronate is generally well tolerated, but is associated with a low yet significant rate of gastrointestinal side effects, including gastroesophageal discomfort and in extreme cases extensive esophageal ulcerations. For this reason, pre-existing upper gastrointestinal symtomatology is a relative contraindication for its use. Bisphosphonates as a group also suffer from very poor absorption, and alendronate requires administration at least 30 minutes before breakfast and before any other medications are taken, since complex formation with divalent ions, particularly calcium, limits absorption. Because of its tendency for esophageal irritation, patients should also be instructed to take alendronate with a large glass of water and to remain upright and not return to bed after taking the drug, so as to reduce reflux. Newer bisphosphonates such as tiludronate and risedronate are currently under study. Whether they prove superior to alendronate in their efficacy and side effect profiles remains to be determined, ideally with head-to-head clinical trials.

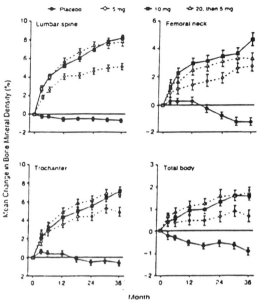

Figure 2. Mean (+/- SE) changes in bone mineral density from baseline values in women with postmenopausal osteoporosis receiving alendronate or placebo for three years. Data are shown for bone mineral density (measured by dual-energy x-ray absorptiometry) of the spine, femoral neck, trochanter, and total body. Data for the alendronate group are shown according to the dose: 5 or 10 mg per day for three years or 20 mg per day for two years followed by 5 mg per day in year 3. (From Liberman UA, Weiss SR, Broll J, et al. Effect of oral alendronate on bone mineral density and the incidence of fractures in postmenopausal osteoporosis. N Engl J Med 1995; 333: 1437-43, with permission.)

The above studies have focused on the efficacy of bisphosphonates in the treatment of established osteoporosis. The FDA recently approved the use of low-dose alendronate (5 mg daily) for prevention of bone loss in early postmenopausal women. This decision was in response to the results of the recent Early Postmenopausal Intervention Cohort (EPIC) Study, which showed that this dose of alendronate after 2 years produced a BMD increase of 5% in the spine and 3% in the total hip, with no difference in the rate of serious side effects with respect to placebo (53). As for ERT, the decision regarding the initiation of such treatment should be made on an individual basis in consultation with the patient.

Calcitonin. Calcitonin remains a therapeutic option in women in whom ERT and alendronate are not satisfactory. Calcitonin has been shown to transiently raise vertebral BMD after 2 years (3% versus 1% for placebo) (54) in women with postmenopausal osteoporosis. This beneficial effect was particularly marked in women with increased bone turnover rates, and is through a direct reduction in osteoclastic activity and number. In addition, calcitonin appears to have significant analgesic effects for painful acute vertebral fractures, possibly mediated through a direct action on the central nervous system. The usual dose is 0.5 ml (100 units) of salmon calcitonin (Calcimar® or Miacalcin®) daily, administered subcutaneously.

In addition to its relatively lower efficacy compared with ERT and alendronate, calcitonin also has the disadvantages of being costly ($1,500 to $3,000 yearly) and requiring parenteral administration. However, calcitonin is now available as an intranasal preparation at a significantly lower cost: Miacalcin® nasal spray, one spray (200 units) daily, all in one nostril, alternating nostrils daily. Nausea and flushing are potential side effects, but are much less common with the nasal spray preparation. Some patients develop resistance to calcitonin either from the development of neutralizing antibodies or possibly via the down-regulation of calcitonin receptors. Because of the potential for inducing secondary hyperparathyroidism, calcium supplements should always be given with calcitonin.

Sodium fluoride. This salt is the only formation-stimulating drug that has been widely tested so far. In two major adequately controlled clinical trials, sodium fluoride at a dose of 75 mg daily substantially improved bone mass, but failed to significantly reduce the rate of vertebral fractures (55, 56). In contrast, a more recent study using a lower dose (50 mg/day) in a delayed release form did indicate a reduction in vertebral fracture rates (15% of 48 women taking fluoride and calcium, 43% of 51 women on placebo and calcium, p<0.001) (57). However, another study using the same dose but without the delayed release formulation failed to confirm these positive results. Moreover, direct studies of bone biopsies from patients treated with a dose of 50 mg per day have indicated decreased trabecular quanlity which could translate to increased fragility of the fluoride-treated bone (58). Thus, the future role of sodium fluoride in the management of postmenopausal osteoporosis is presently unclear, and the FDA is currently reviewing the status of this agent as potential treatment for osteoporosis.

Selective Estrogen Receptor Modulations (SERM's). Tamoxifen, a benzothiophene-derived drug, has partial estrogen agonist/antagonist activity and functions as an antiestrogen in breast tissue. However, it was noted that women who had breast cancer treated with tamoxifen also had reductions in bone loss, and thus tamoxifen appears to have an estrogen-agonist effect in bone (59). Like estrogen, it lowers LDL cholesterol, but tamoxifen does not raise the HDL fraction. Also, the routine use of tamoxifen is limited by significant side effects, such as endometrial hyperplasia, hot flashes and an increased tendency for thrombosis. Nevertheless, women who must receive tamoxifen as cancer treatment and who are not candidates for ERT should be reminded of the beneficial effects of tamoxifen on bone, compared with no treatment. A large-scale trial currently underway aims to determine whether tamoxifen has prophylactic effects against breast cancer. If so, then other estrogen receptor modulators (see below) will likely play a key role in the future osteoporosis treatment armamentarium.

Newer generations of SERM's have estrogen agonist influences on bone, but also have an antiestrogenic effects on uterine tissue as well as on breast, and so could potentially be given without a progestin. Preliminary results from double-blind, placebo-controlled studies indicate that the only FDA-approved SERM, raloxifene, produces lowering in bone remodeling markers similar to that seen with conjugated estrogens, with the same favorable effects on lipids (60). Driloxifene is a similar agent undergoing evaluation. Thus, SERM's show much promise for becoming useful alternatives to estrogens in women prone to complications with ERT, and may find even broader applications if they are demonstrated to reduce the incidence of breast cancer. Along the same vein, with the recognition of the role of androgens in female bone physiology, specific androgen receptor modulators (SARM's) are being examined as a potential treatment modality (see below).

Androgens and synthetic anabolic agents. These drugs probably inhibit resorption like estrogens, and some data also suggests a weak stimulation of bone formation, although this effect is likely quite minor. Because of their relatively low efficacy, masculinizing and hyperlipidemic effects, and tendency to induce hepatic dysfunction when taken orally, androgens have a limited role in the management of osteoporosis in women.

Treatment of the individual patient. Whether the goal is prevention or treatment of osteoporosis, all patients should undergo a thorough review for any lifestyle features that can contribute to additional bone loss (see above), and should be counseled accordingly. This is also an opportune time to search for any secondary medical causes of osteoporosis. At the front-line of pharmacological interventions is the optimization of calcium and vitamin D intakes with supplements as required, unless the patient has any contraindications, such as some forms of nephrolithiasis.

With respect to additional interventions, the mainstay for both prevention and treatment of osteoporosis remains ERT, both for its skeletal and its non skeletal benefits. This is likely to be the case from a medical as well as from a cost-effectiveness standpoint. However, unless the patient chooses ERT also for its other benefits, it is probably unwise to treat all postmenopausal women with ERT exclusively to prevent osteoporosis, because of the side effects and high cost of follow-up. This is where measurement of the BMD becomes useful in determining which patients will benefit the most from antiresorptive therapy.

For those women with established bone loss in whom ERT is contraindicated or intolerable, alendronate is a reasonable alternative. The role of alendronate in osteoporosis may eventually be extended to primary prevention. However, until further clinical experience is accrued, it is probably best to make this decision on an individual basis, in accord with the clinical setting and the patient's preferences. If neither ERT nor alendronate are satisfactory, calcitonin is a feasible third choice for most patients, especially in its intranasal form.

Future Directions

During the last decade, our understanding of bone physiology and pathophysiology has increased drastically and has given rise to a number of exciting new treatment venues for osteoporosis. As this next section will discuss, some are improved versions of agents currently used in clinical practice, while others are bold departures from the beaten path.

Calcitriol analogs. As the crucial importance of vitamin D in bone metabolism has been appreciated, calcitriol analogs have been studied in laboratory animals. These compounds have a wider therapeutic window between ineffective doses and those that induce hypercalcemia, and clinical trials in women with postmenopausal osteoporosis should be soon underway.

Transdermal bisphosphonates. As mentioned above, currently available bisphosphonates suffer from very low gastrointestinal absorption (0.1 to 10% of an oral dose) and from a tendency for gastroesophageal irritation. Zoledronate is the newest and most potent bisphosphonate currently under study, with 10,000 times the potency of etidronate. This high potency results in a greater therapeutic index and makes it possible to administer zoledronate transdermally, thereby circumventing the absorption and irritation problems. A current transdermal zoledronate clinical trial is expected to yield results in the near future.

Intermittent PTH. Persistant high plasma concentrations of parathyroid hormone (PTH) stimulate bone resorption. However, exogenous human PTH (PTH(1-34)) may stimulate bone formation when given intermittently in low doses. This anabolic effect may be mediated by an increase in local production of IGF-I and TGF-β by bone cells. In 3 clinical studies involving women with postmenopausal osteoporosis, PTH(1-34) increased vertebral BMD moderately over 6-24 months, but the effect on fracture rate was not evaluated (61, 62). In one trial (63), the increase in vertebral BMD reached a plateau at 12 months and then began to decrease , while cortical bone mass in the radius decreased progressively throughout the study, despite calcium and vitamin D supplementation. These data indicate that treatment with PTH(1-34) may lead to redistribution of bone from the cortical to the cancellous compartment. Thus, PTH(1-34) may be anabolic or catabolic, depending on the dose, duration and timing of treatment, the method of administration, and most likely other factors. Though PTH(1-34) appears to be a promising formation-stimulating agent, further study is required to combine these variables for optimal benefit in osteoporotic women.

Growth factors. Osteoblastic differentiation and proliferation is stimulated by growth factors secreted in an autocrine fashion. The most important among these appear to be insulin-like growth factors I and II (IGF-I, IGF-II), and TGF-β. There is evidence that an alteration in the production of these growth factors may contribute to the development of osteoporosis. For example, circulating levels of IGF-I decrease by almost 50% with aging, and low levels of IGF-I in young men have also been associated with osteoporosis (64). Additional insight into the possible pathogenesis of osteoporosis has been provided by the discovery of some of the factors which regulate the differentiation of pluripotential bone marrow stem cells into osteoblasts versus adipocytes. Many of these factors are now available in highly purified or recombinant form and may eventually prove most useful in the stimulation of new bone as a treatment for osteoporosis. Unfortunately, they also have potent extraskeletal effects and must be administered parenterally. Various strategies to overcome these limitations are being evaluated. They include confirming the nature of the optimal growth factors, identifying a threshold dose and frequency that affect only bone, targeting the growth factor to bone by conjugating it with a bone-seeking compound, and using drugs that stimulate the local production of growth factors by osteoblasts. Although theoretically attractive, the clinical use of these agents is highly investigational at this point.

Combination treatment. It has already been shown that combinations such as exercise, calcium and ERT are superior to each of these in isolation. Is combining the two currently most effective antiresorptive agents, ERT and alendronate, more

150

effective than either of these agents alone? A clinical trial is currently being performed in an attempt to answer this question. The goal of osteoporosis treatment is to rebalance the bone remodeling cycle, but the slowing of bone resorption also ultimately decreases the rate of bone formation, as evidenced by the reduction in both formation and resorption markers with antiresorptive therapy. Given this, an optimal combination may prove to be an antiresorptive agent with a consistent formation-stimulating agent, once such an agent is found.

Conclusion

Postmenopausal osteoporosis is one of the modern-day scourges of our society. In recent years, significant scientific strides have been made in our understanding of bone turnover regulation, bone loss, and the mechanisms by which these can be manipulated pharmacologically. The latest findings in normal and abnormal bone physiology have opened the door to a host of exciting potential treatment options for osteoporosis, and many of these are likely to become available for clinical use in the near future. In sum, there is every reason to be optimistic that this enormous public health problem can begin to be brought under control within the coming decade.

References

1. Ray NF, Chan JK, Thamer M, Melton LJ III 1997 Medical expenditures for the treatment of osteoporotic fractures in the United States in 1995: Report from the National Osteoporosis Foundation. J Bone Miner Res 12 (1):24-35.

2. Melton LJ III 1995 How many women have osteoporosis now? J Bone Miner Res 10: 175-177.

3. Genant HK, Engelke K, Fuerst T 1996 Noninvasive assessment of bone mineral and structure: State of the art. J Bone Miner Res 11:707-730.

4. Hans D, Dargent-Molina P, Schott AM 1996 Ultrasonographic heel measurements to predict hip fracture in elderly women: The EPIDOS prospective study. Lancet 348:511-514.

5. Rubin SM, Cummings SR 1992 Results of bone densitometry affect women's decisions about taking measures to prevent fractures. Ann Intern Med 116:990-995.

6. Wasnich RD, Ross PD, Heilbrun LK, Vogel JM 1985 Prediction of postmenopausal fracture risk with use of bone mineral measurements. Am J Obstet Gynecol 153:745-751.

7. Hui SL, Slemenda CW, Johnston CC Jr 1989 Baseline measurement of bone mass predicts fracture in white women. Ann Intern Med 111:355-361.

8. Cummings SR, Black DM, Nevitt MC, Browner WS, Cauley JA, Genant HK. Appendicular bone density and age predict hip fracture in women. JAMA 110; 263:665-668.

9.   Kanis JA, Melton LJ III, Christiansen C, Johnston CC, Khaltaev N 1994 The diagnosis of osteoporosis. J Bone Miner Res 9:1137-1141.

10.   Delmas PD 1996 Biochemical markers for the assessment of bone turnover: Clinical usein osteoporosis. In: Osteoporosis: Etiology, Diagnosis, and Management, Second Edition 319-333.

11.   Riggs BL, Melton LJ III, O'Fallon WM 1996 Drug therapy for vertebral fractures in osteoporosis: Evidence that decreases in bone turnover and increases in bone mass both determine antifracture efficacy. Bone 18 (3):Suppl:197S-201S.

12.   Garnero P, Hausherr E, Chapuy MC, Marcelli C, Grandjean H, Muller C, Cormier C, Breart G, Meunier P, Delmas PD 1996 Markers of bone resorption predict hip fracture in elderly women: The EPIDOS prospective study. J Bone Miner Res 11:1531-1538.

13.   Garnero P, Shih WJ, Gineyts E, Karpf DB, Delmas PD 1994 Comparison of new biochemical markers of bone turnover in late postmenopausal osteoporotic women in response to alendronate treatment. J Clin Endocrinol Metab 79:1693-1700.

14.   Riggs BL, Melton LJ III 1990 Clinical heterogeneity in involutional osteoporosis: Implications for preventive therapy. J Clin Endocrinol Metab 70:1229-1232.

15.   Riggs BL, Melton LJ III 1986 Medical progress series: Involutional osteoporosis. N EnglJ Med 314:1676-1686.

16.   Pocock NA, Eisman JA, Yeates MG, Sambrook PN, Eberl S 1986 Physical fitness is a major determinant of femoral neck and lumbar spine bone mineral density. J Clin Invest 78:618-621.

17.   Simkin A, Ayalon J, Leichter I 1987 Increased trabecular bone density due to bone-loading exercises in postmenopausal osteoporotic women. Calcif Tissue Int 40:59-63.

18.   Kanders B, Dempster DW, Lindsay R 1988 Interaction of calcium, nutrition, and physical activity on bone mass in young women. J Bone Miner Res 3:145.

19.   Melton LJ III, Riggs BL 1985 Risk factors for injury after fall. Clin Geriatr Med 1:525-539.

20.   Tinetti T, Speechley M, Ginter SF Risk factors for falls among elderly persons living in the community. N Engl J Med 319:1701-1707.

21.   Ledger GA, Burritt MF, Kao PC, O'Fallon WM, Riggs BL, Khosla S 1995 Role of parathyroid hormone in mediating nocturnal and age-related increases in bone resorption. J Clin Endocrinol Metab 80:3304-3310.

22.   Heaney RP, Gallagher JC, Johnston CC, Neer R, Parfitt AM, Whedon GD 1982 Calcium nutrition and bone health in the elderly. Am J Clin Nutr 36:986-1013.

23.   Epstein S, Bryce G, Hinman JW, Miller ON, Riggs BL, Johnston CC 1986 The influence of age on bone mineral regulating hormones. Bone 7:421-425.

24. Forero MS, Klein RF, Nissenson RA, et al 1987 Effect of age on circulating immunoreactive and bioactive parathyroid hormone levels in women. J Bone Miner Res 2:363-366.

25. Young G, Marcus R, Minkoff JR, Kim LY, Segre GV 1987 Age-related rise in parathyroid hormone in man: The use of intact and midmolecule antisera to distinguish hormone secretion from retention. J Bone Miner Res 2:367-374.

26. Akerstrom G, Rudberg C, Grimelius L, et al 1986 Histologic parathyroid abnormalities in an autopsy series. Hum Pathol 17:520-527.

27. Ledger GA, Burritt MF, Kao PC, et al 1994 Abnormalities in parathyroid secretion in elderly women that are reversible by short term therapy with 1,25-dihydroxyvitamin D3. J Clin Endocrinol Metab 79: 211-216.

28. Riggs BL, Melton LJ III 1992 The prevention and treatment of osteoporosis. N Engl J Med 327:620-627.

29. McKane WR, Khosla S, Egan KS, Robins SP, Burritt MF, Riggs BL 1996 Role of calcium intake in modulating age-related increase in parathyroid function and bone resorption. J Clin Endocrinol Metab 81:1699-1703.

30. Cummings RG 1990 Calcium intake and bone mass: A quantitative review of the evidence. Calcif Tissue Int 47:194-201.

31. Dawson-Hughes B, Harris SS, Krall EA, Dallal GE 1997 The effect of calcium and vitamin D supplementation on bone density in men and women 65 years of age or older. N Engl J Med 337:670-676.

32. NIH Consensus Development Panel 1994 Optimal calcium intake. JAMA 272:1942-1948.

33. Tsai K, Heath H III, Kumar R, Riggs BL 1984 Impaired vitamin D metabolism with aging in women:Possible role in pathogenesis of senile osteoporosis. J Clin Invest 73:1668-1672.

34. Eastell R, Yergey AL, Vieira N, Cedel SL, Kumar R, Riggs BL 1991 Interrelationship among vitamin D metabolism, true calcium absorption, parathyroid function and age in women: Evidence of an age-related intestinal resistance to 1,25 (OH)2D action. J Bone Miner Res 6:125-132.

35. Lips P, Netelenbos JC, Jongen MJM 1982 Histomorphometric profile and vitamin D status in patients with femoral neck fracture. Metab Bone Dis Relat Res 4: 85-93.

36. Chapuy MC, Arlot ME, Duboeuf F 1992 Vitamin D3 and calcium to prevent hip fractures in elderly women. N Engl J Med 327:1637-1642.

37. Grady D, Rubin SM, Petitti DB. 1992 Hormone therapy to prevent disease and prolong life in postmenopausal women. Ann Intern Med 117:1016-1037.

38. McKane RW, Khosla S, Risteli J, Robins SP, Muhs JM, Riggs BL 1997 Role of estrogen deficiency in pathogenesis of secondary hyperparathyroidism and increased bone resorption in elderly women. Proc Assoc Am Physicians 109:174-180.

39. Khosla S, Atkinson EJ, Melton LJ III, Riggs BL 1997 Effects of age and estrogen status on serum parathyroid hormone levels and biochemical markers of bone turnover in women: A population based study. J Clin Endocrinol Metab 82:1522-1527.

40. Eastell R, Delmas PD, Hodgson SF, Eriksen EF, Mann KG, Rigs BL 1988 Bone formation rate in older normal women: Concurrent assessment with bone histomorphometry calcium kinetics, and biochemical markers. J Clin Endocrinol Metab 67:7418.

41. Eriksen EF, Colvard EF, Berg DS 1988 Evidence of estrogen receptors in normal human osteoblast-like cells. Science 241:84-86.

42. Manolagas SC, Jilka RL 1995 Bone marrow, cytokines, and bone remodeling: Emerging insights into the pathophysiology of osteoporosis. N Engl J Med 332:305-311.

43. Turner RT, Riggs BL, Spelsberg TC 1994 Skeletal effects of estrogen. Endocr Rev 15:274-300.

44. Tomkinson A, Reeve J, Shaw RW, Noble BS 1997 The death of osteocytes via apoptosis accompanies estrogen withdrawal in human bone. J Clin Endocrinol Metab 82:3128-3135.

45. Stampfer MJ, Colditz GA, Willett WC 1991 Postmenopausal estrogen therapy and cardiovascular disease: ten-year follow-up from the Nurses' Health Study. N Engl J Med 325: 756.

46. Stevenson JC, Cust MP, Gangar KF, Hillard TC, Lees B, Whitehead MI 1990 Effects of transdermal versus oral hormone replacement therapy on bone density in spine and proximal femur in postmenopausal women. Lancet 336:265-269.

47. Ross D 1997 Randomized cross-over comparison of skin irritation with two transdermal oestradiol patches. BMJ 315:288.

48. Bergkvist L, Persson J 1996 Hormone replacement therapy and breast cancer: A review of current knowledge. Drug Safety 15 (5):360-370.

49. Watts NB, Harris ST, Genant HK 1990 Intermittent cyclical etidronate treatment of postmenopausal osteoporosis. N Engl J Med 323:73-79.

50. Storm T, Thamsborg G, Steiniche T, Genant HK, Sorensen OH 1990 Effect of intermittent cyclical etidronate therapy on bone mass and fracture rate in women with postmenopausal osteoporosis. N Engl J Med 322:1265-1271.

51. Liberman UA, Weiss SR, Broll J 1995 Effect of oral alendronate on bone mineral density and the incidence of fractures in postmenopausal osteoporosis. N Engl J Med 333:1437-1443.

52. Black DM, Cummings SR, Karpf DB 1996 Randomised trial of effect of alendronate on risk of fracture in women with existing vertebral fractures. Lancet 348:1535-1541.

53. Hosking DJ, McClung MR, Ravn P 1996 Alendronate in the prevention of osteoporosis: EPIC study two-year results. J Bone Miner Res S133.

154

54. Overgaard K, Hansen MA, Jensen SB, Christiansen C 1992 Effect of salcatonin given intranasally on bone mass and fracture rates in established osteoporosis: A dose-response study. BMJ 305:556-561.

55. Riggs BL, Hodgson SF, O'Fallon WM 1990 Effect of fluoride treatment on the fracture rate in postmenopausal women with osteoporosis. N Engl J Med 332: 802-809.

56. Kleeekoper M, Peterson EL, Nelson DA 1991 A randomized trial of sodium fluoride as a treatment for postmenopausal osteoporosis. Osteoporos Int 1:155-161.

57. Pak CYC, Sakhaee K, Adams-Huet B, Piziak V, Peterson RD, Poindexter JR 1995 Treatment of postmenopausal osteoporosis with slow-release sodium fluoride. Final report of a randomized controlled trial. Ann Intern Med 123: 401-408

58. Sogaard CH, Mosekilde L, Richards A, Mosekilde L 1994 Marked decrease in trabecular bone quality after five years of sodium fluoride therapy – assessed by biochemical testing of iliac crest bone biopsies in osteoporotic women. Bone 15:393-399.

59. Love RR, Mazess RB, Barden HS, Epstein S, Newcomb PA, Jordan VC 1992 Effects of tamoxifen on bone mineral density in postmenopausal women with breast cancer. N Engl J Med 326:852-856.

60. Draper MW, Flowers DE, Huster WJ, Neild JA, Harper KD, Arnaud C 1196 A controlled trial of raloxifene (LY139481) HCl: Impact on bone turnover and serum lipid profile in healthy postmenopausal women. J Bone Miner Res 11:835-842.

61. Slovik DM, Neer RM, Potts JT Jr 1981 Short-term effects of synthetic human parathyroid hormone (1-34) administration on bone mineral metabolism in osteoporotic patients. J Clin Invest 68:1261-1271.

62. Reeve J, Meunier PJ, Parsons JA 1980 Anabolic effects of human PTH fragment on trabecular bone in involutional osteoporosis: a multicenter trial. BMJ 280:1340-1344.

63. Neer R, Slovik D, Daly M, Lo C, Potts J, Nussbaum S 1990 Treatment of postmenopausal osteoporosis with daily parathyroid hormone plus calcitriol. In: Christiansen C, Overgaard K, eds. Osteoporosis 1990: Proceedings of the Third International Symposium on Osteoporosis, Copenhagen, Denmark, October 14-20, 1990   vol. 3, Copenhagen, Denmark: Osteopress Ass.,:1314-1317.

64. Johansson AG, Lindh E, Ljunghall S 1992 Insulin-like growth factor stimulates bone turnover in osteoporosis. Lancet 339:1619.

10 Individualizing Osteoporosis Therapy

Stuart L. Silverman, M.D.

What every woman should consider

Every woman should consider prevention of postmenopausal osteoporosis at time of menopause with FDA approved antiresorptive therapies and adequate calcium and vitamin D. Every woman with established osteoporosis should consider treatment with antiresorptive therapies and adequate calcium and vitamin D.

Calcium and vitamin D supplementation. All osteoporosis therapies for prevention or treatment should begin with calcium and vitamin D. Calcium supplementation and calcium in the diet are equivalent. As pointed out by Drs. Doran and Khosla in the previous chapter, 1000 mg calcium is suggested for the postmenopausal woman age 50-65 on estrogen and 1500 mg for the woman of the same age not on estrogen supplementation. All women older than 65 are advised to take 1500 mg of calcium regardless of their estrogen status (NIH Consensus Conference 1994). Increased calcium supplementation may be required with some therapies such as PTH and fluoride which may require at least 2500 mg/day (20).

As pointed out by Dr. Davies later in this volume, vitamin D supplementation may play an important role in some patients as it influences calcium absorption. Vitamin D levels are often lower in the elderly who have decreased sun exposure, decreased skin vitamin D synthesis, decreased milk intake as well as other abnormalities of the vitamin D-endocrine system such as decreased responsiveness of renal 1a-hydroxylase to PTH and decreased intestinal mucosal responsiveness to calcitriol (20). The requirement for vitamin D may therefore be increasing with age. Heikinheimo (21) found substantial reduction of fracture rate in an elderly Finnish population given 150,000-300,000 IU vitamin D every autumn.

Chapuy (5) found that supplemental vitamin D3 and calcium can prevent hip fractures in elderly women. Dawson Hughes (10) has reported vertebral fracture reduction with calcium and vitamin D. The doses of vitamin D in the above studies suggest that an intake of 500-800 IU vitamin D may be required in adults (22). This is substantially higher than the current recommended daily allowance (RDA) of 200 IU. This higher intake can be met by use of two multivitamins containing 800 IU vitamin D as a source of 800 IU vitamin D daily; however, this approach may provide an excess of vitamin A.

FDA approved therapies for prevention and treatment of osteoporosis

Current FDA-approved therapies for treatment of osteoporosis at the time of writing this chapter include: estrogen, alendronate, nasal spray and injectable salmon calcitonin. Current FDA approved therapies for prevention of osteoporosis include estrogen, raloxifene and alendronate. All of these therapies should be combined with adequate doses of calcium and vitamin D. All of these drugs inhibit bone resorption, resulting in increased bone mass as well as decreased bone turnover.

Estrogen

Estrogen receptors are present on both osteoclasts and osteoblasts. Estrogen may prevent bone loss by limiting osteoclast lifespan through promotion of apoptosis (25). Estrogen acts on osteoblasts by increasing mRNA levels encoding the type I collagen gene. Furthermore, loss of gonadal function also results in an increase in the sensitivity of osteoclastic precursors to the action of cytokines such as IL-6 (32).

Clinical Efficacy. Estrogen is the gold standard for both the prevention and treatment of osteoporosis. Estrogen results in increases in bone density which are lost on discontinuation of the estrogen. Surprisingly, despite the availability of estrogen for many years now, there is little prospective data on its effects on bone for either prevention or treatment. In the PEPI trial (45) 875 healthy women less than 10 years postmenopausal were randomly allocated to one of five hormone replacement regimens for 3 years. One group received placebo only, another unopposed conjugated equine estrogens (CEE) 0.625 mg/day, and the other three groups were CEE 0.625 mg/day plus one of three progestin schedules: cyclic progesterone 10 mg/d for 12 days each month, continuous progesterone 2.5 mg/d, or micronized progesterone 200 mg/d for 12 days each month. Over 3 years, women receiving unopposed estrogen increased bone (BMD) 4-5% in the spine and 2% in the hip. None of the progestin regimens modified the BMD response at the spine or hip. Only about 8% of the participants were nonresponders. Reduction in hip fracture risk is greater in women who currently use estrogen than never users. Current users have about half the risk of never users, but past users have no protection or show only modest reduction in fracture risk (4). Felson (15) studied the effect of 10 years estrogen therapy after menopause in a cross-sectional study. Estrogen users less than 75 years of age showed 10-12% higher BMD, and estrogen users greater than 75 years had BMD similar to women who had never taken estrogen.

Low-dose estrogen may be an effective alternative for patients unable to tolerate standard doses of estrogen (0.625 mg of conjugated estrogen). 0.3 mg of esterified estrogens or 25 micrograms of transdermal estradiol appear effective in the prevention of postmenopausal bone loss (17). There is a dose-response curve with a serum concentration of about 30 micrograms/ml of estradiol being the threshold for preventing postmenopausal bone loss.

As Drs. Doran and Khosla reminded us in the previous chapter, estrogen has additional benefits which include: relief of menopausal symptoms such as hot flashes and night sweats, correction of postmenopausal genitourinary dysfunction, cardioprotection and a growing body of evidence that estrogen may reduce risk of Alzheimer's disease and have a positive effect on memory (43). Current estrogen users have a 37% lower risk of death (relative risk of 0.63) after adjustment for confounding variables. However, long-term estrogen use reduces mortality by only 20%, because the cardiovascular benefit is offset by thromboembolic events and increased risk of endometrial and breast cancer (14). Therefore, for many women the benefits of hormone replacement may not compensate for the increased risk of breast cancer, especially if the woman is at low cardiovascular risk. Women who have a high risk of breast cancer and a low risk of coronary heart may benefit instead from selective estrogen receptor modulators (SERMs) as discussed below. Despite its global health benefits, the use of estrogen in postmenopausal women is limited due to fear of breast cancer and dislike for reinstituting the menstrual cycle as well as side effects such as mastodynia. Only 20% of patients remain on estrogen replacement long-term ($\geq$3 years). The average woman will only take estrogen 6-12 months to treat symptoms rather than to prevent a silent disease such as osteoporosis. Only 10% will take it for as long as 10 years. These compliance studies were carried out before the use of continuous, low-dose progesterone in hormone replacement regimens. We don't know whether this new approach has improve compliance. The benefit of the estrogen is lost after discontinuation.

Who is the patient of choice for estrogen therapy? Recognizing the many benefits of estrogen therapy, all postmenopausal patients should be educated about the benefits of estrogen replacement for both the prevention and treatment of osteoporosis. Women who are willing to take estrogen should be encouraged to do so. Women who are undecided may benefit from bone density information which may increase their likelihood of filling an estrogen prescription irrespective of the bone density measurement (42). Women who are concerned about reinstitution of menses should be encouraged to use continuous combined estrogen/progesterone therapy, which results in spotting for 6-8 months and then uterine atrophy (37). Women with a strong family history of breast cancer may wish to choose an alternative agent such as a SERM or a bisphosphonate.

Women who are having side effects such as mastodynia may benefit from lowering the dose of estrogen. Women with migraines may also benefit from a lower dose of transdermal estrogen or from a lower dose of progestin. Long cycle estrogen (3 months) with 14 days of 10 mg progesterone may also be considered with endometrial monitoring. Women with high triglycerides may benefit from use of the estrogen patch which avoids the "first pass" through the liver and does not increase triglycerides, however, this route of administration also does not result in a more positive cardiovascular profile.

The older woman in her sixth or seventh decade will also benefit from estrogen. Recent work has shown at least a 5% gain in BMD when estrogen is started 10 or more years after the menopause (7,29,31). Limited studies show that the use of estrogen in older women is associated with fracture reduction (29). This suggests that women older than 65 years who show clinical evidence of osteoporosis, such as height loss, fracture or low BMD, should be targeted for estrogen replacement.

Monitoring therapy. Routine monitoring of bone density has not been recommended for women taking estrogen. However, there is data that as many as 12% of women may not respond to estrogen with an increase in BMD in the hip. This suggests that women may benefit from a bone density measurement several years after starting estrogen. Nonresponders to estrogen may benefit from an increased dose of estrogen. They may also benefit from the addition of bisphosphonate drugs (see below). Of course, annual mammograms and PAP smears should be obtained in any postmenopausal woman on estrogen.

Raloxifene and SERMs

Raloxifene is the first FDA-approved selective estrogen receptor modulator (SERM) approach for the prevention of osteoporosis. SERMs can be distinguished from other estrogens by their activity profile in reproductive tissue, particularly the uterus. For example, tamoxifen (triphenylethylene) a first generation SERM, is a partial agonist for the uterus, while raloxifene (a benzothiophene) is a complete antagonist in the uterus. The precise mechanism for the action of SERMs involves interaction with both of the estrogen receptors ERα and ERβ (3) SERMs affect both osteoclast number and function. Raloxifene, like estrogen, reduces bone resorption and results in a net positive calcium balance (13,18).

Clinical Efficacy. Raloxifene has been approved by the FDA for prevention of postmenopausal osteoporosis as a tablet at the dose of 60 mg per day. Raloxifene showed significant increases over 2 years in postmenopausal women with osteopenia of 2.4% in spine and 2.5% in hip (12). In the MORE trial, an ongoing large, double-blind, randomized study of raloxifene in the treatment of osteoporosis, two dosages of raloxifene (60 and 120 mg) were compared to placebo in 7705 osteoporotic women. In an interim 2 year analysis BMD at the hip and spine increased by 2-3% compared with placebo. There was a significant reduction in the risk of vertebral fracture.

Raloxifene reduced the risk of newly-diagnosed breast cancer and might decrease the risk of newly diagnosed endometrial cancer during two years of use in the MORE trial of 7704 postmenopausal women with osteoporosis who were receiving 60 or 120 mg raloxifene or placebo (9). Compared with the rate in the placebo group after 28.9 months of follow-up there was a decreased relative risk of breast cancer (RR = 0.26) for patients on raloxifene. Compared with placebo the overall relative risk of endometrial cancer was 0.38 (p=0.232). If two cases diagnosed within one month of randomization are excluded, the estimate of relative risk is 0.13 (p=0.045). Using all osteoporosis trials data to date, which includes 14,800 patient-years cumulative exposure to raloxifene and 6,750 patient years cumulative exposure to placebo there was a 58% reduction in breast cancer risk (26). In addition, raloxifene significantly reduced the incidence of both newly diagnosed estrogen receptor-positive tumors (p<0.001) and progesterone receptor positive tumors (p=0.028) without affecting the incidence rate of either ER- or progesterone receptor-negative tumors. These are short term studies, and much longer periods of observation are needed before definitive statements can be made about the effectiveness by Raloxifene on prevention of breast cancer.

Raloxifene increases incidence of hot flashes although it does not influence severity of hot flashes, increases leg cramps and increases the risk of venous thromboembolic disease similar to estrogen (RR=3.4). Raloxifene decreases surrogate cardiovascular markers such as total cholesterol and LDL similar to estrogen but does not increase HDL or triglycerides. It is not yet known, however, if raloxifene decreases the incidence of cardiovascular events. A multicenter study to address cardiovascular outcomes, the RUTH trial, is being organized to address these issues. Prior trials with tamoxifen had suggested a 15-34% reduction in cardiovascular events which was not statistically significant.

Who is the patient of choice for raloxifene? Raloxifene should be considered for osteoporosis prevention. Choices for prevention include estrogen, raloxifene, and the 5 mg dose of alendronate (see below). Raloxifene would not be considered as the agent of choice in the symptomatic woman with hot flashes or night sweats. On the other hand, raloxifene may be the medication of choice for the woman who is at increased risk of breast cancer due to family history or other factors. Raloxifene provides a favorable affect on cardiovascular lipid profile, but it is not known if it reduces cardiovascular events. Data is pending on the effects of raloxifene on cognitive function and Alzheimers disease. Women on raloxifene with vasomotor symptoms may be considered for clonidine (an alpha adrenergic agent) or megace (a progestin) to control symptoms. Data on the safety of combining a low-dose estrogen patch, which may control postmenopausal symptoms, with raloxifene is not available. Raloxifene may be a future option for treatment of patients with osteoporosis pending the third year analysis of the MORE trial which will be available in December 1998.

Monitoring of therapy. Routine monitoring of raloxifene therapy with bone density measurement is not recommended but lack of a uniform individual response monitoring desirable in many instances. The use of bone markers is still experimental. Of course, annual mammograms and PAP smears should be obtained in any postmenopausal woman.

Nasal Calcitonin

Calcitonin is a 32 amino acid polypeptide which is released from the thyroid in mammals in response to hypercalcemia and rapidly lowers plasma calcium and phosphorus by inhibiting bone resorption (33). The action of calcitonin is directed at calcitonin receptors on the osteoclast. Calcitonin directly affects osteoclast activity, and may also inhibit osteoclast formation (33). In the continued presence of calcitonin, "escape" from its inhibitory action may occur, possibly due to downregulation of calcitonin receptors (33). *Clinical Efficacy.* Calcitonin previously required subcutaneous injection but is now available as an intranasal preparation. The dosing of the intranasal preparation is 200 IU/day. Previous data showed modest increases of 2-3% in lumbar spine bone mass of patients with established osteoporosis, with one study (35) showing decreases in vertebral fracture risk. A recent large multicenter study showed significant decreases in new vertebral fracture risk compared to active control (1000 mg calcium and 400 IU vitamin D) at four years (6). No data on nonvertebral or hip fracture efficacy is available. Calcitonin may be beneficial in patients with corticosteroid-induced osteoporosis. Studies have shown increases in lumbar spine bone density (30). Calcitonin nasal spray may have analgesic benefits to the patient with acute vertebral fracture (36). The mechanism of this action may include stimulation of release of endorphins from the pituitary.

Calcitonin is safe. In the multicenter study there was no increased report of adverse events other than rhinitis when calcitonin nasal spray is compared to placebo nasal spray. Unlike injectable calcitonin, there is no increased incidence of nausea or flushing. There is no long-term skeletal retention of nasal calcitonin.

Who is the ideal patient for calcitonin?. Calcitonin nasal spray or injectable should be considered as an alternative to estrogen and alendronate for the treatment of established osteoporosis. Calcitonin has not been proven to be effective in the prevention of postmenopausal osteoporosis. Calcitonin has proven vertebral fracture reduction and should be considered in the patient with vertebral bone loss; however, its fracture efficacy is more modest than estrogen or alendronate. Calcitonin may be preferred in the medically complex patient, the patient with renal failure, the patient with intolerance on contraindications to estrogen or alendronate, the patient who has underlying gastrointestinal problems. Calcitonin may be the agent of choice in the symptomatic patient with established osteoporosis who would benefit from its analgesic effect.

Monitoring of therapy. Routine bone density monitoring of nasal spray calcitonin is not suggested since the bone density increases are so modest that they may not be detected by BMD measurement. In fact, bone density measurement may lead to false conclusions that a patient is not a responder. Similarly changes in bone markers are too modest for monitoring.

Alendronate and Bisphosphonates

Bisphosphonates are synthetic compounds characterized by a P-C-P bond with strong affinity for calcium in bone mineral. In vitro bisphosphonates inhibit bone formation and dissolution of bone mineral (16). Bisphosphonates prevent precipitation of calcium and phosphorus, block transformation of amorphous calcium phosphates in hydroxyapatite, and inhibit aggregation of hydroxyapatite crystals (16). Bisphosphonates inhibit bone resorption through cell-mediated effects on both osteoclasts and osteoblasts. Bisphosphonates promote apoptosis of murine osteoclasts (24). Bisphosphonates also act directly on osteoblasts to produce an inhibitor of osteoclast recruitment (44). Alendronate, the only bisphosphonate yet approved for the treatment of osteoporosis, also causes a dose-dependent inhibition of cytokine production by activated monocytes which may contribute to its inhibitory effect on bone resorption (16). Bisphosphonates may produce an anabolic effect on bone; longer term studies suggest continued increases in bone mineral density (19). About 36-38% of the effects of bisphosphonates can be explained by their antiresorptive effect (19).

Clinical Efficacy. Alendronate is indicated for both the prevention and treatment of osteoporosis. Dosing is 10 mg/day for treatment and 5 mg/day for prevention. Bisphosphonate intestinal absorption is low. Alendronate absorption is maximally 0.7% of the ingested dose and is reduced by simultaneous administration of food or other liquids such as coffee, tea or milk, and especially in the presence of calcium. Bisphosphonates are rapidly cleared from plasma; 20% to 80% are deposited in bone and the remainder excreted in urine. In bone they deposit at sites of mineralization and under osteoclasts. Doses of 10 mg/day given to patients with established osteoporosis result in significant increases in BMD at 3 years as measured by differences between the treatment and placebo groups (1,28). At three years there was an increase of 6.2-8.8% in vertebral BMD, 4.1-5.9% in the femoral neck, and 6.1-7.8% in the trochanter. There was significant reduction in risk of fracture of the spine and hip at 3 years. Alendronate prevents postmenopausal bone loss. In the two year analysis of the EPIC study (Early Postmenopausal Intervention Cohort Study Group) of 1174 postmenopausal women under age 60, women who received placebo lost BMD at all sites whereas women treated with 5 mg alendronate had increases of 3.5% in the lumbar spine, 1.9% at the hip and 0.67% for total body. BMD responses to estrogen and progesterone were 1 to 2 percent higher than that of 5 mg alendronate (23).

There is little clinical data on the use of alendronate in children and adolescents. Brumsen (2) reported on the use of bisphosphonates in 12 patients between ages 10 and 17, and found them to be well tolerated with clinical improvement.

The safety profile of alendronate in randomized clinical trials was excellent with no increased risk of gastrointestinal side effects compared to placebo. However, rare cases of severe esophagitis, gastric ulcer or duodenal ulcer have been reported in patients not taking the prescribed dosing regimen (11). At greatest risk are those patients with active ulcer, acid reflux requiring treatment or esophageal dysmotility. Some women who are intolerant of 10 mg per day may do well on 10 mg every other day or 5 mg daily, still an adequate dose.

Which patients are candidates for alendronate therapy? Alendronate has been FDA approved for both the prevention and treatment of osteoporosis and is a first line therapy. Alendronate is an effective option for the patient who refuses or cannot tolerate estrogen or has a contraindication to estrogen. Alendronate is effective and results in rapid gains in bone mass. In the FOSIT trial there was a gain of 3% in BMD in the first three months, suggesting that alendronate would be an ideal agent even in older populations where time to response is a consideration. Alendronate increases bone density in patients with steroid-induced osteoporosis (39). Alendronate also shows promise in post-transplantation bone disease; alendronate prevents cyclosporin A-induced osteopenia in the rat (40). Alendronate is currently being studied in males with osteoporosis.

Monitoring of therapy. Routine monitoring of alendronate therapy is not recommended as approximately 95% of patients are responders. However, in clinical practice the bone density increases are robust by two to three years, and a bone density measurement may act as reinforcement for increased compliance. Changes in bone density markers are also rapid and significant, with a 60% reduction in urine N-telopeptide excretion; a 60% change does exceed the precision error of the marker measurement. This suggests potential utility for bone marker information for early monitoring of alendronate therapy. A small percentage of patients are nonresponders to bisphosphonates such as alendronate. This nonresponse may be due to poor absorption, poor compliance, or vitamin D deficiency (27).

Combination Therapy

Alendronate and estrogen. Combination therapy with both alendronate and estrogen has been suggested for patients who can only tolerate less than the standard dose of premarin, or who have such severe osteoporosis that combination therapy may be warranted. Such a combination would theoretically provide some of the cardioprotective effects of estrogen, while preventing fracture with alendronate. Data from a two year study will be available at the end of 1998. Until that time, it is not known if there is a beneficial effect of combining the two medications.

References

1. Black DM, Cummings SR, Karpf DB, Cauley JA, Thompson DE, Nevitt MC et al 1996 Randomized trial of effect of alendronate on risk of fracture in women with existing vertebral fractures. Fracture Intervention Trial Research Group. Lancet 348:1535-1541.

2. Brumsen C, Hamdy NA, Papapoulos SE 1997 Long-term effects of bisphosphonates on the growing skeleton. Studies of young patients with severe osteoporosis. Medicine 76:266-283.

3. Bryant HU, Dere WH 1998 Selective estrogen receptor modulators: an alternative to hormonal replacement therapy. Proc Soc Ex Biol Medicine. 217:45-52.

4. Cauley JA, Seeley DG, Ensrud K, Ettinger B, Black D, Cummings SR 1995 For the study of osteoporotic fractures study group estrogen replacement therapy and fractures in older women. Ann Intern Med 122:9-16.

5. Chapuy MC, Arlot ME, Duboeuf F et al 1992 Vitamin D3 and calcium to prevent hip fractures in elderly women. N Engl J Med 328:460-464.

6. Chesnut C, Baylink DJ, Doyle D, Genant H, Harris S, Kiel DP, LeBoff M, Stock JL, Gimona A, Andriano K, Richardson R for the PROOF study group 1998 Salmon calcitonin nasal spray prevents vertebral fractures in established osteoporosis. Further interim results of the PROOF study. In Program/Proceedings of the European Foundation for Osteoporosis, September 11-15; Berlin.

7. Christiansen C, Riis BJ 1990 17-beta estradiol and continuous norethisterone: a unique treatment for established osteoporosis in elderly women. J Clin Endocrinol Metab 71:836-841.

8. Colditz GA, Hankinson SE, Hunter DJ, Willett WC, Manson JF 1995 The use of estrogens and progestins and the risk of breast cancer in postmenopausal women. N Engl J Med 332:1589-1593.

9.   Cummings SR, Norton L, Eckert S, Grady D, Cauley J, Knickerbocker R, Black DM, Nickelsen T, Glusman J, Krueger K for the MORE investigators 1998 Raloxifene reduces the risk of breast cancer and may decrease the risk of endometrial cancer in postmenopausal women. Two year findings from the multiple outcomes of raloxifene evaluation (MORE) trial. (abstract). In Program/Proceedings of the American Society of Clinical Oncology, Thirty-Fourth Annual Meeting, May 16-19; Philadelphia(PA): WB Saunders Company/Mack Printing Group, p 2a. Abstract 3

10. Dawson-Hughes B, Harris SS, Krall EA, Dallal GE 1997 Effect of calcium and vitamin D supplementation on bone density in men and women 65 years of age or older. N Engl J Med 337:670-676.

11. De Groen PC, Lubbe CF, Hirsch LF, Daifotis A, Stephenson W, Freedholm D, Pryor-Tilootson S, Seleznick MJ, Pinkas H, Wang KH 1996 Esophagitis associated with the use of alendronate. N Engl J Med 335:1016-1021.

12. Delmas PD, Bjarnason NH, Mitlak BH et al 1997 Effects of raloxifene on bone mineral density, serum cholesterol concentrations, and uterine endometrium in postmenopausal women. N Engl J Med 337:1641-1647.

13. Draper MW, Flowers DE, Huster WJ et al 1996 A controlled trial of raloxifene (LY139481): impact on bone turnover and serum lipid profile in healthy postmenopausal women. J Bone Miner Res 11:835-842.

14. Ettinger B, Black D, Cummings S, Genant H, Gluer C, Lips P, Knickerbocker R, Eckert S, Nickelsen T, Mitlak B, for the MORE Study Group 1998. Raloxifene reduces the risk of incident vertebral fractures: 24-month interim analyses. In: Program/Proceedings of the European Foundation for Osteoporosis September 11-15; Berlin.

15. Felsen DT, Zhang Y, Hannan MT et al 1993 The effect of postmenopausal estrogen therapy on bone density in elderly women. N Engl J Med 329:1141-1146.

16. Fleisch HA 1997 Bisphosphonates: preclinical aspects and use in osteoporosis. Ann Int Medi 29:55-62.

17. Genant HK, Lucas J, Weiss S, Akin M, Emkey R, et al 1997 Low dose esterified estrogen therapy: effects on bone, plasma estradiol concentrations, endometrium and lipid levels: estratab osteoporosis study group. Arch Int Med 155:2609-2615.

18. Heaney RP, Draper MW 1997 Raloxifene and estrogen: comparative bone remodeling kinetics. J Clin Endocrinol Metab 82:3425-3429.

19. Heaney RP, Yates AJ, Santora AC II 1997 Bisphosphonate effects and the bone remodeling transient. J Bone Miner Res 12:1143-1151.

20. Heaney RP 1998 Nonpharmacologic prevention: nutrition and exercise in Osteoporosis: Diagnosis and Management. Martin Dunitz, Ltd., London.

21. Heikinheimo RJ, Inkovaara JA, Harju EJ et al 1992 Annual injection of vitamin D and fractures of aged bones. Calcif Tissue Int 51:105-110.

22. Holick MF 1994 Vitamin D - new horizons for the 21st century. Am J Clin Nutr 60:619-630.

23. Hosking D, Chilvers CE, Christiansen C, Ravn P, Wasnich R, Ross P, Mc Clung M, Balske A, Thompson D, Daley M, Yates AJ 1998 Prevention of bone loss with alendronate in postmenopausal women under 60 years of age. Early postmenopausal intervention cohort study group. N Engl J Med 338:485-492.

24. Hughes DE, Wright KR, Uy HL, Sasaki A, Yoneda T, Roodman GD, Mundy GR, Boyce BF 1995 Bisphosphonates promote apoptosis in murine osteoclasts in vitro and in vivo. J Bone Mineral Res 10:1478-87.

25. Hughes DE, Dai A, Tiffee JC, Li HH, Mundy GR, Boyce BF 1996 Estrogen promotes apoptosis of murine osteoclasts mediated by TGF-beta. Nature Med 2:1132-1136 .

26. Jordan VC, Glusman JE, Eckert S, Lippman M, Powles T, Costa A, Morrow M, Norton L 1998 Incident primary breast cancers are reduced by raloxifene: integrated data from multicenter, double blind, randomized trials in 12,000 postmenopausal women (abstract). In Program/Proceedings of the American Society of Clinical Oncology, Thirty-Fourth Annual Meeting, May 16-19; Philadelphia(PA): WB Saunders Company/Mack Printing Group, p 122a. Abstract 466.

27. Koster JC, Hacking WH, Mulder H 1996 Diminished effect of etidronate in vitamin D deficient osteopenic postmenopausal women. Eur J Clin Pharm 52:145-147

28. Liberman UA, Weiss SR, Broll J, Minne HW, Quan H, Bell NH, Rodriguez-Portales J, Downs RW Jr, Dequeker J, Favus M 1995 Effect of oral alendronate on bone mineral density and the incidence of fractures in postmenopausal osteoporosis. The Alendronate Phase III Osteoporosis Treatment Study Group. N Eng J Med 333:1437-1443.

29. Lindsay R, Thome JF 1990 Estrogen treatment of patients with established osteoporosis. Obstet Gynecol 76:290-295.

30. Luengo M, Pons F, Martinez de Osaba MJ, Picado C 1994 Prevention of further bone mass loss by nasal calcitonin in patients on long term glucocorticoid therapy for asthma: a two year follow up study. Thorax 49:1099-1102.

31. Lufkin EG , Wahner HW, O'Fallon WM et al 1992 Treatment of postmenopausal osteoporosis with transdermal estrogen. Ann Int Med 117:1-9.

32. Manolagas SC, Bellido T, Jilka RL 1995 New insights into the cellular, biochemical, and molecular basis of postmenopausal and senile osteoporosis: roles of IL-6 and gp130. Int J Immunopharm 17:109-116.

33. Martin TJ, Moseley JM 1990 Calcitonin In Metabolic Bone Disease (L. Avioli and S. Krane, Eds.), Saunders, Philadelphia 131-154.

34. NIH Consensus Conference 1994 Optimal calcium intake. JAMA 272:1942-1948.

35. Overgaard K, Hansen MA, Jensen SB, Christiansen C 1992 Effect of salcatonin given intranasally on bone mass and fracture rate in established osteoporosis: a dose response study. BMJ 305:556-561.

36. Pun KK, Chan LW 1989 Analgesic effect of intranasal salmon calcitonin in the treatment of osteoporotic vertebral fractures. Clin Therap 11:205-209.

37. Rebar RW, Thomas MW, Gass MLS, Liu JH 1990 Problems of hormone therapy: evaluations, follow-up, complications. In the menopause. Serrono Symposium Norwell Massachusetts. 145-156.

38. Reginster JY, Meurmans L, Zegels B, Rovati LC, Minne HW, Giacovelli C, Taquet AN, Setnikar I, Collette J, Gosset C 1998 The effect of sodium fluoromonophosphate plus calcium on vertebral fracture rate in postmenopausal women with moderate osteoporosis. Ann Int Med 129:1-8.

39. Saag KG, Emkey R, Schnitzer TJ, Brown JP, Hawkins F, Goemaere S, Thamsborg G, Liberman UA, Delmas PD, Malice MP, Czachur M, Daifotis AG 1998 Alendronate for the prevention and treatment of glucocorticoid-induced osteoporosis: Glucocorticoid-induced osteoporosis intervention study group. N Engl J Med 339:292-299.

40. Sass DA, Bowman AR, Yuan Z, Ma Y, Jee WS, Epstein S 1997 Alendronate prevents cyclosporin A induced osteopenia in the rat. Bone 21:65-70.

41. Silverman SL, Greenwald M, Klein RA, Drinkwater B 1998 Effect of bone density information on decisions about hormonal replacement therapy: a randomized trial. Obstet Gynecol 89:321-325.

42. Shen V, Dempster DW, Birchman R, Xu R, Lindsay R 1993 Loss of cancellous bone mass and connectivity in ovariectomized rats can be restored by combined treatment with parathyroid hormone and estradiol. J Clin Invest 91:2479-2487.

43. Sherwin B 1997 Estrogenic effects on the central nervous system: clinical aspects. in: estrogens and antiestrogens: basic and clinical aspects. Lindsay R, Dempster D, Jordan V Eds. Lippincott Raven, Philadelphia.

44. Vitte C, Fleisch H, Guenther HL 1996 Bisphosphonates induce osteoblasts to secrete an inhibitor of osteoclast mediated resorption. Endocrinology 137:2324-2333.

45. The Writing Group for the PEPI trial 1996 Effects of hormonal treatment on bone mineral density: results from the postmenopausal estrogen/progestin intervention trial. JAMA 276:1389-1396.

III. Osteoporotic Syndromes of Emerging Impact

11 Fall Prevention and Physical Therapy

Sally Rigler, M.D.
Stephanie Studenski, M.D., M.P.H.

Background

Osteoporosis generally remains silent until fall-related fractures occur. Hip fracture is the main cause of morbidity, mortality, and expense related to osteoporosis, but fractures of the pelvis, proximal humerus, distal wrist, ribs and spine represent other important fall-related events. The public health impact of osteoporosis would be vastly reduced if injurious falls could be largely prevented, even without successful interventions to prevent decline in bone density. Only vertebral compression fractures would remain common manifestations of osteoporosis in such a scenario. Thus, attention to fall prevention should be included in the clinical management of osteoporosis patients to reduce the risk of fracture-related pain, mobility impairment, and disability. Assessment of environmental risks, the underlying extent of gait instability and deconditioning, and the nature of any concomitant physical and cognitive impairments will be necessary to construct appropriate individual care plans.

A review of the prevalence and sequelae of falling will be followed by an outline of important elements of postural control as the basis for clinical assessment. An approach to treatment interventions is suggested, with an emphasis on current knowledge about the role of physical therapy and exercise. Finally, speculations about future directions in fall prevention are offered.

Prevalence and Sequelae of Falling

Fractures occur in about 5% of falls, with hip fracture representing one-quarter of this number.[1] Serious soft tissue injury occurs in another 5% of falls.[1] Inability to get up after a fall is another common consequence with serious ramifications.[1] Since many falls occur without injury, determination of fall characteristics that increase the likelihood of serious injury has been an active area of research. A review of published studies of risk factors for falls and injurious falls demonstrates that varying populations and outcome variables have been examined, but pertinent findings generally fall into the categories of physical function and mobility, gait and balance measures, comorbid medical conditions, sensory impairments, medication utilization, demographic features, and environmental factors.[2]

Another important consequence of falling is a fear-of-falling syndrome in which older adults lose confidence in their ability to carry out daily activities. Self-restriction of physical activity, deconditioning, isolation, loss of important social roles and depression may result. Falls and fractures are feared by older adults because they threaten independence, but loss of perceived self-efficacy due to fear of falling threatens independence as well.[3] Thus, fall prevention interventions should address fear of falling as well because of its own serious sequelae.

Community-Dwelling Older Adults. Patterns of falling among independent older adults differ from those in long-term care. A year-long prospective study of falling among community dwelling adults aged 75 years and older found that 32% fell at least once, with one-quarter of fallers experiencing significant injury (4). Risk factors for falling included sedative use, cognitive impairment, lower extremity disabilities, the presence of a palmomental reflex, abnormalities of balance and gait, and foot problems (4). The likelihood of falling increased with accumulation of these risk factors. Notably, only 10% of falls occurred during acute illness, while 49% were associated with environmental hazards or hazardous activity (4). With median follow up of 31 months, a 49% fall rate was found among community-dwellers (5).

Injurious falls share many risk factors with overall falls, but some additional features are noted. Among fallers, female gender, cognitive impairment, and low body mass index were found to be independent factors predisposing to serious injury, defined as fracture, dislocation, or significant head injury (6). Situational risks for injurious falls were falling on stairs, from at least standing height, and during activities that displaced the center of gravity, such as lifting an object (6). When older subjects were categorized as frail, transitional, or vigorous using defined demographic, physical, and psychological characteristics, it was found that the proportion of falls resulting in serious injury (22%) was greatest among vigorous elderly persons (7), in whom a greater role for home environmental hazards has been noted (7, 8). Recurrent falls among high risk veterans have been found to be influenced by impaired mobility, attitude toward risk, and environmental factors (9).

In summary, functional and environmental factors contribute to the majority of falls among older adults residing in the community. A narrow focus on decompensated medical conditions as the cause of falling will miss the vast majority of potentially preventable falls.

Institutionalized Elderly. Among institutionalized elderly, falls are even more frequent, reported at three times the rate for older adults living at home.10 Risk factors include lower-extremity weakness, gait instability, visual and cognitive impairments, psychotropic medications, and postural hypotension (10). Nursing facility residents with dementia, who are very likely to have osteoporosis, are at very high risk for recurrent falls and fractures for which rehabilitation is difficult.

Approach to Clinical Management

Components of management include the identification of patients at risk for falling, clinical assessment of postural control, and implementation of treatments to reverse, improve, or compensate for these impairments.

Identification of Patients for Fall Prevention Efforts. All osteoporosis patients should receive a fall prevention assessment, including questions about home safety and hazardous activities, screening for fear of falling, and a focused screening evaluation of balance and gait, cognition, strength, vision, postural blood pressure responses, and foot health. Patients who have had prior osteoporotic fractures should receive more intensive preventive efforts, including clarification of the events surrounding prior falls.

Integrated Postural Control as an Organizing Framework. Postural stability requires multiple healthy integrated processes, and lack of such stability is often best thought of as a problem in its own right. By contrast, a disease-based approach to falling is limited by several problems, including highly variable disease expression and the varying impact of comorbid physical and cognitive conditions on functional limitations. In addition, a disease-based approach does not easily incorporate important environmental factors. Finally, normal postural control is underpinned by integrated systems with compensatory back-up mechanisms, so deficits in more than one system are frequently a pre-requisite for impaired postural stability.

Sensory, central processing, and effector functions are key components of postural control and are highlighted next with illustrative concepts. Visual, auditory, vestibular, and peripheral nervous systems provide sensory input that orients individuals to their position in the environment. Visual field cuts, diminished acuity, and other disturbances in eyesight may result in a cautious or uncertain gait, particularly in new environments. Persons of very advanced age often suffer from multiple sensory deficits, particularly of vision and hearing, causing profoundly reduced receipt of environmental information. Symptoms of vestibular impairment, as may occur in benign positional vertigo or Meniere's disease, may include vertigo, dizziness or a feeling of intolerance to movements such as turning over in bed. The presence of nystagmus, or a positive Barany maneuver or Romberg test may suggest vestibular pathology. Peripheral sensory neuropathy is suspected in the context of diabetes, alcoholism, history of familial neuropathy, and a wide range of systemic conditions. Patients may complain that they feel unsteady in the dark and unsure of their footing, especially on uneven outdoor surfaces. Loss of vibratory sense, decreased sensation to pinprick, and any associated motor weakness may be noted on examination.

Even when sensory input is intact, the incoming information from the periphery must be integrated and converted to appropriate motor responses. Dementing illnesses destroy pathways that integrate signals, resulting in gait apraxia and falling. Other mechanisms for impaired central processing include inadequate cerebral perfusion, slowed response time, and primary loss of righting reflexes.

172

Many mechanisms underlie inadequate cerebral perfusion, including the effects of antihypertensive medications, congestive heart failure, dysrhythmia, aortic stenosis, post-prandial hypotension, and autonomic neuropathy. Patients may complain of lightheadedness when rising, near-syncope just before falling, or may experience true syncopal episodes that result frequently in bony or soft tissue injury. Evaluation should include measurement of positional blood pressures and a careful cardiorespiratory examination. However, recent data reveal that, though common, postural dizziness may not correspond to postural blood pressure changes[11], and long-held beliefs implicating thiazide diuretics in falling appear not to have been confirmed in a study of osteoporotic fractures.[12]

Righting reflexes deteriorate in Parkinson's disease and related extrapyramidal syndromes. Unexpected backward falls may occur in the face of little physiologic or mechanical stress. This tendency can be confirmed during examination; a quick backward force applied to the patient's hips may result in a backward fall without evidence of appropriate correcting movements, such as a brisk step backward. Caution is necessary in applying this maneuver and the examiner should be positioned behind the patient for safety.

Slowed corrective responses also occur in numerous medical illnesses of a toxic or metabolic nature, and during use of sedating medications. Patients may feel dizzy, weak, and unsteady. Evaluation may reveal underlying conditions such as hypoxemia, infection, electrolyte or glucose dyscrasia, and renal or hepatic insufficiency. Long-acting benzodiazepines and antipsychotic medications have been associated with increased risk for falling.13 Numerous other medications have been shown to cause sedation in some older persons, such as narcotics, antidepressants, beta-blockers, and drugs with anticholinergic effects(14). Epidemiologic assessments of relationships between falls and medication usage have been confounded by the conditions serving as the indications for various pharmacologic treatments, as well as interactions of medications with physiologic changes of aging (13).

Even when sensory input is intact and properly integrated in the central nervous system, motor output must be effective for maintenance of postural stability. Impairments can occur in endurance, flexibility, and strength, with significant overlap existing among these effector domains.

Deconditioning weakness, cardiovascular insufficiency, and anemia are among the many causes of poor endurance common in cohorts also likely to have osteoporosis. Patients may complain of dyspnea on exertion or intolerance to activity. Other individuals may instead describe poor endurance as a feeling of dizziness or unsteadiness (15), so a careful history is necessary. Observation of quick tiring during office visits, a 6 minute walk distance of less than 500 feet, or similar observations by other health professionals can suggest that endurance is not adequate to meet daily challenges.

Reduced range of motion is a frequent concomitant of arthritis which afflicts more than half of older adults. Contractures and orthopedic injuries are other contributors. Patients may complain of pain or difficulty climbing stairs, getting in and out of a bathtub, or getting up from the floor. Limited range of motion at the neck may decrease visual input from the surroundings. Physical examination should assess the range of motion of the cervical, thoracic, and lumbar spine, shoulder girdle, and lower extremities, and determine if pain occurs during walking.

Strength ranks among the most critical contributors to postural stability, but unfortunately is subject to rapid deterioration during limitation of physical activity. Even brief periods of bed rest can result in significant deconditioning in older adults (16), threatening postural stability and independent function. Cortical pathology, such as stroke, results in subsequent muscle atrophy, while more gradual declines in motor strength may occur with lower motor neuron diseases, spinal stenosis, and radicular pathology. Frequently, a nonspecific process of deconditioning weakness begins with inactivity, initiated by fear of falling, poor cardiorespiratory endurance or pain, which worsens further with the resulting muscle weakness. Identification of this downward cycle of decline is critical since it may be amenable to intervention, but is frequently overlooked in the search for a disease-specific cause.

Clinical Assessment

History and Physical Examination. Features of the medical history will assist the clinician in focusing on pertinent sensory, central, and effector domains requiring increased attention during physical examination. A classic approach to history and physical examination serves well to identify significant abnormalities in many systems, such as decreased cerebral perfusion, sensory deficits, and focal motor weakness. However, accumulated subtle deficits that, in combination, threaten postural control may not be appreciated during routine physical examination of individual organ systems.

Physical Performance of Integrated Tasks Therefore, observation of supplemental tasks that demonstrate integrated functions is required. Simple techniques for office assessment of physical performance have been described and are selectively outlined in **Table 1.** Elements of strength, balance, vision, and foot function are displayed when patients climb on and off the examination table. Normal ambulation should demonstrate symmetric arm swing and a step length of at least twice the foot length. If a cane or walker is used, safety of judgment and technique should be noted. Tandem standing and walking displays integrated balance, sensory and effector functions. If hip girdle strength is minimally adequate, patients should be able to arise from a chair without pushing up using their arms. If stairs are available, health professionals can note whether a normal step-over-step pattern is used, or whether a more cautious single step pattern is preferred.

Table 1: Simple Office Tests of Physical Performance
General Observations:
        Ambulation and turning in office hallways
          Does the patient appear steady?
          Do they use a cane or walker?
    Ability to get on and off examination table
          Is assistance needed?
Specific Tasks of Balance, Strength, Coordination:
        Tandem gait

Can the patient take six continuous heel-to-toe steps?
One-Foot-Standing, with weight-bearing leg flexed at the knee
Can the patient maintain position for 30 seconds?
Chair Rise
Can the patient rise without rocking to get started or
using arms?
Stair ascent and descent
Is a normal step-over-step pattern used?
Obstacle Avoidance
Can the patient step over an obstacle without
hesitation?
Reaching
Can the patient grasp a ruler held a foot beyond their
outstretched arm
without losing balance or taking a step?

Clinical Intervention

Reversible, Modifiable, and Fixed Deficits. Problems identified during clinical assessment of postural stability are of three types: reversible, partially amenable to improvement, and irreversible. Underlying infections, anemia and metabolic disturbances may be treatable, but are unlikely to be the sole cause of falling, particularly when the gait disturbance is chronic. Reduction or elimination of medications that cause orthostasis or impair central processing represents one of the most feasible means of yielding prompt patient benefit. Examples are given in **Table 2**. Chronic conditions that can not be corrected should still be considered for interventions that may reduce instability and risk for falling. For example, patients with arthritis may benefit from improved pain control and exercise programs that improve flexibility and strength. Finally, efforts to compensate for irreversible conditions are often required. For example, individuals with chronic disturbances of balance may require a walker to widen the base of support and appropriate education in its safe use.

Table 2: Mechanisms of Selected Drugs of Potential Importance In Falling

Psychotropic Agents:
Antipsychotics: sedation, extrapyramidal side effects of movement, orthostatic hypotension
Tricyclic antidepressants: sedation; orthostatic hypotension
Benzodiazepines and Alcohol: sedation; increased body sway

Cardiovascular Agents:
Antihypertensives: hypotension; sedation for centrally-acting agents
Beta-Blockers: impaired postural heart rate responses; hypotension; slowing of central processing
Diuretics: orthostatic hypotension

Others:
Metoclopramide: sedation, movement disturbances
Narcotics: sedative effects
Antihistamines: sedation
Cimetidine: sedation

Multi-disciplinary Management. Osteoporosis patients, particularly in older age cohorts, may be found upon comprehensive evaluation to have multifaceted fall risks. Multiple interventions may be needed to maximize patient safety. A multi-disciplinary team may facilitate care planning; contributions from primary and specialty physicians, as well as nursing, physical and occupational therapy, pharmacy, and social work personnel may be needed selectively, depending on individual patient needs. Visual deficits that impact mobility may be modifiable through optometric intervention.20 Podiatrists can address foot disorders that adversely impact gait mechanics. A key component for many patients is a gait safety assessment, followed by prescription of appropriate assistive devices and/or an exercise program individually tailored for deficits in endurance, flexibility, strength, and balance.

Home Safety. Education about home safety can be supplemented by checklists for patients and families (14, 21) **Table 3** outlines common hazards. Higher risk patients may benefit from home safety evaluation by home health or other personnel. Consider having the patient show a therapist around his home, demonstrating how he uses furniture and bathroom facilities. Negotiate with the patient to make the environment more user friendly, eliminating throw rugs and other floor obstacles, and assuring that proper lighting is accessible and stairway rails are in place. Raised toiled seats and grab bars in the bathroom are helpful for persons with impaired mobility or strength. Instruction about behaviors that interact with environmental factors is also important in fall prevention. A study of circumstances surrounding re-enacted falls in the home found collisions in the dark, failure to avoid temporary obstacles, preoccupation with other conditions, and inappropriate environmental use to be among the common fall-producing patterns.22 Finally, coordination of community resources to provide assistance with shopping, home care, bathing and other activities is appropriate for patients who can not safely accomplish these activities independently. A life-line or similar system to call for help can be reassuring and prevent long lies after a fall.

Table 3: Environmental Home Hazards

Stairways that are steep, poorly lit, or lacking sturdy handrails
Home lighting that is too dim or not accessible to turn on when entering
   room
Chairs that are low-seated, lack arm rests, or not sturdy when leaned upon
Obstacles on the floor such as electric or phone cords, raised edges of
   flooring
Throw rugs or loose carpet that may skid when walked upon
High cabinets that can only be reached on a step ladder

Uneven outdoor surfaces, such as cobblestones or broken sidewalk

Primary Prevention for Osteoporosis Patients

Osteoporosis patients who are otherwise healthy and active may not require many of the specific interventions mentioned above. Primary prevention efforts include regular exercise such as walking, adequate food intake for normal body mass index, counseling on home hazards and hazardous activities, and keeping careful track of medication utilization.23   Efforts to educate individuals to avoid potentially hazardous activities must be carefully undertaken to avoid discouraging healthy, active lifestyles. Regular reassessment of the risk of falling is recommended, since significant changes in physical abilities, living environment, and comorbid conditions may occur between visits among older adults.23

The high prevalence of osteoporosis among older adults with dementia and related postural instability unfortunately manifests in frequent falls and fractures.   Gait planning deteriorates irreversibly over time and falls become increasingly common among patients who often pace in their environment until a final bed bound condition is reached.   Weight loss and decreased muscle strength are common, concurrent visual disturbances are frequent, and medications given for attempted behavioral management further slow corrective postural responses.   Although deficits in judgment and motor planning are not amenable to treatment, environmental modifications can reduce visuospatial misperceptions and provide orienting cues. Low beds, carpeting, and avoidance of bed rails can reduce the likelihood of injury when falling does occur. Restraints do not prevent falls, are demeaning and can cause injuries. Restraint reduction in long-term care has not resulted in an increase in injurious falls.   Consensus exists that benefits accrue from continued independent mobility, including prevention of deconditioning, despite the continued propensity to fall.10   Specially designed undergarments to provide additional padding over the trochanter appear promising in a controlled trials of hip fracture prevention in nursing home residents; however, improved designs are necessary to improve feasibility of use of these garments which were frequently not in use among intervention recipients.24

Physical Therapy

Studies have confirmed that impairments in lower extremity function among independent older adults are predictive of subsequent development of disability (25), and intense research efforts are ongoing into interventions to improve strength even among very impaired frail elderly persons. Physical therapy has potential to reduce fall risk in osteoporotic older adults in several domains, including balance, endurance, flexibility, and strength.   A recent review of the role of exercise in older adults found that, though many studies have shown that high and low intensity aerobic exercise programs produce improvement in physiologic measures of aerobic capacity, results have varied for physical performance measurements, such as gait speed (26). Likewise, increased muscle strength can be demonstrated with strength training in healthy and frail older adults, but to what extent these findings are clinically meaningful remains unclear (26). Balance interventions have generally been combined with aerobic and strengthening programs, making it hard to ascertain independent effects of balance training. However, a controlled trial of Tai Chi among community dwellers over the age of 70 found a reduction in the rate of falling and fear of falling in the intervention group (27).   Water exercise also appears to be a promising modality for allowing older adults to safely increase the range of movements they make, thereby practicing postural corrections for movement errors in a safe environment (28).

Many studies have examined the effect of combined aerobic, strengthening, and balance interventions in elderly subjects, but the actual interventions and populations have varied widely (26). Among frail elderly persons who might benefit most, delivery of interventions has been hindered by enrollment challenges, transportation issues, interruption by intercurrent illness, and high drop-out rates resulting in low study power (26). A controlled study of an individualized fall prevention intervention, including exercise as one component, demonstrated a decrease in the rate of falls among recipients, but the individual impact of exercise could not be determined (29).

An additional area of study is the role of divided attention in falling; older adults were more affected than young adults by divided attention in an obstacle-avoidance task (30.) The complex neurocognitive processes that subserve multiple-tasking, such as walking while attending to other environmental information, may be another domain possibly amenable to improvement through physical therapy interventions.

Exercise may have benefits for older adults beyond the realm of fall prevention, requiring a broad approach to outcome assessment. For example, a randomized controlled trial of progressive resistance training among depressed older adults found improvement in depression measures, strength, bodily pain, and social functioning (31.) Nevertheless, it remains to be seen whether improved physiologic and physical performance measures found during structured exercise programs in clinical trials will be maintained and translated into improved daily functioning and fewer falls (26).

Community-Based Efforts to Reduce Falling

Another approach has been to target communities, in addition to individuals, for fall prevention efforts. Unfortunately, insufficient power has plagued many studies attempting to find efficacy for community-based efforts to prevent injurious falls (23). Various programs focusing on home safety improvements, group meetings for education and exercise, and discussion of behaviors that may represent increased risk for falling have, in general, not demonstrated improved fall-injury outcomes. The randomized controlled trial of multifactorial, targeted prevention mentioned above which showed a 30% reduction in fall rates among the intervention group29 was found to be most cost-effective to the health maintenance organization when the higher risk subgroup was analyzed separately (32.) The FICSIT (Frailty and Injuries: Cooperative Studies of Intervention Techniques), a group of differing trial methodologies and populations, showed a reduction in fall incidence in meta-analysis for balance and general exercise interventions, but likewise lacked sufficient power to draw conclusions about injurious falls (33).

Future Direction in Fall Prevention

What can be anticipated in fall prevention for older adults in the years to come? We expect that larger trials of exercise interventions will confirm efficacy and cost-effectiveness in decreasing fall related injury among frail older adults and those with partial impairments in mobility. Health plans and life care communities will increase their interest in fall prevention in an attempt to reduce the impending enormity of the costs of hip fracture and subsequent dependency in the growing elderly population. Active older enrollees may be provided behavioral hazards counseling, home safety evaluations, and osteoporosis treatment. Senior groups or health plans may offer programs using Tai Chi or similar activities that provide socialization while also improving balance and confidence. Virtual reality games, tailored for older adults, may provide enjoyable challenges that improve obstacle avoidance and physical performance during attention distractions. We anticipate that intensive multidisciplinary fall-reduction programs, while helpful for frail individuals or those with histories of falling, will not be found cost-effective in otherwise healthy osteoporosis patients.

Medication reduction strategies will continue to be a fruitful area for primary prevention and for clinical management of patients who fall. Quality improvement monitoring will focus on physician prescribing patterns regarding medications known to be related to risk of injurious falls. Public health strategies might be employed to educate older patients and their families that familiar medications prescribed in the past for sleep, anxiety, or pain may not be current optimal choices, in an attempt to decrease consumer demand for drugs known to impair stability. Controlled trials of new drugs currently seldom include physically frail or medically complex older adults, and even large trials face a low rate of injury falls and fractures as potential endpoints. While it is hoped that such patients will be included in more randomized clinical trials of new medications in the future, challenges will remain. Therefore, large national data bases may prove to be useful sources of ecologic data about associations between specific drugs utilization and fall-related injury. We also expect that pharmaceutical manufacturers will examine the impact of new medications on balance, gait safety and cognition in older adults, using performance measures that will have been shown to be linked to clinically meaningful outcomes.

Summary

Fractures sustained during falls from standing heights account for the vast majority of osteoporosis-related morbidity, mortality, and expense. Hip fracture looms as a justifiably feared threat to independent function among older adults. Osteoporosis management should include assessment of sensory, central, or effector contributions to postural instability and interventions targeted to reverse, improve, or compensate for these conditions. The multifactorial nature of most falling syndromes requires a multifaceted care plan with participation of health care personnel from different disciplines. Physical therapy programs may improve strength, endurance and balance measures, but the actual impact on fracture rate largely remains to be determined. Falling among patients with dementia remains particularly problematic, but restraints do not serve to reduce injurious falls. Protective hip padding appears to be a promising area for further study among dementia victims. It is anticipated that fall prevention efforts by health plans and public health organizations will be

Table 4   Clinical Interventions in Fall Prevention

1.   Treatment of reversible conditions:
            Correction of metabolic, infectious, or cardiorespiratory derangements

2.   Improvement of modifiable conditions:
            Medication review and reduction efforts
            Exercise programs for balance, strength, endurance
            Improved pain control in musculoskeletal disease
            Correction of visual impairments
            Attention to podiatric problems

3.   Compensation for fixed deficits:
            Assistive devices where appropriate, with training in their use

4.   Environmental modification

5.   Education on modification of risky behaviors

180

intensified, and greater attention will be paid to the impact of new medications on postural stability when tested in older adults.

References

1. King MB, Tinetti ME 1995 Falls in community-dwelling older persons. J Am Geriatr Soc 43:1146-1154.

2. Myers AH, Young Y, Langlois JA 1996 Prevention of falls in the elderly. Bone 18:87S-101S.

3. Tinetti ME, Mendes de Leon CF, Doucette JT 1994 Fear of falling and fall-related efficacy in relationship to functioning among community-living elders. J Gerontol Med Sci 49:M140-147.

4. Tinetti ME, Speechley M, Ginter SF 1988 Risk factors for falls among elderly persons living in the community. N Eng J Med 1701-1707.

5. Tinetti ME, Doucette J, Claus E 1995 Risk Factors for serious injury during falls by older persons in the community. J Am Geriatr Soc 43:1214-1221.

6. Tinetti ME, Doucette JT, Claus EB 1995 The contribution of predisposing and situational risk factors to serious fall injuries. JAm Geriatr Soc 43:1207-1213.

7. Speechley M, Tinetti M 1991 Falls and injuries in frail and vigorous community elderly persons. J Am Geriatr Soc 39:46-52.

8. Northridge ME, Nevitt MC, Kelsey JL 1995 Home hazards and falls in the elderly: The role of health and functional status. Am J Public Health 85:509-515.

9. Studenski S, Duncan PW, Chandler J 1994 Predicting falls: the role of mobility and nonphysical factors. J Am Geriatr Soc 42:297-302.

10. Rubenstein LZ, Josephson KR, Robbins AS 1994 Falls in the nursing home. Ann Int Med 121:442-451.

11. Ensrud KE, Nevitt MC, Yunis C 1992 Postural hypotension and postural dizziness in elderly women. The study of osteoporotic fractures research group. Arch Int Med 152:1058-1064.

12. Cauley JA, Cummings SR, Seeley DG 1993 Effects of thiazide diuretic therapy on bone mass, fractures, and falls. The study of osteoporotic fractures research group. Ann Int Med 118:666-673.

13. Monane M, Avorn J 1996 Medications and falls: causation, correlation, and prevention. Clin Geriatr Med 12:847-858.

14. Hindmarsh JJ, Estes EH 1989 Falls in older persons: causes and interventions. Arch Int Med 149:2217-2222.

15. Sloane PD 1996 Evaluation and management of dizziness in the older patient. Clin Geriatr Med 12:785-802.

16. Creditor MC 1993 Hazards of hospitalization of the elderly. Ann Int Med 118:219-223.

17. Sudarsky L 1990 Geriatrics: gait disorders in the elderly. N Eng J Med 322:1441-1445.

18. Studenski S 1992 Falls. In Practice of Geriatrics, Calkins, Ford, Katz, eds. W. B. Saunders Co. 213-129.

19. Berg K, Norman KE 1996 Functional assessment of balance and gait. Clin Geriatr Med 12:705-723.

20. Maino JH 1996 Visual deficits and mobility: Evaluation and Management. Clin Geriatr Med 12:803-824.

21. Rubenstein LZ, Robbins AS, Schulman BL 1988 Falls and instability in the elderly. J Am Geriatr Soc 36:266-278.

22. Connell BR, Wolf SL for the Atlanta FICSIT Group 1997 Environmental and behavioral circumstances associated with falls at home among healthy elderly individuals. Arch Phys Med Rehabil 78:179-186.

23. King MB, Tinetti ME 1996 A multifactorial approach to reducing injurious falls. Clin Geriatr Med 12:745-760.

24. Lauritzen JB, Petersen MM, Lund B 1993 Effect of external hip protectors on hip fractures. Lancet 341:11-13.

25. Guralnik JM, Ferrucci L, Simonsick EM 1995 Lower extremity function in persons over the age of 70 years as a predictor of subsequent disability. N Engl J Med 45:239-243.

26. Chandler JM, Hadley EC 1996 Exercise to improve physiologic and functional performance in old age. Clin Geriatr Med 12:761-784.

27. Wolf SL, Barnhart HX, Kutner NG and the Atlanta FICSIT Group 1996 Reducing frailty and falls in older persons: an investigation of Tai Chi and computerized balance training. J Am Geriatr Soc 44:489-497.

28. Simmons V, Hansen PD 1996 Effectiveness of water exercise on postural mobility in the well elderly: an experimental study on balance enhancement. J Gerontol Med Sci 51A:M233-M238.

29. Tinetti ME, Baker DI, McAvay G 1994 A multifactorial intervention to reduce the risk of falling among elderly people living in the community N Engl J Med 331:821-827.

30. Chen HC, Schultz AB, Ashton-Miller JA 1996 Stepping over obstacles: dividing attention impairs performance of old more than young adults. J Gerontol Med Sci 51A:M116-M122.

31. Singh NA, Clements KM, Fiatarone MA 1997 A randomized controlled trial of progressive resistance training in depressed elders. J Gerontol Med Sci 52A:M27-M35.

32. Rizzo JA, Baker DI, McAvay G 1996 The cost-effectiveness of a multifactorial targeted prevention program for falls among community elderly persons. Med Care 34:954-969.

33. Province MA, Hadley EC, Hornbrook MC for the FICSIT Group 1995 The effects of exercise on falls in elderly patients: a pre-planned meta-analysis of the FICSIT trials. J Am Med Assoc 273:1341-1347.

12 Diagnosis and Treatment of Male Osteoporosis

Eric S. Orwoll, M.D.

The earliest reports of the epidemiology of fractures associated with osteoporosis revealed that the classical age-related increase in fractures seen in women is evident in men as well. Only in the last few years has it been recognized that the problem of osteoporosis in men represents an important public health issue, and that it also presents a unique array of scientific challenges and opportunities (1-3).

Epidemiology of Fractures in Men

In women, the relationship between bone mass and fracture risk has become increasingly clear, and it is possible to confidently discuss the epidemiology of osteoporosis as defined either by the presence of atraumatic fractures or low bone mass (4, 5). In men there is less information available regarding the causation of fracture, and hence a discussion of osteoporosis epidemiology must be primarily related to fracture patterns.

The incidence of all fractures is higher in men than women early in life, probably as a result of serious trauma (6, 7). At about age 40-50 years there is a reversal of this trend, with fractures in general, but in particular those of the pelvis, humerus, forearm, and femur becoming much more common in women. Nevertheless, the incidence of fractures due to minimal-to moderate trauma (particularly hip and spine) also increases rapidly with aging in men (6), and reflects an increasing prevalence of skeletal fragility. Some fractures are due to excessive trauma or local bone pathology, but in older men most cannot be attributed to these factors and are probably osteoporotic. Recently, the Dubbo Osteoporosis Epidemiology Project (8) has raised the possibility that low trauma fracture rates in men may be greater than previously recognized, and data from that study suggests that the lifetime risk of an atraumatic fracture is about 25% in an average 60 year old man.

Proximal Femur The incidence if hip fracture rises exponentially in men with aging, as it does in women. However, the age at which the increase begins is slightly older (~5-10 years) in men (9). In U.S. men older than 65 years, the incidence of hip fracture is 4-5/1000 (10, 11), compared with 8-10/1000 in similarly aged U.S. women. A similar 2:1 female:male ratio has been reported in Northern Europe and Australia (12), although in other geographic areas the ratio has been noted to be much lower (13). In Southern Europe and other areas (*e.g.* Asia), the incidence of hip fracture is relatively lower in both sexes, and men have as many hip fractures as do women (14-17). Since there are fewer older men than women, the absolute number of hip fractures tends to be proportionally less in men (of those experiencing their first hip fracture 65 years or older, 165,000 are in men vs. 580,000 in women in the U.S. in 1984-87, or 22% of the total in men) (11). In the U.S (Rochester) the lifetime risk of a hip fracture at age 50 has been calculated to be 6% in men and 17.5% in women (18), and 2.4% in men and 9% in women in Canada (Saskatchewan and Manitoba) (19). It is estimated that approximately 30% of hip fractures worldwide will occur in men (20).

Perhaps as a result of a higher prevalence of concomitant disease (21), the mortality associated with a hip fracture in elderly men (>75 yrs) is considerably higher than in women (30% vs. 9%) (22, 23). In Europe the incidence of fracture is at least twice as great in women, but the death rates for femoral neck fractures are approximately equal, again suggesting a greater risk of mortality in men (24). One of the strongest predictors of mortality after a hip fracture is gender (25).

Unfortunately, the number of hip fractures is projected to increase dramatically as the elderly population expands (26). Compounding matters, the age-adjusted incidence of hip fractures is also increasing in many areas. On a positive note, hip fracture rates in Rochester MN are declining in both men and women (27).

Racial differences in the incidence of hip fracture in men are substantial. For instance, African-American men experience hip fractures at a rate of only half that of Caucasians (11). Interestingly, whereas African-American women are at significantly lower risk for hip fracture than Caucasian women, African-American men and Caucasian men are at similar risk, as are African-American women and men (9). There are not extensive comparative data concerning other races, but one study clearly suggests a lower rate of hip fracture in Japanese compared to Caucasian men from the U.S. (28).

Vertebral Fractures. Previously considered uncommon in men, recent information suggests that the incidence of clinically apparent osteoporotic vertebral fracture in U.S. men is about half that in women (similar to hip fractures) (28-32). In other studies, the prevalence of vertebral fracture is actually higher in men than women (33-35). It has been assumed that this represents an increase in the occurrence of early life trauma in men (32, 36). On the other hand, men with vertebral fractures clearly have lower bone density than controls, suggesting that osteopenia contributes to vertebral fracture risk in men as well (29). Fractures are primarily in low thoracic vertebrae in men, but are found at all levels. Most fractures are anterior compression in type (29) with vertebral crush fractures occurring less frequently than in women. Vertebral epiphysitis (Scheuermann=s disease) is an uncommon cause of significant vertebral deformity in men (29).

Other Fractures Other fractures (radius/ulna, humerus, pelvis, femoral shaft) share a common epidemiological pattern. Men experience more of these fractures in youth, but with unusual exceptions (e.g. humerus) the incidence remains relatively stable during mid-life, while rising markedly in women (7, 37, 38). It is only later (>75 years) that the incidence of limb fractures begins to rise in men, and it then does so rapidly (7). This increase is due primarily to a rise in lower limb fractures, while upper extremity fractures do not change as much. Importantly, the occurrence of a distal forearm fracture (39) or a tibial fracture (40) in a man indicated a considerably increased risk of subsequent hip fracture, presumably as a result of low bone mass and/or an increased risk of falling.

Determinants of Fracture in Men: Bone Mass

Age-related changes in bone mass in men. The pattern of osteoporotic fractures is intimately related to aging, and changes in bone mass with age clearly contribute to that association. The decline in axial bone density was initially considered to be relatively slow in men, primarily because of the results of cross-sectional studies using techniques that assess total spinal bone mass (dual photon absorptiometry [DPA]). Vertebral cancellous bone density as measured by quantitative computed tomography QCT, however, suggested a much more rapid rate of bone loss with aging in normal men (41). Subsequently, the results derived from DPA were shown to be influenced by artifacts introduced by extra-vertebral calcifications. If men with such calcifications are excluded, the relationship of spinal bone density to age is similar in men and women (29). Longitudinal studies verify a more rapid rate of vertebral bone loss with aging in normal men (42). In cross-sectional studies the negative slope of density with age at proximal femoral sites is similar, albeit somewhat less, in men compared to women (43-45). Moreover, bone volume in the iliac crest declines at very similar rates in both men and women.

In cortical bone the pattern of age-related loss also affects eventual fracture risk. Cortical bone mass in young men is much greater than in women, probably accounting in part for the lower incidence of cortical bone fractures in men. Cross-sectional studies suggest that age is associated with a fairly linear decrease in cortical bone mass (42, 43, 46-49) but some also indicate the BMD: age slope becomes more negative in men after 50 years (42, 48, 50, 51). This slope is not quite as steep as that in women (49), thereby accentuating the sexual differences in cortical mass present in early adulthood. However, the rate of loss of cortical bone mass in men as reported in longitudinal studies is considerably more rapid (5-10%/decade) (42, 48, 50, 51) than previously estimated from cross-sectional studies (1-3%/decade) (43, 44, 47). The differences noted in longitudinal vs. cross-sectional studies may reflect the difficulty in adequately estimating time-dependent processes by cross-sectional methods, but also suggest that an increasingly greater rate of bone loss in men has taken place over the last several decades. This possibility is in accord with an apparent increase in fracture incidence (17).

Sex steroid levels. Clinical hypogonadism is a well established cause of osteoporosis in men. Bone loss results from the appearance of hypogonadism in adults, and a failure to achieve peak bone mass is a consequence of hypogonadism before the onset of puberty (52, 53). It has become quite clear that testosterone replacement therapy has beneficial effects on bone mass in men with established gonadal failure, sometimes to the extent that bone mass is normalized (54-57).

Because testicular and adrenal androgen concentrations decline in men with aging, an important issue is whether the decline in androgen levels with aging contributes to the fall in bone mass and the increase in fracture risk that occur concomitantly. A number of studies have examined the relationship between androgen levels and bone mass in non-hypogonadal men, but the results have been inconclusive. In some, there has been a correlation (albeit weak) between androgen levels and measures of bone density (58-61), but in other reports when age is considered in the statistical model it is not possible to document a clear influence of androgen levels on bone (62-64). Unfortunately, these studies have utilized small numbers of subjects and have been cross sectional in design. There have been few attempts to more directly assess the influence of androgens in elderly men. In one notable report, Tenover found that a three month period of testosterone supplementation in a small group of elderly men with low normal testosterone levels at baseline was associated with a significant decline in urinary hydroxyproline excretion (although there was no change in osteocalcin levels) (65). In sum, the issue of whether declines in androgen activity with aging have a clear impact on skeletal health remains unresolved. Important questions include whether there is a threshold level of androgen activity which is necessary for the maintenance of skeletal health, whether some skeletal compartments are more affected than others by changes in androgen levels, whether androgens may affect the skeleton via indirect effects on other tissue (*e.g.* muscle or body composition), and whether androgen supplementation is capable of preventing or reversing age-related changes in skeletal mass.

Although attention has until recently focused on the role of androgens in men, reports of severe osteopenia in several men with estrogen deficiency (estrogen receptor abnormality or absent aromatase activity) (66) have raised the question of the role of estrogens. Aromatase activity is present in bone (67). In transsexuals, estrogens are capable of maintaining bone mass in the absence of androgens (68), and two recent cross-sectional studies have suggested that bone density in older men may be more closely related to estrogen than to androgens (69, 70). Studies in experimental animals and in osteoblastic cells in vitro indicate that non-aromatizable androgens are potent modulators of skeletal homeostasis (71-74), but the role of estrogens now must also be systematically evaluated

Other causes of low bone mass in men. Although important, age-related bone loss explains only part of the problem of osteoporosis in men. Genetic determinates are undoubtedly important in both sexes (75, 76). Weight contributes substantially to the variation in bone mass, with heavier men having greater bone (8, 77), and weight loss seems to be associated with greater rates of bone loss in older men (8). Tobacco smoking exerts a negative effect on bone (8, 78, 79). Particularly in younger men, idiopathic osteoporosis represents an important fraction of the overall problem. Kelepouris et al. found that approximately 1/3 of osteoporotic men have idiopathic disease (80). Recently a link between idiopathic osteoporosis and low levels of insulin like growth factor -1 (IGF-1), or IGF-1 binding protein 3 (IGFBP-3) levels, has been postulated (81, 82), but there remains little understanding of the importance of those relationships.

Especially consequential are systemic diseases, medications and lifestyles that may increase the risk of bone loss (**Table 1**). The frequency with which these conditions contribute to the etiology of osteoporosis in men is illustrated by several series in which the majority of men with osteoporotic fractures were found to have secondary causes of metabolic bone diseases (80, 83). In clinical situations, success in the prevention and treatment of osteoporosis depends heavily upon the recognition of these conditions.

Table 1

Causes of Osteoporosis in Men

I. Primary
  Aging
  Idiopathic
  Genetic
II. Secondary
  Hypogonadism
  Glucocorticoid excess
  Alcoholism
  Gastrointestinal disorders
  Hypercalciuria
  Anticonvulsants
  Thyrotoxicosis
  Immobilization
  Osteogenesis imperfecta
  Homocystinuria
  Systemic mastocytosis
  Neoplastic diseases
  Rheumatoid arthritis

The relationship between bone mass and fracture in men. There are few data available, but those available are consistent with the inverse relationship of bone mass and fracture. For instance, spinal fractures in men are related to femoral cortical area and Singh grade (84), proximal femoral bone mass (8, 29), and vertebral bone mass (42, 85-87). As in women, there is a clear overlap of bone density in men with vertebral fractures and nonfractured control subjects, indicating that bone density is not the sole determinant of vertebral fracture risk. There are few specific data concerning the measurement of bone mass in men with hip fracture, although several reports have recently observed that hip and spine bone mass are clearly reduced in a series of men with hip fracture when compared with age-matched controls (88-90). In a prospective study, Gardsell *et al.* showed that forearm bone density measurers at both proximal and distal sites are lower in men who go on to sustain osteoporotic fractures (vertebrae, hip, proximal humerus, forearm, pelvis and tibial condyle) in the subsequent ten year study period (91). Moreover, in the Dubbo Osteoporosis Epidemiology Study it was found that femoral bone density measures were quite predictive of subsequent atraumatic fractures (although spinal BMD was not) (89).

Finally, studies of bone density in men with vertebral or femoral fractures suggest that the average bone density in fractured men is somewhat higher than that previously reported in similar studies in women (29, 89, 92). This finding argues that the association between measures of bone density and fractures must be independently evaluated in men and women. Unfortunately, the relationship between absolute values of bone mass and fracture risk has not been explored in men. Thus, whereas the results of prospective, longitudinal trials are available to guide clinical decisions in older women, the specific levels of bone mass that should prompt more aggressive diagnostic or therapeutic measures in men remain conjectural. This issue has major personal and public health implications. For instance, a recent analysis reveals that the number of men considered at risk for fracture based on bone mass measures is tremendously affected by the criteria used to designate the diagnosis (93).

Falls

In addition to bone mass, the risk of falling has been identified as a major determinant of fracture in women. In men, there are few prospective data that directly relate to fall propensity to subsequent fractures, but a variety of factors indirectly related to risk of falling are associated with fracture. For instance Nguyen et al. found that men who had experienced a nontraumatic fracture exhibit more body sway and lower grip strength (as well as lower bone density) than nonfracture controls (89). Similarly, in a study of men with hip fractures (94) a number of factors associated with falls were found to be more prevalent than in controls. These included neurological disease, confusion, Ambulatory problems, and alcohol use. As in women, the use of several classes psychotropic drugs is associated with hip fracture risk (95, 96). Finally, men with hip fracture are of lower weight, have lower fat and lean body mass, and more commonly live alone than control subjects (88). These differences suggest a body habitus and lifestyle more conducive to falls and injury, as well as the possibility that there are other interacting risk factors (nutritional deficiencies, comorbidities). These impressions were recently substantiated in an epidemiological study of the factors associated with hip fracture in men (Table 2) (97). The characteristics of falls may be different in men and women. Some (98), but not all (99, 100) suggest that falls are less common in older men than women, and when they fall, women may more often fall on their hip (99).

The Evaluation of Osteoporosis in Men

Guidelines for the most efficient, cost-effective approach for the evaluation of the patient with osteoporosis, or the patient suspected of having osteoporosis, are poorly validated for either sex. Recommendations are therefore based on existing knowledge of disease epidemiology and clinical characteristics (101, 102) rather than upon models that have been carefully tested in prospective studies. Within these constraints, it is possible to formulate an approach to the male osteoporotic (**Figure 1**).

Table 2 Some Factors Associated with Hip Fractures in Men

Metabolic Disorders
        Thyroidectomy
        Gastrectomy
        Pernicious anemia
        Chronic respiratory diseases

Disorders of movement and balance
        Hemiparesis/hemiplegia
        Parkinsonism Dementia
        Other neurological diseases
        Vertigo
        Alcoholism
        Anemia
        Blindness
        Use of cane or walker

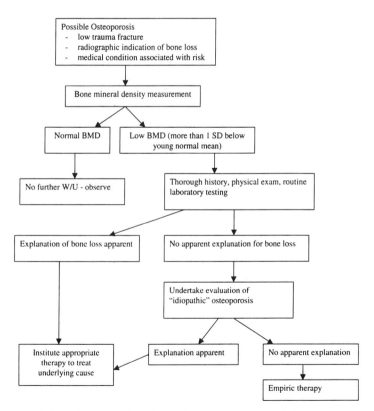

Figure 1 Schematic approach to the evaluation of osteoporosis in men.

There are several clinical situations in which the presence of osteoporosis should be considered likely. These include the occurrence of fractures with little trauma, the radiographic finding of low bone mass or vertebral deformity, and the presence of conditions known to be associated with osteoporosis. In these circumstances further diagnostic steps are appropriate.

Men with fractures. The diagnosis of osteopenic metabolic bone disease should be strongly suspected in men with a history of low traumatic fractures in the absence of any evidence of a focal process (malignancy, infection, Paget=s disease). A wide variety of fractures (101, 102) are associated with low bone mass in women (103). In men there are fewer data, but the reports that have examined the relationships between bone mass, bone structure, mechanical strength and fracture in men suggest similar associations (91, 104). Hence the presence of a low trauma fracture should raise the probability of metabolic bone disease and prompt further evaluation (i.e., quantitative bone mass measurement). Even incidentally discovered vertebral deformities have been shown to be associated with low bone mass (29), and should raise the suspicion of metabolic bone disease.

Radiographic evidence of reduced bone mass. Radiographic signs of reduced bone mass, even in the absence of a fracture, is of concern, and should be verified by a quantitative assessment.

Clinical conditions associated with osteoporosis. There is a spectrum of secondary causes of osteoporosis in men, including glucocorticoid excess, alcoholism, and hypogonadism (7, 40) (**Table 1**). The presence of one, or particularly several, of these conditions should prompt the consideration for additional diagnostic evaluation.

Bone Mass Measurements

In men who present with findings that suggest the presence of metabolic bone disease (low trauma fractures, radiographic criteria indicating the presence of a reduction in bone mass, or conditions associated with bone loss), the measurement of bone mass should be strongly considered. Bone mass determinations in men can be useful in several ways, including cementing the diagnosis of low bone mass, gauging severity, and serving as a baseline from which to judge progression/improvement of the disease. Although this contention is derived from studies in women, its basic underpinnings should be applicable in men as well. Specifically, 1) bone mass is related to fracture risk, 2) bone mass can be accurately and conveniently measured, 3) knowledge of bone mass may influence the diagnostic or therapeutic approach, and 4) treatment of osteoporosis affects fracture risk.

There have been few prospective attempts to relate bone mass to eventual fracture risk in men, and hence the implications of a specific level of bone density are uncertain. The World Health Organization has proposed that in women osteopenia should be identified when density is more than 1.5 standard deviations below the young normal mean, and osteoporosis when the density is more than 2.5 standard deviations below (5). Whether a similar approach can be taken in the diagnosis of osteopenia and osteoporosis in men is unknown. Looker et al. have recently attempted to apply the 1 and 2.5 standard deviation criteria derived from young normal male density levels to identify what proportion of the overall U.S. male population would have osteopenia or osteoporosis (105). They found that 47% of men aged 50 or more would have osteopenia at the femoral neck measurement site, and 6% would have osteoporosis using these criteria. The usefulness of the application of these criteria is yet to be established.

The use of screening bone mass measures is controversial, but as practical, inexpensive methods become available and are validated this application will become more attractive. Two groups of men may be considered reasonable candidates for screening measures: those with conditions associated with low bone mass (**Table 1**) and the elderly (>75 years).

Differential Diagnosis

If a man is determined to be osteopenic or osteoporotic, an evaluation should be considered to determine with reasonable certainty the cause of the disorder. In women with low trauma fractures, the vast majority has histological osteoporosis, but a small proportion is found to be osteomalacic (106-108). Similarly, a fraction of men with fracture have osteomalacia (106-108). Osteomalacia is estimated to be present in <4% to 47% of men with femoral fractures, with most reports being 20% (106-110). Since food is fortified with vitamin D, occult osteomalacia may be less frequent in the U.S. than in other areas (e.g. Northern Europe). Increasing age is associated with an increasing prevalence of osteomalacia (108). Thus far, the only patients who have been carefully surveyed are those with femoral fractures, and it is not known whether populations with other fractures (vertebral) would include similar proportions of osteoporotic and osteomalacic individuals. Some have suggested that women with femoral fracture are more frequently osteomalacic than men (106, 107), but others report no distinction (108). Although the exact magnitude of the problem presented by osteomalacia in men is uncertain, it is clear that any differential diagnosis of low bone mass and fractures in men must consider the possibility. This becomes particularly imperative because the treatment for osteomalacia differs considerably from that of osteoporosis (111).

Initial Evaluation of Osteoporosis: History, Physical, Routine Biochemical Measures

The history, physical and routine biochemical profile can be very helpful in directing a focused evaluation of a man with low bone mass. A variety of approaches for the differential diagnosis of low bone mass have been suggested using standard clinical and biochemical information (105, 106, 112). The goals of this stage of the evaluation should be to determine the specific diagnosis (what is the cause of the low bone mass - osteoporosis or osteomalacia?), and to identify contributing factors in the genesis of the disorder. Of particular importance in the history and physical, therefore, are clinical signs of genetic, nutritional/environmental, social (alcohol, tobacco), medical, or pharmacological factors that may be present to aid in these goals. Routine laboratory testing should include levels of serum creatinine, calcium, phosphorus, alkaline phosphatase, and liver function tests, as well as a complete blood count. If, on the basis of these tests, there is evidence for medical conditions associated with, bone loss (alcoholism, hyperparathyroidism, malignancy, Cushing=s syndrome, thyrotoxicosis, malabsorption, etc.) a definitive diagnosis should be pursued with appropriate testing.

Evaluation Of The Patient With Idiopathic Osteoporosis

In men with reduced bone mass in whom no clear pathophysiology is identified by the routine methods above, it has been considered appropriate to be diagnostically aggressive, primarily because the potential for occult, secondary causes of osteoporosis may be higher in men. However, the incidence of occult causes of osteoporosis in men, or whether it is greater than in women, is poorly studied. The diagnostic yield and cost effectiveness of extensive biochemical studies in the man with apparently idiopathic osteoporosis is thus unknown. Nevertheless, lacking this information, a reasonable evaluation of the man without a clear etiology for osteoporosis might include:

-   24-hour urine calcium and creatinine, to identify hypercalciuria
-   24-hour urine cortisol
-   serum 25-hydroxyvitamin D level
-   serum testosterone
-   serum thyroid stimulating hormone level
-   serum protein electrophoresis (in those >50 years to exclude   multiple myeloma)

Histomorphometric Characterization

Transiliac bone biopsy is a safe and effective means of assessing skeletal histology and remodeling characteristics (113). Some have suggested a transiliac bone biopsy is indicated in those men in whom a thorough biochemical evaluation has failed to reveal an etiology for osteoporosis (114). The rationale for this approach is based on the need to accomplish several objectives: 1) ensure that occult osteomalacia is not present; 2) identify unusual causes of osteoporosis that may be revealed only by a histological analysis, such as mastocytosis (115, 116) and 3) to yield information concerning the remodeling rate, which in turn may further direct the differential diagnosis (e.g. unappreciated thyrotoxicosis or secondary hyperparathyroidism suggested by the presence of increased turnover) or may be helpful in designing the most appropriate therapeutic approach.

Considerable histological heterogeneity exists among men with osteoporosis. Whether distinct histological patterns represent different stages of a single disease entity, separate subtypes of the disease, or simply an arbitrary subdivision of a normal distribution of remodeling rates is unknown. Realistically, the cost and invasiveness of a bone biopsy, coupled with the uncertain likelihood of detecting useful information (in addition to that available from noninvasive testing) has relegated the procedure to only the most unusual situations.

A more reasonable approach to the evaluation of remodeling dynamics in men with idiopathic osteoporosis may be to utilize the advantages of biochemical markers of bone turnover. In women, biochemical indices of remodeling have frequently been found to correlate with histological measures of bone turnover, rates of bone loss, and the risk of fracture. Although similar studies are not available in men, the presence of an increase in biochemical indices of remodeling may indicate one of those conditions associated with higher bone turnover (early hypogonadism, thyrotoxicosis, mastocytosis, etc.). Even if no obvious etiology is discovered, the increase in biochemical markers can help judge the effectiveness of subsequent therapy. The presence of normal or low levels of markers is less helpful.

Prevention/Therapy

Therapy of osteoporotic disorders in men is virtually unexplored, and in the U.S. there are no approved pharmacological therapies for osteoporosis in men. Recommendations must come from assumptions based on the much larger knowledge base in women. Certainly, any of the conditions associated with excessive bone loss (**Table 1**) should be aggressively treated, to both prevent and treat osteoporosis.

Exercise

Whereas an exercise prescription is difficult to generate with currently available information, activity is probably beneficial in several ways. Reductions in strength and coordination contribute to fracture via an increased risk of falling (117). In addition, inactivity is associated with bone loss, and exercise may increase or maintain bone mass (118). Specific exercise prescriptions to accomplish these goals have not been confirmed in men or women, although it is clear that strength can be dramatically increased, and risk of falls reduced, in the elderly with achievable levels of exercise (117). That fracture rates are lower in elderly men who exercise modestly buttresses this contention (119).

Supplements and Therapeutic Agents

Calcium/vitamin D. An area of obvious interest is the influence of aging in calcium economy. Calcium intake is probably important in the achievement of optimal peak bone mass in boys (120), as well as the prevention and therapy of osteoporosis later in life. Calcium absorption declines with aging in men as in women, particularly after the age of 60, and well documented changes in mineral metabolism occur concomitantly with age in men (83). These data suggest both that optimal levels of calcium intake may change with age, and that inadequate calcium nutrition can have an adverse effect on skeletal mass. However, the level of calcium intake that should be recommended is unclear, as few prospective studies have addressed this issue. No benefit from calcium/vitamin D supplementation was observed in a very well-nourished population (dietary calcium intake >1000 mg/day) (42). In a recent report (121), healthy older men were found to improve their bone mass in the. with a calcium and vitamin D supplement, while placebo treated men lost bone. The Institute of Medicine recently recommended that men should have a calcium intake of 1200 mg/day, and a vitamin D intake of 800 IU. A reasonable approach, therefore, is to suggest a calcium intake of at least 1200 mg/day in both preventative as well as therapeutic situations. The appropriate level of intake may actually be higher. A NIH Consensus Development Conference has recommended a calcium intake of 1500 mg/day in men after 65 years (122). One theoretical concern regarding dietary calcium supplementation has been the precipitation of calcium stones in susceptible individuals. Recent data, though, suggest dietary calcium intake actually correlated negatively with the risk of nephrolithiasis in men (123), potentially by increasing gastrointestinal oxalate binding.

Calcitonin. There has been one trial of calcitonin therapy in a small group of men with idiopathic osteoporosis (124) in which total body calcium tended to increase during a 24 month treatment interval (100 IU administered subcutaneously each day with a calcium and vitamin D supplement. However, the change was not significantly different from that observed in the control groups (receiving calcium plus vitamin D supplements, or vitamin D alone), and there were no changes in radial bone mass. Men have been included in several other trials of calcitonin therapy, but the results in men are not separable from those in women subjects. There are no published studies of the effectiveness of intranasal calcitonin in men. Although there are little data, theoretically calcitonin should be effective in reducing osteoclastic activity in at least some patients with osteoporosis or at the risk of continuing bone loss.

Bisphosphonates. There have been no trails of any bisphosphonate performed exclusively in men. Male patients with osteoporosis have been included in mixed patient populations and have seemed to experience beneficial effects on calcium balance and lumbar spine bone density during treatment with pamidronate (125), and were specifically reported to benefit (increased vertebral bone density, with no change in femoral density) from etidronate treatment in a 12 months study (126). Although specific data are lacking, there is no conceptual barrier to the use of bisphosphonates in men. Dose response relationships and the frequency of complications in men are unknown.

Thiazide diuretics. Evidence supports a beneficial effect of thiazide administration on bone mass, rates of bone loss, and hip fracture risk in men. For instance, the use of thiazides reduced calcaneal bone mass loss rates by 49% compared to controls (127) and the relative risk of hip fracture was halved by exposure to thiazides for more than 6 years (128). Other diuretics did not seem to impart the same benefits. The nature of the effect is unclear, but it has been postulated to stem from the hypocalciuric effects of thiazides.

Fluoride. The use of fluoride in the therapy of osteoporosis remains controversial. Although consistent and sometimes dramatic increases in vertebral bone mass can be achieved with supplemental fluoride, the effectiveness of fluoride therapy in reducing fracture rates is uncertain. Nevertheless, there is an active interest in refining the formulation and dose of fluoride in the hope of taking better advantage of its anabolic properties. In fact, a recent evaluation of cyclically administered slow-release form of fluoride was reported to increase bone mass and reduce fracture rates in older women (129). As with many of the other therapies discussed, there have been no specific trials of fluoride administration in men. In some studies, osteoporotic men have been included in the treatment groups but it is difficult to ascertain whether responses were in any way sex-specific.

Emerging therapies. Parathyroid hormone administration to osteoporotic subjects has been shown to increase trabecular bone formation and bone volume in concert with an increase in calcium balance. Slovic et al. reported that in a small group of men with idiopathic osteoporosis, combined PTH and 1,25-dihydroxyvitamin D administration increased trabecular (spinal) bone mass and improved intestinal calcium absorption (130). Although the role of parathyroid hormone administration in the treatment of osteoporosis, either alone or in concert with other agents, remains unclear, its potential appears similar in men and women.

Growth hormone may have anabolic actions on the skeleton in the elderly and in subjects with osteoporosis, but the available data are inconclusive (29). Low levels of IGF-I have been reported to be present in men with idiopathic osteoporosis (131), and in a study of healthy older men with low IGF-I levels, Rudman et al. (58) found that in addition to positive effects on lean mass, fat mass, and skin thickness, vertebral bone mass was increased slightly (1.6%) by the administration of growth hormone for 6 months. Radial and proximal femoral densities were unaffected. In either sex, growth hormone therapy may thus be of potential, but as yet unproved usefulness.

Summary

Osteoporosis in men is a substantial public health problem. Although in many ways similar to the disease in women, the character and pathophysiology of osteoporosis in men is unique. Recently, information concerning the risk factors for osteoporosis in men has begun to emerge, and it is finally possible to formulate some reasonable clinical approaches for its detection, evaluation and prevention. The treatment of established osteoporosis in men remains problematic, as there are still no studies available to guide the use of available therapies. Nevertheless, such trials have begun, and we can look forward to the emergence of more information in the next several years.

References

1. Niewoehner C 1993 Osteoporosis in men: Is it more common than we think? Postgrad Med 93:59-60 and 63-70.

2. Scane AC, Sutcliffe AM, Francis RM 1992 Osteoporosis in men. Clin Rheum 7:589-601.

3. Seeman E 1993 Osteoporosis in men: epidemiology, pathophysiology, and treatment possibilities. Am J Med 95:22S-28S.

4. Melton LJI 1995 How many women have osteoporosis now? J Bone Miner Res 10:175-177.

5. World Health Organization 1994 Assessment of fracture risk and its application to screening for postmenopausal osteoporosis (report of a WHO study group) Geneva, Switzerland: World Health Organization.

6. Donaldson LJ, Cook A, Thomson RG 1990 Incidence of fractures in a geographically defined population. J Epi Comm Health 44:241-245.

7. Garraway WM, Stauffer RN, Kurland LT, O'Fallon WM 1979 Limb fractures in a defined population. I. Frequency and distribution. Mayo Clin Proc 54:701-707.

8. Nguyen TV, Eisman JA, Kelly PJ, Sambrook PN 1996 Risk factors for osteoporotic fractures in elderly men. Am J Epidemiol 144(3):258-261.

9. Farmer ME, White LR, Brody JA, Bailey KR 1984 Race and sex differences in hip fracture incidence. Am J Public Health 74:1374-1380.

10. Bacon, WE, Smith GS, Baker SP 1989 Geographic variation in the occurrence of hip fractures among the elderly white US population. Am J Public Health 79:1556-1558.

11. Jacobsen SJ, Goldberg J, Miles TP, Brody JA, Stiers W, Rimm AA 1990 Hip fracture incidence among the old and very old: a population-based study of 745,435 cases. Am J Public Health 80:871-873.

12. Jones G, Nguyen T, Sambrook PN, Kelly PJ, Gilbert C, Eisman JA 1994 Symptomatic fracture incidence in elderly men and women: The Dubbo osteoporosis epidemiology study (DOES). Osteoporosis Int 4:277-282.

13. Gallagher, JD, Melton LJ, Riggs BL 1980 Epidemiology of fracture of the proximal femur in Rochester, MN. Clin Orthop & Rel Res 150:163-171.

14. Kanis, JA 1993 The incidence of hip fracture in Europe. Osteoporosis Int S10-S15.

15. Chalmers, J, Ho KC 1970 Geographical variations in senile osteoporosis: The association with physical activity. J Bone Joint Surg 2B:667-675.

16. Solomon, L 1968 Osteoporosis and fracture of the femoral neck in the South African Bantu. J Bone Joint Surg 50B:2-13.

17. Elffors I, Allander E, Kanis JA 1994 The variable incidence of hip fracture in Southern Europe: The MEDOS study. Osteoporosis Int 4:253-263.

18. Melton LJ, III, Chrischilles EA 1992 Perspective: how many women have osteoporosis? J Bone Miner Res 7:1005-1010.

19. Martin AD, Silverthorn KG, Houston CS, Bernhardson S, Wajda A, Roos LL 1991 The incidence of fracture of the proximal femur in two million Canadians from 1972 to 1984. Clin Orthop Rel Res 266:111-118.

20. Cooper, C, Melton LJI 1992 Epidemiology of osteoporosis. Trends Endocrinol Metab 3:224-229.

21. Poor, G, Atkinson EJ, O'Fallon WM, Melton LJ 1995 Determinants of reduced survival following hip fractures in men. Clin Ortho Rel Res 319:260-265.

22. Melton, LJ, III, Riggs BL 1983 Epidemiology of age-related fractures. In: Avioli LV, ed. The Osteoporotic Syndrome. N.Y.:Grune & Stratton 45-72.

23. Myers AH, Robinson EG, Van Natta ML, Michelson JD, Collins K, Baker SP 1991 Hip fractures among the elderly: Factors associated with in-hospital mortality. Am J Epidemiol 134:1128-1137.

24. Heyse, SP 1993 Epidemiology of hip fractures in the elderly: a cross-national analysis of mortality rates for femoral neck fractures. Osteoporosis Int 1:S16-S19.

25. Schurch MA, Rizzoli R, Mermillod B, Vasey H, Michel JP 1996 A prospective study on socioeconomic aspects of fracture of the proximal femur. J Bone Miner Res 11:1935-1942.

26. Schneider EL, Guralnik JM 1990 The aging of America: impact on health care costs. JAMA 263:2335-2340.

27. Melton LJ, Atkinson EJ, Madhok R 1996 Downturn in hip fracture incidence. Public Health Reports 111:146-150.

28. Ross PD, Norimatsu H, Davis JW 1991 A comparison of hip fracture incidence among native Japanese, Japanese Americans, and American Caucasians. Am J Epidemiol 133:801-809.

29. Mann T, Oviatt SK, Wilson D, Nelson D, Orwoll ES 1992 Vertebral deformity in men. J Bone Miner Res 7:1259-1265.

30. Cooper C, Campion G 1992 Hip fractures in the elderly: a world-wide projection. Osteoporosis Int 2:285-289.

31. Cooper C, Atkinson EJ, O'Fallon WM, Melton LJ 1992 Incidence of clinically diagnosed vertebral fractures: a population-based study in Rochester, Minnesota, 1985-1989. J Bone Miner Res 7:221-227.

32. Kanis JA, McCloskey EV 1992 Epidemiology of vertebral osteoporosis. Bone 13:S1-S10.

33. Davies KM, Stegman MR, Recker RR 1993 Preliminary vertebral deformity analysis for a rural population of older men and women. J Bone Miner Res 8:S331.

34. O'Neill TW, Felsenberg D, Varlow J, Cooper C, Kanis JA, Silman AJ 1996 The prevalence of vertebral deformity in european men and women: The eurpoean vertebral osteoporosis study. J Bone Miner Res 11:1010-1018.

35. Santavirta S, Konttinen YT, Heliovaara M, Knekt P, Luthje P, Aromaa A 1992 Determinants of osteoporotic thoracic vertebral fracture. Acta Orthop Scand 63(2):198-202.

36. Silman AJ, O'Neill TW, Cooper C, Kanis J, Felsenberg D 1997 Influence of physical activity on vertebral deformity in men and women: Results from the European vertebral osteoporosis study. J Bone Miner Res 12:813-819.

37. Melton LJ, III, O'Fallon WM, Riggs BL 1987 Clinical investigations: secular trends in the incidence of hip fractures. Calcif Tiss Int 41:57-64.

38. Buhr AJ, Cooke AM 1959 Fracture patterns. Lancet I:531-536.

39. Mallmin H, Ljunghall S, Persson I, Naessen T, Krusemo UB, Bergstrom R 1993 Fracture of the distal forearm as a forecaster of subsequent hip fracture: a population-based cohort study with 24 years follow-up. Calcif Tissue Int 52:269-272.

40. Karlsson M, Hasserius R, Obrant EJ 1993 Individuals who sustain nonosteoporotic fractures continue to also sustain fragility fractures. Calcif Tissue Int 53:229-231.

41. Meier DE, Orwoll ES, Jones JM 1984 Marked disparity between trabecular and cortical bone loss with age in healthy men: measurement by vertebral computed tomography and radioal photon absorptiometry. Ann Int Med 101:605-612.

42. Orwoll ES, Oviatt SK, McClung MR, Deftos LJ, Sexton G 1990 The rate of bone mineral loss in normal men and the effects of calcium and cholecalciferol supplementation. Ann Int Med 112:29-34.

43. Hannan MT, Felson DT, Anderson JJ 1992 Bone mineral density in elderly men and women: results from the Framingham osteoporosis study. J Bone Miner Res 7:547-553.

44. Riggs BL, Wahner HW, Dunn WL, Mazess RB, Offord KP, Melton LJI 1981 Differential changes in bone mineral density of the appendicular and axial skeleton with aging. J Clin Invest 67:328-335.

45. Elliott JR, Gilchrist NL, Wells JE 1990 Effects of age and sex on bone density at the hip and spine in a normal Caucasian New Zealand population. NZ Med J 103:33-37.

46. Gotfredsen A, Hadberg A, Nilas L, Christiansen C 1987 Total body bone mineral in healthy adults. J Lab Clin Med 110:362-368.

47. 47.Mazess RB, Barden HS, Drinka PJ, Bauwens SF, Orwoll ES, Bell NH 1990 Influence of age and body weight on spine and femur bone mineral density in U.S. white men. J Bone Miner Res 5:645-652.

48. Davis JW, Ross PD, Vogel JM, Wasnich RD 1991 Age-related changes in bone mass among Japanese-American men. Bone and Mineral 15:227-236.

49. Garn SM, Sullivan TV, Decker SA, Larkin FA, Hawthorne VM 1992 Continuing bone expansion and increasing bone loss over a two-decade period in men and women from a total community sample. Am J Human Biol 4:57-67.

50. Tobin JD, Fox KM, Cejku ML 1993 Bone density changes in normal men: a 4-19 year longitudinal study. J Bone Miner Res 8:102.

51. Slemenda CW, Christian JC, Reed T, Reister TK, Williams CJ, Johnston CCJ 1992 Long-term bone loss in men: effects of genetic and environmental factors. Ann Int Med 117:286-291.

52. Stepan JJ, Lachman M 1989 Castrated men with bone loss: effect of calcitonin treatment on biochemical indices of bone remodeling. J Clin Endocrinol Metab 69:523-527.

53. Finkelstein JS, Neer RM, Biller BMK, Crawford JD, Klibanski A 1992 Osteopenia in men with a history of delayed puberty. N Engl J Med 326:600-604.

54. Finkelstein JS, Klibanski A, Neer RM 1989 Increase in bone density during treatment of men with idiopathic hypogonadotropic hypogonadism. J Clin Endocrinol Metab 69(4):776-783.

55. Guo CY, Jones H, Eastell R 1997 Treatment of isolated hypogonadotropic hypogonadism effect on bone mineral density and bone turnover. J Clin Endocrinol Metab 82(2):658-665.

56. Wang C, Eyre DR, Clark D 1996 Sublingual testosterone replacement improves muscle mass and strength, decreases bone resorption, and increases bone formation markers in hypogonadal men- A clinical research center study. J Clin Endocrinol Metab 81(10):3654-3662.

57. Katznelson L, Finkelstein JS, Schoenfeld DA, Rosenthal DI, Anderson EJ, Klibanski A 1996 Increase in bone density and lean body mass during testosterone administration in men with acquired hypogonadism. J Clin Endocrinol Metab 81(12):4358-4365.

58. Rudman D, Feller AG, Hoskote S 1990 Effects of human growth hormone in men over 60 years old. New Engl J Med 323:1-6.

59. McElduff A, Wilkinson M, Ward P, Posen S 1988 Forearm mineral content in normal men: relationship to weight, height and plasma testosterone concentrations. Bone 9:281-283.

60. Murphy S, Khaw KT, Cassidy A, Compston JE 1993 Sex hormones and bone mineral density in elderly men. J Bone Miner Res 20:133-140.

61. Kelly PJ, Pocock NA, Sambrook PN, Eisman JA 1990 Dietary calcium, sex hormones, and bone mineral density in men. Br Med J 300:1361-1364.

62. Meier DE, Orwoll ES, Keenan EJ, Fagerstrom RM 1987 Marked decline in trabecular bone mineral content in healthy men with age: lack of association with sex steroid levels. J Am Geriatr Soc 35:189-197.

63. Drinka PJ, Olson J, Bauwens S, Voeks S, Carlson I, Wilson M 1993 Lack of association between free testosterone and bone density separate from age in elderly males. Calcif Tissue Int 52:67-69.

64. Wishart JM, Need AG, Horowitz M, Morris HA, Nordin BEC 1995 Effect of age on bone density and bone turnover in men. Clin Endocrinol 42:141-146.

65. Tenover JS 1992 Effects of testosterone supplementation in the aging male. J Clin Endocrinol Metab 75(4):1092-1098.

66. Morishima A, Grumbach MM, Simpson ER, Fisher C, Qin K 1995 Aromatase deficiency in male and female siblings caused by a novel mutation and the physiological role of estrogens. J Clin Endocrinol Metab 80:3689-3698.

67. Sasano H, Uzuki M, Sawai T 1997 Aromatase in human bone tissue. J Bone Miner Res 12:1416-1423.

68. Van Kesteren P, Lips P, Deville W 1996 The effect of one-year cross-sex hormonal treatment on bone metabolism and serum insulin-like growth factor-1 in transsexuals. J Clin Endocrinol Metab 81(6):2227-2232.

69. Slemenda CW, Longcope C, Zhou l, Hui S, Peacock M, Johnston CC 1997 Sex steroids and bone mass in older men. Positive associations with serum estrogens and negative associations with androgens. J Clin Invest 100:1755-1759.

70. Greendale GA, Edelstein S, Barrett-Connor E 1997 Endogenous sex steroids and bone mineral density in older women and men: The Rancho Bernardo study. J Bone Miner Res 12:1833-1843.

71. Goulding A, Gold E 1993 Flutamide-mediated androgen blockade evokes osteopenia in the female rat. J Bone Miner Res 8:763-769.

72. Wiren KM, Zhang X, Chang C, Keenan E, Orwoll E 1997 Transcriptional up-regulation of the human androgen receptor by androgen in bone cells. Endocrinology 138:2291-2300.

73. Wakley GK, Schutte HDJ, Hannon KS, Turner RT 1991 Androgen treatment prevents loss of cancellous bone in the orchidectomized rat. J Bone Miner Res 6:325-330.

74. Mason RA, Morris HA 1997 Effects of dihydrotestosterone on bone biochemical markers in sham and oophorectomized rats. J Bone Miner Res 12:1431- 1437.

75. Evans RA, Marel GM, Lancaster EK, Kos S, Evans M, Wong SYP 1988 Bone mass is low in relatives of osteoporotic patients. Ann Intern Med 109:870-873.

76. Diaz, MN, O'Neill TW, Silman AJ 1997 The influence of family history of hip fracture on the risk of vertebral deformity in men and women: The European vertebral osteoporosis study. Bone 20:145-149.

77. Felson DT, Zhang Y, Hannan MT, Kiel DP, Wilson PWF, Anderson JJ 1993 The effect of postmenopausal estrogen therapy on bone density in elderly women. N Engl J Med 329:1141-1146.

78. Vogel JM, Davis JW, Nomura A, Wasnich RD, Ross PD 1997 The effects of smoking on bone mass and the rates of bone loss among elderly japanese-american men. J Bone Miner Res 12:1495-1501.

79. Nguyen TV, Kelly PJ, Sambrook PN, Gilbert C, Pocock NA, Eisman JA 1994 Lifestyle factors and bone density in the elderly: Implications for osteoporosis prevention. J Bone Miner Res 9:1339-1346.

80. Kelepouris N, Harper KD, Gannon F, Kaplan FS, Haddad JG 1995 Severe osteoporosis in men. Ann Int Med 123:452-460.

81. Kurland TS, Rosen CJ, Cosman F 1997 Insulin-like growth factor-I in men with idiopathic osteoporosis. J Clin Endocrinol Metab 82:2799-2805.

82. Johansson AG, Eriksen EF, Lindh E 1997 Reduces serum levels of the growth hormone-dependent insulin-like growth factor binding protein and a negative bone balance at the level of individual remodeling units in idiopathic osteoporosis in men. J Clin Endocrinol Metab 82:2795-2798.

83. Orwoll ES, Klein RF. 1995 Osteoporosis in men. Endocrine Rev. 16:87-116.

84. Francis RM, Peacock M, Marshall DH, Horsman A, Aaron JE 1989 Spinal osteoporosis in men. Bone and Mineral 5:347-357.

85. Genant HK, Gordan GS, Hoffman PGJ 1983 Osteoporosis Part I. Advanced radiologic assessment using quantitative computed tomography - Medical Staff Conference, University of California, San Francisco. West J Med 139:75-84.

86. Resch A, Schneider B, Bernecker P 1995 Risk of vertebral fractures in men: relationship to mineral density of the vertebral body. AJR 164:1447-1450.

87. Riggs BL, Wahner HW, Seeman E 1982 Changes in bone mineral density of the proximal femur and spine with aging. J Clin Invest 70:716-723.

88. Karlsson MK, Johnell O, Nilsson BE, Sernbo I, Obrant KJ 1993 Bone mineral mass in hip fracture patients. Bone 14:161-165.

89. Nguyen T, Sambrook P, Kelly P, Jones G, Lord S, Freund J 1993 Prediction of osteoporotic fractures by postural instability and bone density. BMJ 307:1111-1115.

90. Chevalley T, Rizzoli R, Nydegger V 1991 Preferential low bone mineral density of the femoral neck in patients with a recent fracture of the proximal femur. Osteoporosis Int 1:147-154.

91. Gardsell P, Johnell O, Nilsson BE 1990 The predictive value of forearm bone mineral content measurements in men. Bone 11:229-232.

92. Greenspan SL, Myers ER, Maitland LA, Kido TH, Krasnow MB, Hayes WC 1994 Trochanteric bone mineral density is associated with type of hip fracture in the elderly. J Bone Miner Res 9(12):1889-1894.

93. Looker AC, Orwoll ES, Johnston CC 1997 Prevalence of low femoral bone density in older U.S. adults from NHANES III. J Bone Miner Res 12:1761-1768.

94. Grisso JA, Chiu GY, Maislin G, Steinmann WC, Portale J 1991 Risk factors for hip fractures in men: a preliminary study. J Bone Miner Res 6:865-868.

95. Ray WA, Griffin MR, Schaffner W, Baugh DK, Melton III LJ 1987 Psychotropic drug use and the risk of hip fracture. N Engl J Med 316:363-370.

96. Ray WA, Griffin MR, Downey W 1989 Benzodiazepines of long and short elimination half-life and the risk of hip fracture. JAMA 262:3303-3307.

97. Poor G, Atkinson EJ, O'Fallon WM, Melton JL 1995 Predictors of hip fractures in elderly men. J Bone Miner Res 10(2):1902-1905.

98. Hindmarsh JJ, Estes EH 1989 Falls in older persons: Causes and interventions. Arch Intern Med 149:2217-2222.

99. O'Neill TW, Varlow J, Reeve J 1995 Fall frequeny and incidence of distal forearm fracture in the UK. J Epidemiol Com Health 49(6):597-598.

100. Tinetti ME, Speechley M, Ginter SF 1988 Risk factors for falls among elderly persons living in the community. N Engl J Med 319:1701-1707.

101. Eastell R, Riggs BL 1980 Diagnostic evaluation of osteoporosis. Endocrinol Metab Clin North Am 17:547-571.

102. Lane JM, Vigorita VJ. 1984 Osteoporosis. Orthop Clin North Am. 15:711-728.

103. Seeley DG, Browner WS, Nevitt MC, Genant HK, Scott JC, Cummings SR 1991 Which fractures are associated with low appendicular bone mass in elderly women? Ann Int Med 115:837-842.

104. Mosekilde L 1989 Sex differences in age-related loss of vertebral trabecular bone mass and structure - biomechanical consequences. Bone 10:425-432.

105. Looker AC, Johnston CC, Wahner HWJ 1995 Defining low femur bone density levels in men. In: Drezner MC, ed. 17th Annual Meeting of the American Society for Bone and Mineral Research. Baltimore, MD: Blackwell Science, Inc S468.

106. Campbell GA, Hosking DJ, Kemm JR, Boyd RV 1984 How common is osteomalacia in the elderly? Lancet II:386-388.

107. Aaron JE, Stasiak L, Gallagher JC 1974 Frequency of osteomalacia and osteoporosis in fractures of the proximal femur. Lancet I:229-233.

108. Hordon LD, Peacock M 1990 Osteomalacia and osteoporosis in femoral neck fracture. J Bone Miner Res 11:247-259.

109. Sokoloff L 1978 Occult osteomalacia in America (USA) patients with fracture of the hip. Am J Surg Pathol 2:21-30.

110. Wilton TJ, Hosking DJ, Pawley E, Stevens A, Harvey L 1987 Osteomalacia and femoral neck fractures in the elderly patient. J Bone Joint Surg 69-B:388-390.

111. Marel GM, McKenna MJ, Frame B 1986 Osteomalacia. In: Peck WA, ed. Bone and Mineral Res/4. Vol. 4. Amsterdam:335-413.

112. Johnston CCJr, Slemenda CW, Melton LJ III 1991 Clinical use of bone densitometry. N Engl J Med 324:1105-1109.

113. Klein RF, Gunness M 1992 The transiliac bone biopsy: When to get it and how to interpret it. Endocrinologist 2:158-168.

114. Jackson JA, Kleerekoper M 1990 Osteoporosis in men: diagnosis, pathophysiology, and prevention. Medicine 69:137-152.

115. Chines A, Pacifici R, Avioli LA, Korenblat PE, Teitelbaum SL 1993 Systemic mastocytosis and osteoporosis. Osteoporosis Int 1:S147-S149.

116. Chines A, Pacifici R, Avioli LV, Teitelbaum SL, Korenblat PE 1991 Systemic mastocytosis presenting as osteoporosis: a clinical and histomorphometric study. J Clin Endocrinol Metab 72:140-144.

117. Rubenstein LZ, Josephson KR 1992 Causes and prevention of falls in elderly people. In: Vellas B, Toupet M, Rubenstein L, Albarede JL, Christen Y, eds. Falls, Balance and Gait Disorders in the Elderly. Paris: Elsevier.

118. Fujimura R, Ashizawa N, Watanabe M 1997 Effect of resistance exercise training on bone formation and resorption in young male subjects assessed by biomarkers of bone metabolism. J Bone Miner Res 12:656-662.

119. Paganini-Hill A, Chao A, Ross RK, Henderson BE 1991 Exercise and other factors in the prevention of hip fracture: The Leisure World study. Epidemiology 2:16-25.

120. Johnston CC, Miller JZ, Slemenda CW 1992 Calcium supplementation and increases in bone mineral density in children. N Engl J Med 327:82-87.

121. Dawson-Hughes B, Harris SS, Krall EA, Dallal GE 1997 Effect of calcium and vitamin D supplementation on bone density in men and women 65 years of age or older. N Engl J Med. 337:670-702.

122. NIH. 1994 NIH Consensus statement(Number 4 ed.). Vol. 12. Bethesda, MD: National Institutes of Health.

123. Curhan GC, Willett WC, Rimm EB, Stampfer MJ 1993 A prospective study of dietary calcium and other nutrients and the risk of symptomatic kidney stones. N Engl J Med 328:833-838.

124. Agrawal R, Wallach S, Cohn S 1981 Calcitonin treatment of osteoporosis. In: Pecile A, ed. Calcitonin. Vol. 540. Amsterdam: Exerpta Medica 237.

125. Valkema R, Vismans F-JFE, Papapoulos SE, Pauwels EKJ, Bijvoet OLM. 1989 Maintained improvement in calcium balance and bone mineral content in patients with osteoporosis treated with the bisphosphonate APD. Bone Miner 5:183-192.

126. Orme SM, Simpson M, Stewart SP 1994 Comparison of changes in bone mineral in idiopathic and secondary osteoporosis following therapy with cyclical disodium etidronate and high dose calcium supplementation. Clin Endocrinol 41(2):245-250.

127. Wasnich R, Davis J, Ross P, Vogel J 1990 Effect of thiazide on rates of bone mineral loss: a longitudinal study. Br Med J 301:1303-1305.

128. Ray WA, Griffin MR, Downey W, Melton LJI 1989 Long-term use of thiazide diuretics and risk of hip fracture. Lancet I:687-690.

129. Pak CYC, Sakhaee K, Piziak V 1994 Slow-release sodium fluoride in the management of postmenopausal osteoporosis: a randomized controlled trial. Ann Int Med 120:625-632.

130. Slovik DM, Rosenthal DI, Doppelt SH. 1986 Restoration of spinal bone in osteoporotic men by treatment with human parathyroid hormone (1-34) and 1,25-dihydroxyvitamin D. J Bone Miner Res 1:377-381.

131. Ljunghall S, Johansson AG, Burman P, Kampe O, Lindh E, Karlsson FA 1992 Low plasma levels of insulin-like growth factor 1 (IGF-1) in male patients with idiopathic osteoporosis. J Intern Med 232:59-64.

13 Diagnosis and Treatment of Renal Osteodystrophy

Dean T. Yamaguchi, M.D., Ph.D.

Arnold J. Felsenfeld, M.D.

Introduction

Bone disease develops as a consequence of renal failure. Alterations in phosphate clearance and calcium metabolism brought on by loss of functional nephrons affect homeostatic mechanisms such as parathyroid hormone secretion and vitamin D metabolism aimed at normalization of serum calcium levels. The chronic metabolic acidosis seen with advanced renal disease also likely plays a major contributory role in the bone disease of renal failure since bone is a major buffering site for acid in the body. These hormonal and physicochemical changes induced by renal disease lead to a spectrum of bone abnormalities that appear to change as therapies for both renal failure and the associated pathophysiologic processes are implemented.

Pathogenesis of Renal Osteodystrophy

The genesis of the bone disease observed with renal failure results from changes in circulating hormones such as parathyroid hormone (PTH), and the most active form of vitamin D, 1,25 dihydroxyvitamin D_3 (calcitriol), and in calcium and phosphorus metabolism. The "trade-off" hypothesis advanced by Bricker (1, 2) was a concept to explain the development of renal osteodystrophy. Essentially, Bricker suggested that the increase in serum phosphorus levels in renal failure reduced serum calcium levels resulting in an increase in PTH secretion to keep serum calcium levels as close to normal as possible. With a decline in renal function, phosphorus excretion by the kidneys becomes impaired resulting in a transient hyperphosphatemia. While there may not be an identifiable change in blood ionized calcium due to the increase in PTH in early renal failure, the increase in PTH results in an increased reabsorption of calcium from remaining functioning nephrons and release of calcium from bone. Thus more PTH is needed to maintain the same serum calcium; moreover, the increase in PTH secretion has a phosphaturic effect which returns serum phosphorus towards normal and improves the decreased calcemic response to PTH. The "trade-off" in early to moderate renal failure is an increase in PTH levels to maintain a normal serum calcium. However, this leads to increased bone turnover with subsequent development of osteitis fibrosa. Thus, the initial response in renal failure is an increase in PTH which functions to maintain normal serum calcium, phosphorus, and calcitriol levels. As renal failure advances, PTH levels increase further but can no longer maintain homeostasis of calcium due to an increasing phosphorus burden, a reduction in calcitriol levels, and azotemia. Thus in advanced renal failure, hypocalcemia, hyperphosphatemia, and a deficiency of calcitriol are commonly observed despite marked elevations in PTH.

Serum phosphorus has thus been the primary factor central to the development of secondary hyperparathyroidism and renal bone disease. Phosphorus excesses affect all the counter-regulatory mechanisms by which PTH maintains calcium homeostasis. Phosphorus retention inhibits calcitriol production, exacerbates resistance to the calcemic actions of PTH, and may directly stimulate PTH secretion. The former two factors counteract the ability of PTH to restore a normal serum calcium.

Elevations in serum phosphorus have been shown to stimulate PTH secretion independent of decreases in ionized calcium levels in hemodialysis patients (3). Further supporting the critical role of phosphorus are the data from a dog model of renal failure in which it was shown that a low phosphorus, low calcium diet resulted in lower PTH levels than dogs fed a high calcium, normal phosphorus diet; ionized calcium and calcitriol levels were similar in both groups suggesting that phosphorus independently reduced PTH levels in animals with renal failure (4). In vitro studies in rat parathyroid glands have demonstrated that PTH secretion is stimulated by high phosphate medium under conditions of controlled medium calcium. Moreover, parathyroid cells were less sensitive to inhibition by calcium (5). Pre-pro parathyroid hormone mRNA was found to be greater in normal rats fed a high phosphorus diet (1.2% phosphorus, 0.6% calcium) compared to rats fed a standard diet (0.6% phosphorus, 0.6% calcium). Morphological examination of parathyroid glands from high phosphorus-fed rats showed evidence of hyperplasia (6). Parathyroid cell proliferation and PTH mRNA were increased when rats in which chronic renal failure was induced were fed a high phosphate diet (7). Conversely, a low phosphorus diet decreased serum PTH levels and PTH mRNA. The effect of a low phosphorus diet to decrease PTH mRNA levels was at a post-transcriptional level. (8). Finally, increases in serum phosphorus can inhibit the conversion of 25-hydroxyvitamin D3 to calcitriol by the 1-α-hydroxylase resulting in decreased levels of calcitriol (9-12).

It is well-known that renal failure induces a resistance to the action of PTH on bone. One likely reason for this skeletal resistance to PTH is a uremic-induced down-regulation of the PTH receptor at the level of PTH/PTHrP receptor mRNA in kidney and bone (13, 14). It has also been suggested that calcitriol may independently decrease bone remodeling even with high PTH levels (15). Calcitriol suppresses PTH secretion as well as rendering bone unresponsive to the effect of PTH by the down regulation of the PTH/PTHrP receptors on osteoblasts (16). Finally, uremic toxins such as a low molecular weight inhibitor of osteoblast function described by Andress, et. al. (17) may contribute to the resistance of osteoblasts to PTH action.

Classification of Renal Osteodystrophy: Criteria to Distinguish Among the Renal Bone Disease Types

The spectrum of renal bone disease can be generally classified as follows: high turnover bone disease characterized by markedly increased levels of PTH associated with an increase in both bone resorption and the bone formation rate and characterized by increased numbers of osteoclasts and osteoblasts; low turnover bone disease characterized by normal to minimally increased PTH levels, diminished bone formation rate and either an increase in osteoid (osteomalacia) or normal amounts of osteoid (adynamic bone disease) and both with minimal osteoblast and osteoclast cellularity; mixed bone disease with mild to moderate elevations of PTH and having characteristics of a normal bone formation rate, an increase in osteoid, and a moderate increase in the numbers of osteoblasts and osteoclasts.

A number of hormonal and biochemical tests are available to assess bone disease in renal failure. In addition to total and serum ionized calcium and phosphorus levels, assessment of PTH levels is crucial. With respect to PTH assay the intact molecule (PTH 1-84) assayed by a two-site immunoradiometric method has become the preferred method in renal failure patients (18-21).

In general biochemical tests have been divided into markers for bone resorption and for bone formation. The bone resorption markers include collagen cross-link molecules, pyridinoline, deoxypyridinoline, and type I collagen cross-linked telopeptide (ICTP). In contrast to non-azotemic individuals in whom these tests are in general performed in urine, tests in azotemic patients must be performed in the serum. Bone formation markers include procollagen type I C-terminal propeptide (PICP), alkaline phosphatase and osteocalcin. In general however in renal disease, bone formation and resorption markers often correlate with each other because bone formation and resorption are matched. Urena, et. al. (22) reported that serum pyridinoline levels determined by an enzyme immunoassay were positively correlated with bone resorption parameters of osteoclast surface and osteoclast number but also with bone formation parameters including osteoblast surface and bone formation rate. In hemodialysis patients, serum pyridinoline levels were higher than in normal individuals, some of which may be due to the failure of diseased kidneys to excrete pyridinoline. However, serum pryidinoline levels were found to be higher in chronic hemodialysis patients with osteitis fibrosa than in patients with normal or low-turnover bone disease (23). Serum ICTP is also increased in chronic renal failure, but in initial studies, it has not been shown to be useful as a marker for bone resorption in renal disease (23).

Procollagen type I carboxy-terminal extension peptide (PICP) which is not cleared by the kidney but via the mannose 6-phosphate receptor on endothelial cells in the liver was initially thought to potentially be a good marker of bone formation. In predialysis patients, PICP levels correlated with the bone formation rate. In patients on dialysis, the role of PICP as a bone formation marker has been less clear, and more work is needed to clarify the utility of this marker in end-stage renal disease (24, 25).

Elevation of total alkaline phosphatase has been observed in bone disease, especially, high turnover disease (osteitis fibrosa). However, tissue-specific forms of alkaline phosphatase are found in liver, kidney, intestine, and placenta in addition to being found in bone. Thus elevations of total alkaline phosphatase in dialysis patients may be due to concomitant liver abnormalities and thus could even be seen in patients with normal or low-turnover bone disease (26). Determination of (gamma-glutamyltranferase would be a reasonable approach to distinguish between total alkaline phosphatase derived from bone versus liver as elevated (gamma-glutamyltranferase levels would suggest a hepatic source of alkaline phosphatase. The development of an immunoradiometric assay for bone-specific alkaline phosphatase has helped to distinguish bone disease in hemodialysis patients. Bone formation rate and histomorphometric parameters of increased bone turnover were better correlated to bone alkaline phosphatase than to total alkaline phosphatase. These investigators concluded that bone alkaline phosphatase levels > 20 ng/ml had a sensitivity and specificity of 100% and positive predictability of 84% for high turnover bone disease. The prediction of normal or low-turnover bone disease resulted in 100% sensitivity, 100% specificity, and 100% positive predictability when bone alkaline phosphatase was <20 ng/ml. However, these initial results using bone alkaline phosphatase to predict normal or low-bone turnover disease need further confirmation. Others using total alkaline phosphatase level of >200 IU/liter or <200 IU/liter in children on peritoneal dialysis showed lesser specificity, sensitivity and positive predictive value for both high- and low-bone turnover disease, respectively (27). However, normal bone alkaline phosphatase was noted in some patients with mild high turnover bone disease.

Osteocalcin, a vitamin K-dependent protein rich in (gamma-carboxyglutamic acid residues, comprises 20 to 25% of non-collagen bone protein and is synthesized exclusively by osteoblasts and odontoblasts and incorporated into bone matrix and dentin, respectively. Joffe, et. al. (28) using an ELISA for serum osteocalcin in CAPD patients, found that serum osteocalcin correlated significantly with bone formation parameters including bone formation rate and osteoid thickness. However, significant correlations were also found between serum osteocalcin and bone eroded surface and osteoclast surface, indicators of bone resorption. Additionally, the correlation of serum osteocalcin with histomorphometric parameters was similar to that of PTH. Others have also found that in hemodialyzed patients serum osteocalcin > 8 nmole/liter correlated with high-turnover bone disease while serum osteocalcin levels < 4 nmole/liter correlated with low-turnover bone disease (29).

Despite attempts to utilize serum markers of both bone resorption and bone formation, the "gold standard" for the diagnosis of the various forms of renal osteodystrophy remains the bone biopsy. An excellent review of the techniques for both the procedure itself and the histologic examination of bone specimens has recently been published by Malluche and Monier-Faugere (30). Bone histomorphometric nomenclature has been standardized (31). **Table 1** shows common bone histomorphometric parameters used to distinguish the various forms of renal osteodystrophy.

Histomorphometric parameters can help to define the different forms of renal osteodystrophy. The spectrum of renal osteodystrophy includes 1) high-turnover predominant hyperparathyroid bone disease (osteitis fibrosa)(**Figure 1**), 2) low-turnover disease which includes osteomalacia (**Figure 2**) and adynamic renal bone disease, and 3) mixed renal osteodystrophy encompassing features of increased bone resorption and normal mineralization and increased osteoid. Osteoid volume depends on the relative relationship between osteoid deposition by osteoblasts and the bone formation rate. Thus as shown in **Figure 3**, the osteoid volume will be increased whenever osteoid deposition by osteoblasts exceeds the bone formation rate. This may occur in osteomalacia and mixed renal osteodystrophy. Normal osteoid volume can result from proportionate increases or decreases in osteoid deposition and bone formation rate as seen in osteitis fibrosa and adynamic bone, respectively.

Aluminum deposition in bone can be found in low-turnover osteomalacia, adynamic bone disease, mixed renal osteodystrophy, and to a lesser extent, in high turnover hyperparathyroid disease. Generally, surface staining of aluminum > 25% in bone biopsy specimens showing either aplastic lesion or osteomalacia meets the criteria for aluminum bone disease (32-34

High-turnover Bone Disease

[1]Histomorphometric Criteria in Renal Osteodystrophy				
	Bone Formation Rate $\mu m^3/mm^2$ of tissue area/day	Osteoid Area % of total bone area	Marrow Fibrosis % of tissue area	Relative Osteoclast number	Relative Osteoblast number
[1]CHILDREN	97-613	1-12	0	++	++
Osteitis Fibrosa	>613	<12	++	++++	++++
Osteomalacia	<97	>12	0	+	+
Adynamic Bone	<97	<12	0	+	+
Mixed	97-613	>15	+	++	++
[2]ADULTS	108-500	1-7	0	+ / ++	+ / ++
Osteitis Fibrosa	>500	<15	>0.5%	+++ / ++++	+++ / ++++
Osteomalacia	<108	≥15	<0.5%	+	+
Adynamic Bone	<108	<15	<0.5%	+	+
Mixed	108-500	≥15	≥0.5%	++ / +++	++ / +++

Table 1. The usual parameters determined include double tetracycline labeled surface expressed as the fraction of trabecular bone surface, mineralizing surface defined as the total extent of double label plus half of the extent of single label and expressed as the fraction of the bone surface; mineral

210

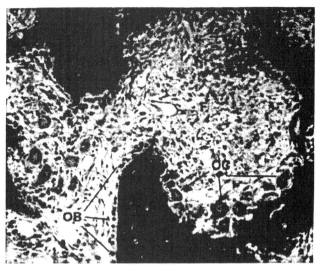

Figure 1: Osteitis Fibrosa
Histologic section of iliac crest biopsy from hemodialysis patient stained with Goldner's trichrome stain. The red areas are osteoid while the blue-green stained areas are mineralized bone. A substantial number of osteoclasts (OC) together with a large number of osteoblasts (OB) indicative of increased bone resorption and bone matrix production, respectively, is characteristic of this high turnover disease. Extensive marrow space fibrosis (F) is noted.

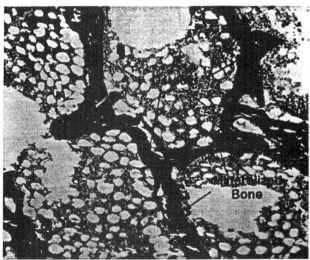

Figure 2: Osteomalacia
Histologic section of iliac crest biopsy from hemodialysis patient stained with Goldner's trichrome stain. The red areas are osteoid while the blue-green stained areas are mineralized bone. The volume of osteoid is great compared to that of mineralized bone. Correlated with the severity of high-turnover bone disease is the appearanceof marrow fibrosis. All of these histologic features are the result of overproduction of PTH.

appositional rate expressed as mm/day; bone formation rate in mm3/mm2 per day after tetracycline labeling; trabecular bone volume as a percentage of trabecular space; osteoid volume as a percentage of trabecular bone volume; osteoid surface as a percentage of trabecular bone surface; osteoblast surface expressed as the osteoid surface covered with active osteoblasts and expressed as the percentage of trabecular bone surface; osteoid thickness in mm; osteoclast surface expressed as the fraction of trabecular bone surface covered with osteoclasts; osteoclast number per mm2 of tissue section; and aluminum surface expressed as the fraction of trabecular bone surface covered by aluminum (assessed by aurin tricarboxylic-acid method).

[1]Parfitt, *et. al.*, 1987 (31)

[2]Mathias, *et. al.*, 1993 (35); Salusky, *et. al.*, 1994 (21)

[3]Sherrard, *et. al.*, 1993 (20); Pei, *et. al.*, 1995 (19)

Histologically, high-turnover bone disease (osteitis fibrosa) displays features of both increased bone resorption as well as bone formation (**Figure 1**). This is manifested by increases in the number of osteoclasts and their associated resorption pits and increased numbers of actively matrix secreting osteoblasts. Additionally, dynamic bone parameters show an increased bone formation rate. The organization of newly synthesized collagen is frequently haphazard resulting in the formation of woven bone which is structurally inferior to lamellar bone.

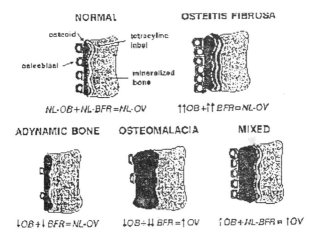

Figure 3: Schematic Representation Showing Relationship of Osteoblast Number and Bone Formation Rate to Osteoid Volume. Osteoid volume (OV) is proportional to the number of osteoblast (OB) secreting osteoid and the bone formation rate (BFR) determined by double tetracycline labeling shown as the wavy dark lines. In osteitis fibrosa, an increase in osteoblast number and an increased in bone formation rate result in normal osteoid volume while in adynamic bone, decreased osteoblast number is matched by decreased bone formation rate also resulting in normal osteoid volume. In osteomalacia, a marked decrease in bone formation rate with a lesser decrease in osteoblast number results in an increased osteoid volume. Mixed disease is characterized by an increase in osteoblast number but a normal bone formation rate resulting in an increased osteoid volume.

The increase in circulating PTH in chronic renal failure as stated above results from a number of factors in which hyperphosphatemia plays a prominent role. Additionally, calcitriol production by the kidney is reduced in renal failure due to the reduction in functional renal mass and moreover, the hyperphosphatemia inhibits the conversion of 25-dihydroxyvitamin D3 to calcitriol. Investigation into PTH secretion in chronic renal disease have generally concluded that there may be alterations in the mechanism of calcium-mediated PTH release from parathyroid cells as well as increased PTH secretion simply due to an increased mass of parathyroid tissue (36).

Controversy has developed regarding calcium-stimulated PTH secretion and alteration in the set-point of calcium for PTH secretion. While earlier studies suggested that the set-point for PTH secretion was decreased in low versus high turnover bone disease thus reflecting the magnitude of hyperparathyroidism, others have reported that the set-point for calcium was not different in the different forms of renal osteodystrophy (37, 38). Initially, the discrepancy in findings was attributed to different methodologies for reporting the set-point for PTH secretion. While Felsenfeld and Rodriguez defined the set-point as the calcium concentration at which 50% of maximal PTH secretion was inhibited, Goodman and Salusky have defined the set-point as the calcium concentration at which PTH values are midway between the maximum and minimum levels of PTH secretion induced by low and high calcium concentrations, respectively. However, set-point determinations by both methods are well-correlated. More recent studies by Pahl, et. al., (39) and Rodriguez, et. al., (40) have shown that PTH secretion may adapt to ambient serum calcium concentration. Thus these studies suggest that the differences reported in previous studies may have been due to differences in the ambient serum calcium concentration. One mechanism by which PTH secretion per cell could be altered is by changing the ability of the parathyroid cell to sense changes in extracellular calcium. A G-protein-linked seven transmembrane spanning calcium receptor protein has been cloned (41). Recently it has been reported that in both primary and secondary hyperparathyroidism, there is decreased expression of calcium receptor protein (42) and mRNA in the nodular areas of hyperplastic parathyroid glands (43).

In addition to regulation by changes in secretion by the amount of calcium receptors, circulating PTH levels can also be regulated at the level of synthesis by parathyroid glands. PTH synthesis has been shown to be regulated by calcitriol. Calcitriol inhibits pre-proPTH mRNA transcription (42, 43). In renal failure, calcitriol receptor concentrations in parathyroid glands are decreased (44), which could potentially account for a diminished response to calcitriol resulting in uncontrolled PTH synthesis. Recently, Patel, et. al.(45) confirmed that calcitriol receptor protein is down-regulated while calcitriol receptor mRNA is increased in a rat renal failure model. Additionally in that same study, infusion of uremic ultrafiltrate to normal rats mimics the effects on calcitriol receptor protein and mRNA seen in renal failure rats.

In addition to regulating the synthesis of PTH, calcitriol has been shown to inhibit proliferation of parathyroid cells (46). As parathyroid gland mass resulting from hyperplasia is an important determinant of the circulating level of PTH, understanding how calcitriol regulates parathyroid cell proliferation is a key concern. A review of in vitro studies of calcitriol action on parathyroid cell proliferation suggests that calcitriol may prevent the increase in c-myc protooncogene and stimulate expression of the cyclin kinase inhibitor p21 resulting in decreased proliferation (47). Thus a deficiency of calcitriol and calcitriol receptor as found in renal failure could lead to increased parathyroid cell proliferation.

In a concise review on the role of parathyroid gland size, Parfitt (48) stated that hyperplasia rather than hypertrophy is the major determinant of parathyroid enlargement in chronic renal failure and that regulation of parathyroid cell proliferation rather than PTH secretion was of paramount importance in the treatment of hyperparathyroidism in renal disease. Cell turnover is normally low in parathyroid glands in vivo, and any increase in cell number by proliferation may in part be offset by apoptosis of parathyroid cells to keep cell numbers constant. In renal failure, hypocalcemia induced by hyperphosphatemia increases parathyroid cell proliferation as well as increased PTH secretion.

Histologically, parathyroid hyperplasia can be categorized as diffuse or nodular. Nodular hyperplasia consists of densely packed cells which are actively cycling in distinct, usually well-demarcated nodules. Nodular hyperplastic cells demonstrate lower calcium receptor numbers and a greater proliferative capacity (43, 45). It is unclear if nodular hyperplasia results from a single cell (monoclonality) or from a group of adjacent cells (multiclonal). A high proliferative rate may predispose to mutations in one cell resulting in an adenoma with possible subsequent malignant transformation to carcinoma (48, 50).

Management of Secondary Hyperparathyroidism in the Dialysis Patient.

Treatment of secondary hyperparathyroidism has been aimed at decreasing PTH levels or preventing excessive increases in PTH levels that would be detrimental to bone metabolism. Thus therapy can involve the inhibition of PTH synthesis and secretion on a per cell basis and/or control of parathyroid cell proliferation to decrease PTH secretion due to bulk mass of cells. Drueke (51) reviewed the three main factors leading to excessive PTH production which included calcitriol deficiency, hypocalcemia and hyperphosphatemia. In addition other factors such as metabolic acidosis, uremic toxins, aluminum, and other hormones such as catecholamines, glucocorticoids, estrogens, and retinoids were mentioned as having potential effects either on PTH secretion or end-organ effects of PTH. Bover, et. al (11) showed that the increase in PTH levels in experimental renal failure is dependent on the amount of dietary calcium and phosphate ingested. Thus in a renal failure model in rats given a high phosphate diet, hypocalcemia, phosphorus retention, calcitriol deficiency, and decreased calcemic response to PTH contributed to development of secondary hyperparathyroidism. In a high calcium diet group, calcitriol deficiency was the most important factor for the development of secondary hyperparathyroidism, while in a moderate calcium and phosphorus diet group, a decreased calcemic response to PTH seemed to contribute most to the development of secondary hyperparathyroidism. Hence consideration should be given as to dietary control of phosphorus intake as well as judicious use of calcium salts to bind phosphorus as the first step in the early treatment of secondary hyperparathyroidism. Also the use of low-dose calcitriol in early renal failure may be important to prevent the development of more severe secondary hyperparathyroidism (52).

Phosphorus Control. As uncontrolled hyperphosphatemia is a central factor in the pathogenesis of renal osteodystrophy resulting from alterations in PTH and calcitriol, secretion initial therapy should be aimed at keeping serum phosphorus to levels < 6.0 mg/dl and preferably in the 5 mg/dl range (53). It has been shown that when serum phosphorus levels exceed 7 mg/dl, the effectiveness of calcitriol to decrease PTH levels is impaired (Rodriguez, et. al., 1991; Quarles, et. al., 1994).

Previous to the recognition of aluminum-induced low-turnover osteomalacia, aluminum hydroxide phosphate binders were used as the primary phosphorus binders. Other complications of aluminum phosphate binders included dialysis dementia, microcytic anemia, and hypercalcemia which have been reviewed in detail elsewhere (56). Since approximately the mid to late 1980s, calcium carbonate has been consistently used as first-line therapy for phosphorus control in patients with chronic renal failure (57, 32, 58, 59). In addition to being efficacious in binding phosphorus in the gut and to suppress excessive PTH secretion by both lowering phosphorus levels as well as increasing the ionized calcium concentration, calcium carbonate may be helpful in correcting the negative calcium balance that is associated with severe renal failure. Bone calcium loss in advanced renal disease can occur by chronic metabolic acidosis usually associated with advanced renal failure. The alkalinizing effect of calcium carbonate helps to correct acidosis (59). Other forms of calcium salts such as calcium citrate and calcium acetate have been used to bind phosphorus. Calcium carbonate has a higher calcium content (40%) than does calcium citrate (21%) or calcium acetate (23%). It has been suggested that calcium acetate is as effective as calcium carbonate in complexing phosphorus using approximately half the usual dose of calcium carbonate since calcium acetate perhaps may be better solubilized at the alkaline pH of the intestine. The theoretical advantage of calcium acetate would be in lowering the incidence of hypercalcemia, especially in those dialysis patients receiving calcitriol. However, while lower doses of elemental calcium in the form of calcium acetate were found to be as effective as almost twice the elemental calcium dose from calcium carbonate, the incidence of hypercalcemia was unchanged (60, 59). In cases where hypercalcemia is a complicating issue in dialysis patients taking calcium salts as phosphorus binders, it is now recommended that dialysate calcium be adjusted to 2.5 meq/L for hemodialysis and from 1.0 meq/L up to 1.75 meq/L for peritoneal dialysis when calcium salt phosphorus binders are used (61, 59, 62). Thus the overall goal would be to adjust dialysate calcium so that hypercalcemia does not develop with calcium salt therapy for hyperphosphatemia. Additionally, caution should be exercised to not allow excessive PTH secretion with chronic low dialysate calcium or excessive PTH suppression using a high dialysate calcium in combination with calcium salt phosphorus binders that may lead to adynamic bone (63). Calcium citrate should be used with caution as it may increase absorption of aluminum. A suggested alternative to dialysis patients who develop hypercalemia during therapy with calcitriol and calcium carbonate is the combination of magnesium carbonate and a low magnesium dialysate (0.6 mg/dL). Such a combination may allow for decreasing the dose of calcium carbonate (64).

Use of Calcitriol, Other Vitamin D Analogs, and Calcium Receptor Agonists. Due to its ability to inhibit PTH synthesis and parathyroid cell proliferation, calcitriol has been used for the treatment of secondary hyperparathyroidism. The use of calcitriol should be considered in those patients with moderate to severe secondary hyperparathyroidism. Since there is a high degree of correlation with the level of intact circulating PTH and bone-specific alkaline phosphatase activity and histomorphometric changes of osteitis fibrosa shown by increased bone formation rate and increased numbers of osteoclasts and osteoblasts, PTH has been used as an indicator for bone disease. Coburn and Frazao (61) have categorized patients with mild, moderate, and severe secondary hyperparathyroidism as having approximate ranges of intact PTH levels of 200-400 pg/mL, 300-800 pg/mL, and greater than 800 pg/mL, respectively. The patients at the higher end of moderate and severe disease deserve a trial of calcitriol. PTH levels below 100 pg/mL are suggestive of adynamic bone in dialysis patients while PTH levels between 150 to 350 pg/mL are probably associated with a "normal" bone turnover rate and osteoblast surface. It is necessary to note that PTH levels higher than normal (10-65 pg/mL with the immunoradiometric assay) are probably needed due to the relative resistance of bone to PTH in renal failure. Thus in adynamic bone disease and in patients with mild elevations of PTH up to 200-250 pg/mL, calcitriol therapy should not be instituted.

In patients with moderate to severe secondary hyperparathyroidism that are not hypercalcemic and have controlled serum phosphorus levels, a trial of calcitriol therapy is warranted. Various routes of administration (oral versus intravenous/intraperitoneal) and dosing levels and dosing schedules have been used (65, 66, 67, 27, 61). The following conclusions can be drawn from these publications: 1) despite differences in pharmacokinetics of intravenous/intraperitoneal versus oral calcitriol, effects on PTH suppression appear to be similar; 2) there is little difference between intermittent versus continuously administered calcitriol (at least with oral therapy) as judged by the fall in serum PTH and complications of hypercalcemia and hyperphosphatemia (68); 3) a threshold dose of calcitriol leading to PTH suppression is likely to be between 0.75 and 0.87 µg per dialysis treatment which is equivalent to approximately 2.25 mg of calcitriol per week (61, 65); 4) the response to calcitriol depends on the degree of secondary hyperparathyroidism in which there has been a good response in moderate secondary hyperparathyroidism (Levine and Song, 1996) but a poor response in severe secondary hyperparathyroidism (66).

Recently, at least in some animal studies, 1,25(OH)2-22-oxa-vitamin D3 (OCT), has been shown to be as effective as calcitriol in decreasing circulating PTH levels in uremic rat models 69, 70, 71, 72). However, Kubrusly, et. al.(73) reported that OCT was less potent than calcitriol in suppressing PTH levels. These authors suggested that OCT may not be as effective as calcitriol in severe secondary hyperparathyroidism due to its shorter plasma half-life as a result of less binding to the vitamin D binding protein, and thus more frequent dosing of OCT is necessary for maximal inhibition. Similar to calcitriol, OCT also inhibits pre-pro PTH mRNA levels. The advantage of OCT over calcitriol has been postulated that it has a lesser calcemic and phosphatemic effect than calcitriol. However, investigation has shown that OCT does have calcemic activity via bone (76) and duodenal calcium absorption (73). Both OCT and calcitriol were found to up-regulate the vitamin D receptor in parathyroid glands in uremic rats although the potency of OCT to do so was less than for calcitriol. The presence of vitamin D receptor is necessary for the action of calcitriol and OCT to inhibit PTH mRNA synthesis, and decreased vitamin D receptor density is present in secondary hyperparathyroidism and contributes to the resistance of calcitriol to suppress PTH mRNA transcription and therefore PTH synthesis. It has been suggested that early use of vitamin D metabolites in renal failure may be beneficial in controlling parathyroid gland hyperplasia and worsening of secondary hyperparathyroidism (72).

Other vitamin D analogs are presently under study for their ability to suppress PTH synthesis without the untoward effects of hypercalcemia. Such compounds include 19-nor-1,25-dihydroxyvitamin D2 and 1-α(-hydroxyvitamin D2 (61, 74). Clinical trials using this latter compound in hemodialysis patients have shown that total weekly doses of approximately 15 mg of 1-α(-hydroxyvitamin D2 progressively lowered serum PTH levels over a 12 week period (74). Mild hypercalcemia was noted in some of the patients during treatment but no significant changes in serum phosphorus were noted in patients on therapy compared to a washout, pre-therapy period.

Calcium Receptor Agonests. Development of calcium receptor agonists to antagonize PTH secretion is currently underway. NPS R-568 is such a calcium receptor agonist that can mimic the effects of extracellular calcium to bind to the G-protein-coupled calcium receptor on parathyroid cells, increase cytosolic calcium concentrations, and inhibit PTH secretion (75). In a rat model of secondary hyperparathyroidism, NPS R-568 acutely decreased PTH secretion (76).

Surgical Therapy of High Turnover Bone Disease. The criteria for surgical management of high turnover bone disease have not been uniformly set, and various indications for parathyroidectomy have been advocated. Medical therapy of secondary hyperparathyroidism may be unsuccessful in dialysis patients with high PTH levels and/or the detection of markedly enlarged parathyroid glands by imaging techniques. Thus severe secondary hyperparathyroidism that has not responded to a trial of calcitriol should be considered for parathyroidectomy (77). Hypercalcemia, uncontrolled hyperphosphatemia, severe symptoms of bone and joint pain, muscle weakness, and pathologic fractures with marked elevations of PTH are clinical findings that would favor surgical removal of the parathyroid glands (78). Calciphylaxis, the appearance of ischemic skin lesion associated with vascular calcifications, with marked increase in PTH would be another indication for parathyroidectomy in the dialysis patient (79). Finally, the nodular form of parathyroid hyperplasia which has been correlated to length on dialysis, the magnitude of hyperparathyroidism, and the size of the parathryoid glands does not respond as well to calcitriol therapy, and would best be handled surgically. It should also be emphasized that the risk of recurrence after parathyroidectomy is increased in glands with nodular hyperplasia (80, 81).

There is divided opinion whether parathyroid gland localization should be used pre-operatively. Use of ultrasound to assess gland size has been advocated even during medical management of the patient as a means to follow response to calcitriol therapy (82). However, neck exploration by an experienced surgeon is a common approach for the first parathyroid surgery, while the use of imaging techniques to localize parathyroid glands used for cases of recurrent hyperparathyroidism which may occur in 5-15% of cases (77). Other modes of parathyroid localization such as computerized tomography and nuclear magnetic resonance have been advocated to localize ectopic parathyroid tissue that can be found spanning the superior thyroid pole to the thymus and superior mediastinum. Function tests such as 99mTc-sestamibi scans which may be an indicator metabolic activity of cells may prove useful (82), but more comparisons to other imaging techniques and biochemical markers of PTH hypersecretion need to be done.

The surgical approaches are subtotal parathyroidectomy versus total parathyroidectomy and immediate autotransplantation of parathyroid fragments into forearm pockets in the brachioradialis muscle. The efficacy of parathyroidectomy in diminishing bone mineral loss in the midshaft and distal radius in dialysis patients has been shown. However, with respect to bone mineral loss, older patients and those patients who have undergone oophorectomy without estrogen replacement may not benefit from parathyroidectomy (83). Leaving remnant functioning parathyroid tissue has been advocated to prevent severe hypoparathyroidism and hypocalcemia but also to ensure that PTH is present to function in normal bone turnover to prevent the development of adynamic bone disease. The different surgical approaches (subtotal parathyroidectomy versus total parathyroidectomy with autotransplantation) does not seem to matter with respect to the efficacy of correction of and recurrence rate of severe secondary hyperparathyroidism (80, 77). However, it is the presence of nodular hyperplasia that is correlated with recurrence of the hyperparathyroidism (78, 80, 77). Thus it is important that the auto-transplanted or remnant tissue be from areas of the glands that do not contain nodular hyperplasia. Frozen histologic sections may aid in this determination. Finally, the development of rapid techniques to determine calcitriol receptor and calcium receptor densities may be helpful. Pre-operative or intraoperative knowledge of areas of parathyroid tissue with diminished calcitriol and calcium receptors should help in avoiding those areas for use in auto-transplantation as these areas would likely stem from domains of nodular hyperplasia.

Adynamic Bone Disease

Adynamic bone disease is one of the low-turnover bone diseases and is histomorphometrically characterized by a paucity of both osteoblasts and osteoclasts and a low bone formation rate. In general, there is a normal osteoid volume due to a proportional decrease in the deposition of osteoid by osteoblasts and the bone formation rate. A review of a number of series by Felsenfeld (84) concluded that histomorphometric criteria for adynamic bone has not been strictly defined. Most series tend to use an osteoid volume of less than 12-15% as a major criteria for the separation of adynamic bone and osteomalacia while the study by Llach, et. al. (85), often used as a standard for comparison with more recent studies used an osteoid volume of less than 5% as a criteria for adynamic bone. Such differences in criteria would affect the reported incidence of adynamic bone disease as osteoid volumes of >5% would be reported as osteomalacia in this latter study while osteomalacia would not be reported until the osteoid volume exceeded 12-15% in the former studies. The incidence of adynamic bone disease has been reported to be approximately 20% in all dialysis patients as reported by Malluche and Monier-Faugere (86) or 49.4% as reported by Hercz, et. al., 1993). However, adynamic disease has been observed at a higher incidence in patients on peritoneal dialysis compared to patients on hemodialysis (20, 87).

Pathogenesis. The development of adynamic bone disease has been ascribed to or associated with 1) aluminum deposition along the mineralizing front, 2) peritoneal dialysis, 3) diabetes mellitus, 4) calcium loading either by oral intake of calcium or by high dialysate calcium concentration, 5) calcitriol treatment, 6) older age, 7) acidosis, and 8) cytokines such as interleukins 4 and 11, and osteogenic protein-1 (88).

Increases in serum ionized calcium due to ingestion of calcium-containing phosphate binders, increased gut absorption of calcium by calcitriol, and the continuous exposure of chronic ambulatory peritoneal dialysis patients to high dialysate calcium (3.5 mEq/L) suppresses PTH secretion (20). As higher PTH levels are necessary to sustain bone turnover in patients with chronic renal failure due to skeletal resistance to PTH, the relative "lack" of PTH may be a factor in the generation of adynamic bone. When dynamic PTH secretion as a function of serum ionized calcium was examined, Sanchez, et. al. (89) found that while the setpoint for PTH secretion was unchanged, the slope of the

PTH/ionized calcium curve was less in adynamic bone lesion patients compared to those with secondary hyperparathyroidism. The authors concluded that the attenuated PTH secretory response in patients with adynamic disease suggests less sensitivity of the parathyroid glands to changes in serum ionized calcium. Goodman, et. al. (15) showed that when 14 children and adolescents on peritoneal dialysis and who had either osteitis fibrosa or mild lesions of secondary hyperparathyroidism by bone biopsy were treated with calcitriol, adynamic bone was seen in 6 patients after one year of therapy. Six other patients reverted to normal bone histology. PTH levels declined in the patients developing adynamic bone. However, bone formation rate decreased even in those patients having increased PTH levels that did not change after treatment with calcitriol. Thus calcitriol may reduce bone turnover independent of PTH suppression. Calcitriol has been shown to inhibit proliferation and decrease collagen synthesis in osteoblasts and thus have the potential to lead to adynamic bone. Finally, diabetes mellitus may predispose renal failure patients to adynamic bone disease of aluminum or non-aluminum etiology by the suppression of PTH secretion by hyperglycemia and insulin deficiency (33). The lack of appropriate levels of PTH leads to low bone turnover and an inability to extract aluminum from the mineralizing front.

Whether adynamic bone in the absence of stainable aluminum as demonstrated by bone biopsy is pathological is still unclear. Indeed in a recent review Musci and Hercz (90) stated that while in their earlier study patients with adynamic bone without aluminum accumulation were asymptomatic (32), their more recent data from suggested that there may be an increase in musculoskeletal symptoms. However, others have not reported that adynamic bone was associated with clinical symptomatology in the absence of aluminum bone disease (75). It has been suggested that at least in children, reduction of bone formation and bone turnover may adversely affect longitudinal bone growth during skeletal maturation (37). In adults it has been shown that adynamic bone has a very low capacity to buffer calcium by incorporation of serum calcium into bone matrix after a calcium load. This observation is the likely explanation for the increased frequency of hypercalcemia in patients with adynamic disease (91).

Management of Adynamic Bone

Although it is unclear if adynamic bone is truly pathologic, patients with this lesion are at risk for hypercalcemia and may develop musculoskeletal symptomatology (90). Since a relative deficiency of PTH may be central to the pathogenesis of adynamic bone, it would seem prudent to maintain PTH levels at 100-200 pg/ml in hemodialysis patients and 100-300 pg/ml in peritoneal dialysis patients (32, 75). Vitamin D analogs should not be used until PTH levels are above four to six times the upper limit of the normal range. Furthermore, dialysate calcium should be individually tailored so that adequate amounts of calcium phosphate binders can be used to effectively control serum phosphorus levels (lowering dialysate calcium if necessary to prevent hypercalcemia when calcium phosphate binders are used). In those patients with low PTH levels who are currently being treated with vitamin D metabolites, it is suggested that the vitamin D metabolites be discontinued to allow PTH levels to rise. While the temporary use of aluminum gels to control phosphorus levels may be necessary if calcium phosphate binders need to be stopped, it may be prudent to consider the use of magnesium salts and low magnesium dialysate in place of the aluminum gels. Finally, at least in diabetic patients with adynamic bone disease, tight glucose control with appropriate insulin regimens would be in order.

Contribution of Acidemia to Bone Loss. Bone mineral is composed of hydroxyapatite (Ca10(PO4)6(OH)2) and serves as a buffer for hydrogen ions. A decrease in systemic pH leads to an increased exchange of hydrogen ions for sodium and potassium and sodium from bone mineral surface. Additionally, bone contains 80% of the total pool of CO3-2, HCO3--, and CO2 in the body. Approximately one-third of this pool consists of HCO3- located in the hydration shell of hydroxyapatite and is readily accessible to the systemic circulation where protons can complex with HCO3-. Thus the net result with prolonged acidemia is the loss of base and the leaching of calcium, sodium, and potassium from bone (**Figure 4**).

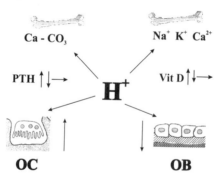

Figure 4: Schematic Representation of the Effects of Acidosis on Bone. Protons (H+) can be exchanged with sodium (Na+), potassium (K+), and calcium (Ca2+) at the surface of bone or complexed with carbonate (CO3) deeper within bone which would buffer protons generated in metabolic acidosis. At least in vitro, metabolic acidosis can cause increased osteoclastic bone resorption (OC) and a decrease in bone protein matrix production by osteoblasts (OB). The effects of metabolic acidosis have been reported to increase, decrease, or cause no change in PTH and vitamin D levels.

The loss of bone in states of chronic acidemia is due to both a physicochemical effect of bone mineral dissolution (92, 93) as well as the stimulation of the cell-mediated process of osteoclastic bone resorption (94). The physicochemical effects on calcium release from bone are more immediate while cell-mediated calcium release occurs with more chronic exposure to acidosis. Moreover, chronic metabolic acidosis in in vitro studies has also been shown to decrease osteoblastic activity which results in a decrease in collagen synthesis (95) and inhibition of mineralized bone nodule formation (96). Interestingly in this latter study, metabolic acidosis had a greater effect on bone nodule inhibition than did respiratory acidosis. Differences in the degree of calcium loss from bone with metabolic versus respiratory acidosis may be due to differences in intracellular pH and calcium. Ori, et. al. (97) reported that similar decrements in pH in respiratory acidosis decreased intracellular pH more as compared to metabolic acidosis; moreover, initial changes in cytosolic calcium were higher in respiratory acidosis than in metabolic acidosis. How these intracellular ionic changes affect bone cell function remain to be elucidated.

While in vivo observations in azotemic humans with metabolic acidosis have suggested that the dominant histologic finding is osteomalacia (98, 99), animal studies have not been able to demonstrate that metabolic acidosis results in osteomalacia (100, 101). The data regarding the effect of metabolic acidosis on PTH levels suggest that correction of metabolic acidosis may decrease PTH levels. Lefebvre, et. al (102) reported that PTH levels were increased in dialysis patients who had predialysis bicarbonate levels of approximately 16 mEq/L and that PTH levels decreased when supplemental bicarbonate was added to the dialysis bath and the predialysis bicarbonate was increased to 24 mEq/L. Lu, et. al. (103) treated predialysis chronic renal failure patients with bicarbonate infusion while serum ionized calcium levels were clamped at constant values and found that correction of the metabolic acidosis decreased PTH levels.

The effect of metabolic acidosis on the PTH-ionized calcium curve is less clear. Correction of acidosis in hemodialysis patients has also been reported to shift the PTH-ionized calcium curve downward and to the left suggesting PTH suppression by increased sensitivity of the parathyroid glands to a given ionized calcium level (104). However, Ouseph, et. al. (105) could not find a difference in the PTH / ionized calcium curves in dialysis patients that had serum bicarbonate levels either less than 20 mEq/l (metabolic acidosis group) or greater than 22 mEq/L (normal group). Similarly, de Precigout, et. al. (106) could not find a difference in PTH or vitamin D metabolite levels in dialysis patients whose metabolic acidosis was corrected; PTH-ionized calcium curves were also not different prior to or after correction of metabolic acidosis. Thus an increase, decrease, or no change in serum levels have been reported and these have probably been confounded by concomitant hyperphosphatemia (107), chronicity of the acidosis, and various assays for PTH and vitamin D metabolites (101, 108). What can be concluded however, is that metabolic acidosis in chronic renal failure may worsen renal osteodystrophy. How specific forms of renal osteodystrophy (high turnover versus low turnover) diseases are affected by superimposed metabolic acidosis needs to be further investigated.

Correction of Acidosis. The previous discussion on the effects of acidemia on bone concluded that chronic acidemia from renal failure can lead to a loss of calcium from bone and the depletion of bone buffering stores of HCO3-. Ritz, et. al. (52) also advocated correction of metabolic acidosis as there appears to be a positive correlation between metabolic acidosis and PTH levels. Clearly, it is imperative that the acidemia of renal failure be treated. Bushinsky has suggested that the serum HCO3- concentration be kept within the normal range (109). This can be accomplished by adjusting the HCO3- concentration in the dialysate bath of hemodialysis patients. Oettinger and Oliver (110) found that a high-bicarbonate dialysate (42 mEq/L) corrected pre-dialysis acidosis in 75% of their hemodialysis patients without causing pre-dialysis alkalemia or changes in ionized calcium and phosphorus. However, post-dialysis alkalemia resulted with pH of 7.50 and serum HCO3- concentration of approximately 34 mM. The use of exogenous sodium bicarbonate has also been advocated with the caveat that doing so may increase the sodium load to the patient (109, 111). In predialysis patients, natriuresis resulting from increased sodium ingestion may also result in calciuria with further loss of body calcium. Additionally, the use of loop diuretics in predialysis patients with renal failure may also result in enhanced calciuresis. Thus further investigation is warranted prior to settling on the most appropriate avenue to adequately correct acidosis in dialysis patients without subjecting them to problems attendant with post-dialysis alkalemia.

In postmenopausal women without renal failure, oral potassium bicarbonate has been shown to neutralize endogenous acid production, decrease bone resorption, and to decrease calcium and phosphorus loss (112). The use of calcium carbonate as a phosphorus binder is also efficacious in neutralizing acids. Consideration should be given to the protein load in dialysis and predialysis patients as endogenous acid production of approximately 1 mEq/L per kg body weight occurs as a result of protein intake. (113). Thus at least in predialysis patients, there is probably a need to decrease protein load from the standpoint of lessening glomerular hyperfiltration but also the concept that protein loading increases acid production which results in bone mineral losses is also important. In the dialysis patient, while limitation of protein should theoretically limit acid production, the feasibility of such an approach would be limited if protein restriction resulted in malnourished dialysis patients with increases in morbidity and mortality. However, as reviewed by Barzel (113), ingestion of vegetable protein rather than animal protein may decrease acid production and calcium loss, and thus be the preferred type of protein in patients with chronic renal disease.

In summary, there are a number of issues that still need to be resolved. Although it has been suggested that acidosis in renal failure be corrected to prevent bone mineral loss, whether normalization of pre-dialysis serum HCO3- levels in dialysis patients will alter the course or histologic patterns of renal osteodystropy and/or exacerbate bone loss remain to be investigated. Similarly, in vivo effects of acute and chronic acidosis on osteoblast function and bone formation remain to be detailed as are the issues regarding the effects of acidosis on vitamin D and PTH synthesis and metabolism in vivo.

References

1. Bricker, NS 1972 On the pathogenesis of the uremic state: An exposition of the "trade-off hypothesis." N Engl J Med 286:1093-1099.

2. Delmez, JA 1993 Long-term complications of dialysis: Pathogenetic factors with special reference to bone. Kidney Int 43(Suppl 41):S116-S120.

3. Fine, A, Cox, D, Fontaine, B 1993 Elevation of serum phosphate affects parathyroid hormone levels in only 50% of hemodialysis patients, which is unrelated to changes in serum calcium. J Am Soc Nephrol 3:1947-1953.

4. Lopez-Hilker, S, Dusso, A, Rapp, N, Martin, KJ, Slatopolsky, E 1990 Phosphorus restriction reverses hyperparathyroidism in uremia independent of changes in calcium and calcitriol. Am J Physiol 259:F432-F437.

5. Almaden, Y, Canalejo, A, Hernandez, A, Ballesteros, E, Garcia-Navarro, S, Torres, A, Rodriguez, M 1996 Direct effect of phosphorus on PTH secretion from whole rat parathyroid glands in vitro. J Bone Miner Res 11:970-976.

6. Hernandez, A, Concepcion, MT, Rodriguez, M, Salido, E, Torres, A 1996 High phosphorus diet increases preproPTH mRNA independent of calcium and calcitriol in normal rats. Kidney Int 50:1872-1878.

7. Naveh-Many, T, Rahaminov, R, Livni, N, Silver, J 1995 Parathyroid cell proliferation in normal and chronic renal failure rats. The effects of calcium phosphate and vitamin D. J Clin Invest 96:1786-1793.

8. Kilav, R, Silver, J, Naveh-Many, T 1995 Parathyroid hormone gene expression in hypophosphatemic rats. J Clin Invest 96:327-333.

9. Portale, AA, Booth, BE, Halloran, BP, Morris, RC Jr 1989 Physiologic regulation of the serum concentration of 1,25-dihydroxyvitamin D by phosphorus in normal men. J Clin Invest 83:1494-1499.

10. Rodriguez, M, Felsenfeld, AJ, Williams, C, Pederson, JA, Llach, F 1991 The effect of long-term intravenous calcitriol administration on parathyroid function in hemodialysis patients. J Am Soc Nephrol 2:1014-1020.

11. Bover, J, Rodriguez, M, Trinidad, P, Jara, A, Martinez, ME, Machado, L, Llach, F, Felsenfeld, AJ 1994 Factors in the development of secondary hyperparathyroidism during graded renal failure in the rat. Kidney Int 45:953-961.

12. Tallon, S, Berdud, I, Hernandez, A, Concepcion, MT, Almaden, Y, Torres, A, Martin-Malo, A, Felsenfeld, AJ, Aljama, P, Rodriguez, M 1996 Relative effects of PTH and dietary phosphorus on calcitriol production in normal and azotemic rats. Kidney Int 49:1441-1446.

13. Urena, P, Kubrusly, M, Mannstadt, M, Hruby, M, Tan, M-M TT, Silve, C, Lacour, B, Abou-Samra, A-B, Segre, GV, Drueke, T 1994 The renal PTH/PTHrP receptor is down-regulated in rats with chronic renal failure. Kidney Int 45:605-611.

224

14. Urena, P, Mannstadt, M, Hruby, M, Ferreira, A, Schmitt, F, Silve, C, Ardaillou, R, Lacour, B, Abou-Samra, A-B, Segre, GV, Drueke, T 1995 Parathyroidectomy does not prevent the renal PTH/PTHrP receptor down-regulation in uremic rats. Kidney Int 47:1797-1805.

15. Goodman, WG, Ramirez, JA, Belin, TR, Chon, Y, Gales, B, Segre, GV, Salusky, IB 1994 Development of adynamic bone in patients with secondary hyperparathyroidism after intermittent calcitriol therapy. Kidney Int 46:1160-1166.

16. Gonzalez, EA, Martin, KJ 1996 Coordinate regulation of PTH/PTHrP receptors by PTH and calcitriol in UMR 106-01 osteoblast-like cells. Kidney Int 50:63-70.

17. Andress, DL, Howard, GP, Birnbaum, RS 1991 Identification of a low molecular weight inhibitor of osteoblast mitogenesis in uremic plasma. Kidney Int 39:942-945.

18. Cohen-Solalm ME, Sebert, JL, Boudailliez, B, Marie, A, Moriniere, P, Gueris, J, Bouillon, R, Fournier, A 1991 Comparison of intact, midregion, and carboxy-terminal assays of parathyroid hormone for the diagnosis of bone disease in hemodialyzed patients. J Clin Endocrinol Metab 73:516-524.

19. Pei, Y, Hercz, G, Greenwood, C, Segre, G, Manuel, A, Saiphoo, C, Fenton, S, Sherrard, D 1995 Risk factors for renal osteodystrophy: A multivariate analysis. J Bone Miner Res 10:149-156.

20. Sherrard, DJ, Hercz, G, Pei, Y, Maloney, NA, Greenwood, C, Manuel, A, Saiphoo, C, Fenton, SS, Segre, GV 1993 The spectrum of bone disease in end-stage renal failure--An evolving disorder. Kidney Int 43:436-442.

21. Salusky, IB, Ramirez, JA, Oppenheim, W, Gales, B, Segre, GV, Goodman, WG 1994 Biochemical markers of renal osteodystrophy in pediatric patients undergoing CAPD/CCPD. Kidney Int 45:253-258.

22. Urena, P, Ferreira, A, Kung, VT, Morieux, C, Simon, P, Ang, KS, Souberbielle, JC, Segre, GV, Drueke, TB, de Vernejoul, M-C 1995 Serum pyridinoline as a specific marker of collagen breakdown and bone metabolism in hemodialysis patients. J Bone Miner Res 10:932-939.

23. Schmidt-Gayk, H, Drueke, T, Ritz, E 1996 Non-invasive circulating indicators of bone metabolism in uraemic patients: can they replace bone biopsy? Nephrol Dial Transplant 11:415-418.

24. Coen, G, Mazzaferro, S 1994 Bone metabolism and its assessment in renal failure. Nephron 67:383-401.

25. Fournier, A, Porisiu, R, Said, S, Sechet, A, Ghazali, A, Marie, A, el Esjer, I, Brazier, M, Archard, JM, Moriniere, P 1997 Invasive versus non-invasive diagnosis of renal bone disease. Current Opinion in Nephrol Hyperten 6:333-348.

225

26. Urena, P, Hruby, M, Ferreira, A, Ang, KS, de Vernejoul, M-C 1996 Plasma total versus bone alkaline phosphatase as markers of bone turnover in hemodialysis patients. J Am Soc Nephrol 7:506-512.

27. Salusky, IB, Goodman, W 1996 Skeletal response to intermittent calcitriol therapy in secondary hyperparathyroidism. Kidney Int 49(Suppl 53):S135-S139.

28. Joffe, P, Heaf, JG, Hyldstrup, L 1994 Osteocalcin: A non-invasive index of metabolic bone disease in patients treated by CAPD. Kidney Int 46:838-846.

29. Sperschneider, H, Abendroth, K, Gunther, K, Stein, G 1992 Significance of osteocalcin in diagnosis of renal bone disease in hemodialysis patients. Klin Lab 38:202-210.

30. Malluche, HH, Monier-Faugere-Monier, M-C 1994 The role of bone biopsy in the management of patients with renal osteodystrophy. J Am Soc Nephrol 4:1631-1642.

31. Parfitt, AM, Drezner, MK, Glorieux, FH, Kanis, JA, Malluche, HH, Meunier, PJ, Ott, SM, Recker, RR 1987 Bone histomorphometry: standardization of nomenclature, symbols, and units. J Bone Miner Res 2:595-610.

32. Hercz, G, Pei, Y, Greenwood, C, Manuel, A, Saiphoo, C, Goodman, WG, Segre, GV, Fenton, S, Sherrard, DJ 1993 Aplastic osteodystrophy without aluminum: The role of "suppressed" parathyroid function. Kidney Int 44:860-866.

33. Pei, Y, Hercz, G, Greenwood, C, Segre, G, Manuel, A, Saiphoo, C, Fenton, S, Sherrard, D 1993 Renal osteodystrophy in diabetic patients. Kidney Int 44:159-164.

34. Frazao, JM, Coburn, JW 1996 Aluminum toxicity in patients with end-stage renal disease: Diagnosis, treatment, and prevention. Rev Port Nefrol Hipert 10(Suppl 1):S85-S112.

35. Mathias, R, Salusky, I, Harman, W, Paredes, A, Emans, J, Segre, G, Goodman, W 1993 Renal bone disease in pediatric and young adult patients on hemodialysis in a Children's Hospital. J Am Soc Nephrol 3:1938-1946.

36. Indridason, OS, Heath, H III, Khosla, S, Yohay, DA, Quarles, LD 1996 Non-suppressible parathyroid hormone secretion is related to gland size in uremic secondary hyperparathyroidism. Kidney Int 50:1663-1671.

37. Goodman, WG, Belin, T, Gales, B, Juppner, H, Segre, GV, Salusky, IB 1995 Calcium-regulated parathyroid hormone release in patients with mild or advanced secondary hyperparathyroidism. Kidney Int 48:1553-1558.

38. Pahl, M, Jara, A, Bover, J, Rodriguez, M, Felsenfeld, AJ 1996 The set point of calcium and the reduction of parathyroid hormone in hemodialysis patients. Kidney Int 49:226-231.

39. Rodriguez, M, Caravaca, F, Fernandez, E, Borrego, MJ, Lorenzo, V, Cubero, J, Martin-Malo, A, Betriu, A, Rodriguez, AP, Felsenfeld, AJ 1997 Evidence for both abnormal set point of

226

PTH stimulation by calcium and adaptation to serum calcium in hemodialysis patients with hyperparathyroidism. J Bone Miner Res 12:347-355.

40. Brown, EM, Hebert, SC 1996 A cloned extracellular Ca2+-sensing receptor: Molecular mediator of the actions of extracellular Ca2+ on parathyroid and kidney cells? Kidney Int 49:1042-1046.

41. Silver, J, Russell, J, Sherwood, LM, 1985 Regulation by vitamin D metabolites of messenger ribonucleic acid for preproparathyroid hormone in isolated bovine parathyroid cells. Proc Natl Acad Sci (USA) 82:4270-4273.

42. Silver, J, Naveh-Many, T, Mayer, H, Schmelzer, HJ, Popovtzer, MM 1986 Regulation by vitamin D metabolites of parathyroid hormone gene transcription in vivo in the rat. J Clin Invest 78:1296-1301.

43. Brown, AJ, Dusso, A, Lopez-Hilker, S, Lewis-Finch, J, Grooms, P, Slatopolsky, E 1989 1,25(OH)2D receptors are decreased in parathyroid glands from chronically uremic dogs. Kidney Int 35:19-23.

44. Patel, SR, Ke, HQ, Hsu, CH 1994 Regulation of calcitriol receptor and its mRNA in normal and renal failure rats. Kidney Int 45:1020-1027.

45. Szabo, A, Merke, J, Beier, E, Mall, G, Ritz, E 1989 1,25(OH)2 vitamin D3 inhibits parathyroid cell proliferation in experimental uremia. Kidney Int 35:1049-1056.

46. Silver, J, Bar Sela, S, Naveh-Many, T 1997 Regulation of parathyroid cell proliferation. Current Opinion in Nephrol Hyperten 6:321-326.

47. Parfitt, AM 1997 The hyperparathyroidism of chronic renal failure: A disorder of growth. Kidney Int 52:3-9.

48. Fukuda, N, Tanaka, H, Tominaga, Y, Fukagawa, M, Kurokawa, S, Seino, Y 1993 Decreased 1,25-dihydroxyvitamin D3 receptor density is associated with a more severe form of parathyroid hyperplasia in chronic uremic patients. J Clin Invest 92:1436-1442.

49. Arnold, A, Brown, MF, Urena, P, Gaz, RD, Sarfati, E, Drueke, TB 1995 Monoclonality of parathyroid tumors in chronic renal failure and in primary parathyroid hyperplasia. J Clin Invest 95:2047-2053.

50. Drueke, TB 1995 The pathogenesis of parathyroid gland hyperplasia in chronic renal failure. Kidney Int 48:259-272.

51. Ritz, E, Matthias, S, Seidel, A, Reichel, H, Szabo, A, Horl, WH 1992 Disturbed calcium metabolism in renal failure--Pathogenesis and therapeutic strategies. Kidney Int 42(Suppl. 38):S37-S42.

52. Felsenfeld. AJ 1997 Considerations for the treatment of secondary hyperparathyroidism in renal failure. J Am Soc Nephrol 8:993-1004.

53. Rodriguez, M, Martin-Malo, A, Martinez, ME, Torres, A, Felsenfeld, AJ, Llach, F 1991 Calcemic response to parathyroid hormone in renal failure: Role of phosphorus and its effect on calcitriol. Kidney Int 40:1055-1062.

54. Quarles, LD, Yohay, DA, Carroll, BA, Spritzer, CE, Minda, SA, Bartholomay D, Lobaugh, BA 1994 Prospective trial of pulse oral versus intravenous calcitriol treatment of hyperparathyroidism in ESRD. Kidney Int 45:1710-1721.

55. Jara, A, Bover, J, Felsenfeld, AJ, Nemeh, M, Levine, BS 1995 Divalent Ion Metabolism in Current Nephrology, Volume 18, Ed. H Gonick, Mosby Year Book, Inc, pp.133-182.

56. Fournier, A, Moriniere, P, Sebert, JL, Dkhissi, H, Atik, A, Leflon, P, Renaud, H, Gueris, J, Gregoire, I, Idrissi, A 1986 Calcium carbonate, an aluminum-free agent for control of hyperphosphatemia, hypocalcemia, and hyperparathyroidism. Kidney Int 29:S114-S119.

57. Slatopolsky, E, Weerts, C, Lopez-Hilker, S, Norwood, K, Zink, M, Windus, D, Delmez, J 1986 Calcium carbonate as a phosphate-binder in patients with chronic renal failure undergoing dialysis. N Engl J Med 315:157-161.

58. Fournier, A, Moriniere, P, Ben Hamida, F, el Esjer, N, Shenovda, M, Ghazali, A, Bouzernidj, M, Archard, JM, Westeel, PF 1992 Use of alkaline calcium salts as phosphate binder in uremic patients. Kidney Int 42(Suppl 38):S50-S61.

59. Delmez, JA, Tindira, CA, Windus, DW, Norwood, KY, Giles, KS, Nighswander, TL, Slatopolsky, E 1992 Calcium acetate as a phosphorus binder in hemodialysis patients. J Am Soc Nephrol 3:96-102.

60. Coburn, JW, Frazao, J 1996 Calcitriol in the management of renal osteodystrophy. Seminars in Dialysis 9:316-326.

61. Oettinger, CW, Oliver, JC, Macon, EJ 1992 The effects of calcium carbonate as the sole phosphate binder in combination with low calcium dialysate and calcitriol therapy in chronic hemodialysis patients. J Am Soc Nephrol 3:995-1001.

62. Fernandez, E, Borras, M, Pais, B, Montoliu, J 1995 Low-calcium dialysate stimulates parathormone secretion and its long-term use worsens secondary hyperparathyroidism. J Am Soc Nephrol 6:132-135.

63. Delmez, JA, Kelber, J, Norwood, KY, Giles, KS, Slatopolsky, E 1996 Magnesium carbonate as a phosphorus binder: A prospective, controlled, crossover study. Kidney Int 49:163-167.

64. Gallieni, M, Brancaccio, D, Padovese, P, Rolla, D, Bedani, P, Colantonio, G, Bronziere, C, Bagni, B, Tarolo, G 1992 Low-dose intravenous calcitriol treatment of secondary hyperparathyroidism in hemodialysis patients. Kidney Int 42:1191-1198.

65. Levine, BS, Song, M 1996 Pharmacokinetics and efficacy of pulse oral versus intravenous calcitriol in hemodialysis patients. J Am Soc Nephrol 7:488-496.

66. Quarles, LD, Yohay, DA, Carroll, BA, Spritzer, CE, Minda, SA, Lobaugh, BL 1994 Prospective trial of pulse oral versus intravenous calcitriol treatment of hyperparathyroidism in ESRD. Kidney Int 45:1710-1721.

67. Hermann, P, Ritz, E, Schmidt-Gayk, H, Schafer, I, Geyer, J, Nonnast-Daniel, B, Koch, K-M, Weber, U, Horl, W, Haas-Worle, A, Kuhn, K, Bierther, B, Schneider, P 1994 Comparison of intermittent and continuous oral administration of calcitriol in dialysis patients: A randomized prospective trial. Nephron 67:48-53.

68. Slatopolsky, E, Berkoben, M, Kelber, J, Brown, A, Delmez, J 1992 Effects of calcitriol and non-calcemic vitamin D analogs on secondary hyperparathyroidism. Kidney Int 42(Suppl 38):S43-S49.

69. Finch, JL, Brown, AJ, Mori, T, Nishii, Y, Slatopolsky, E 1992 Suppression of PTH and decreased action on bone are partially responsible for the low calcemic activity of 22-oxacalcitriol relative to 1,25-(OH)2D3. J Bone Miner Res 7:835-839.

70. Finch, JL, Brown, AJ, Kubodera, N, Nishii, Y, Slatopolsky, E 1993 Differential effects of 1,25-(OH)2D3 and 22-oxacalcitriol on phosphate and calcium metabolism. Kidney Int 43:561-566.

71. Denda, M, Finch, J, Brown, AJ, Nishii, Y, Kubodera, N, Slatopolsky, E 1996 1,25-Dihydroxyvitamin D3 and 22-oxacalcitriol prevent the decrease in vitamin D receptor content in the parathyroid glands of uremic rats. Kidney Int 50:34-39.

72. Kubrusly, M, Gagne, E-R, Urena, P, Hanrotel, C, Chabanis, S, Lacour, B, Drueke, TB 1993 Effect of 22-oxa-calcitriol on calcium metabolism in rats with severe secondary hyperparathyroidism. Kidney Int 44:551-556.

73. Tan, Jr, AU, Levine, BS, Mazess, RB, Kyllo, DM, Bishop, CW, Knutson, JC, Kleinman, KS, Coburn, JW 1997 Effective suppression of parathyroid hormone by 1a-hydroxyvitamin D2 in hemodialysis patients with moderate to severe secondary hyperparathyroidism. Kidney Int 51:317-323.

74. Fournier, A, Oprisiu, R, Yverneau-Hardy, P, Ghazali, A, el Esjer, N, Moriniere, P 1996 Vitamin D and renal osteodystrophy: From basic science to clinical practice. Rev Port Nefrol Hipert 10(Suppl 1):S9-S36.

75. Fox, J, Hadfield, S, Petty, BA, Conklin, RL, Nemeth, EP 1993 NPS R-568 inhibits parathyroid hormone secretion and stimulates calcitonin secretion in hyperparathyroid rats with chronic renal failure. J Am Soc Nephrol 4:719.

76. Drueke, TB, Zingraff, J 1994 The dilemma of parathyroidectomy in chronic renal failure. Current Opinion in Nephrol Hyperten 3:386-395.

77. Tominaga, Y, Numano, M, Tanaka, Y, Uchida, K, Takagi, H 1997 Surgical treatment of renal hyperparathyroidism. Seminars Surg Oncology 13:87-96.

78. Gallieni, M, Brancaccio, D 1994 Which is the preferred treatment of advanced hyperparathyroidism in a renal patient? I. Medical intervention is the primary option in the treatment of advanced hyperparathyroidism in chronic renal failure. Nephrol Dial Transplant 9:1816-1821.

79. Gagne, E-R, Urena, P, Leite-Silva, S, Zingraff, J, Chevalier, A, Sarfati, E, Dubost, C, Drueke, TB 1992 Short- and long-term efficacy of total parathyroidectomy with immediate autografting compared with subtotal parathyroidectomy in hemodialysis patients. J Am Soc Nephrol 3:1008-1017.

80. Ritz, E 1994 II. Early parathyroidectomy should be considered as the first choice. Nephrol Dialy Transplant 9:1816-1821.

81. Fukagawa, M, Kitaoka, M, Inazawa, T, Kurokawa, K 1997 Imaging of the parathyroid in chronic renal failure: diagnostic and therapeutic aspects. Current Opinion in Nephrology and Hypertension 6:349-355.

82. Copley, JB, Hui, SL, Leapman, S, Slemenda, CW, Johnston, Jr, CC 1993 Longitudinal study of bone mass in end-stage renal disease patients: Effects of parathyroidectomy for renal osteodystrophy. J Bone Miner Res 8:415-422.

83. Felsenfeld, AJ 1996 Adynamic bone: Possible causes and possible strategies. Rev Port Nefrol Hipert 10(Supl 1):S59-S72.

84. Llach, F, Felsenfeld, AJ, Coleman, MD, Keveney, JJ, Pederson, JA, Medlock, TR 1986 The natural course of dialysis osteomalacia. Kidney Int 29(Suppl 18):S74-S79.

85. Malluche, HH, Monier-Faugere, M-C 1992 Risk of adynamic bone disease in dialyzed patients. Kidney Int 42(Suppl 38):S62-S67.

86. Hercz, G, Kraut, JA, Andress, DA, Howard, N, Roberts, C, Shinaberger, JH, Sherrard, DJ, Coburn, JW 1986 Use of calcium carbonate as a phosphate binder in dialysis patients. Miner Electrol Metab 12:314-319.

87. Hruska, KA, Teitelbaum, SL 1995 Renal osteodystrophy. N Engl J Med 333:166-174.

88. Sanchez, CP, Goodman, WG, Ramirez, JA, Gales, B, Belin, TR, Segre, GV, Salusky, IB 1995 Calcium-regulated parathyroid hormone secretion in adynamic renal osteodystrophy. Kidney Int 48:838-843.

89. Musci, I, Hercz, G 1997 Adynamic bone disease: pathogenesis, diagnosis and clinical relevance. Current Opinions in Nephrol Hyperten 7:356-361.

90. Kurz, P, Monier-Gaugere, M-C, Bognar, B, Werner, E, Roth, P, Vlachojannis, J, Malluche, HH 1994 Evidence for abnormal calcium homeostasis in patients with adynamic bone disease. Kidney Int 46:855-861.

91. Bushinsky, DA, Wolbach, W, Sessler, NE, Mogilevshy, R, Levi-Setti, R 1993 Physicochemical effects of acidosis on bone calcium flux and surface ion composition. J Bone Miner Res 8:93-102.

92. Bushinsky, DA, Sessler, NE, Glena, RE, Featherstone, JDB 1994 Proton-induced physicochemical calcium release from ceramic apatite disks. J Bone Miner Res 9:213-220.

93. Shibutani, T, Heersche, JNM 1993 Effect of medium pH on osteoclast activity and osteoclast formation in cultures of dispersed rabbit osteoclasts. J Bone Miner Res 8:331-336.

94. Kreiger, NS, Sessler, NE, Bushinsky, DA 1992 Acidosis inhibits osteoblastic and stimulates osteoclastic activity in vitro. Am J Physiol 262:F442-F448.

95. Sprague, SM, Kreiger, NS, Bushinsky, DA 1994 Greater inhibition of in vitro bone mineralization with metabolic than respiratory acidosis. Kidney Int 46:1199-1206.

96. Ori, Y, Lee, SG, Kreiger, NS, Bushinsky, DA 1995 Osteoblastic intracellular pH and calcium in metabolic and respiratory acidosis. Kidney Int 47:1790-1796.

97. Cunningham, J, Fraher, LJ, Clemens, TL, Revell, PA, Papapoulos, SE 1982 Chronic acidosis with metabolic bone disease: effect of alkali on bone morphology and vitamin D metabolism. Am J Med 73:199-204.

98. Mora-Palma, FJ, Ellis, HA, Cook, DB, Dewar, JH, Ward, MK, Wilkinson, R, Kerr, DNS 1983 Osteomalacia in patients with chronic renal failure before dialysis or transplantation. Quart J Med, New Series LII 207:332-348.

99. Chan, Y-L, Savdie, E, Mason, RS, Posen, S 1985 The effect of metabolic acidosis on vitamin D metabolites and bone histology in uremic rats. Calcif Tissue Int 37:158-164.

100. Kraut, JA 1995 The role of metabolic acidosis in the pathogenesis of renal osteodystrophy. Adv Renal Replacement Therapy 2:40-51.

101. Lefebvre, A, De Vernejoul, C, Gueris, J, Goldfarb, B, Graulet, AM, Morieux, C 1989 Optimal correction of acidosis changes progression of dialysis osteodystrophy. Kidney Int 36:1112-1118.

102. Lu, K-C, Shieh, S-D, Li, B-L, Chu, P, Jan, S-Y, Lin, Y-F 1994 Rapid correction of metabolic acidosis in chronic renal failure: Effect on parathyroid hormone activity. Nephron 67:419-424.

103. Graham, KA, Hoenich, NA, Tarbit, M, Ward, MK, Goodship, THJ 1997 Correction of acidosis in hemodialysis patients increases the sensitivity of the parathyroid glands to calcium. J Am Soc Nephrol 8:627-631.

104. Ouseph, R, Leiser, JD, Moe, SM 1996 Calcitriol and the parathyroid hormone-ionized calcium curve: a comparison of methodologic approaches. J Am Soc Nephrol 7:497-505.

105. de Precigout, V, Combe, C, Blanchetier, V, Larroumet, N, Pommereau, A, Potaux, L, Aparicio, M 1995 Correction of chronic metabolic acidosis in haemodialyzed patients by acetate-free biofiltration does not influence parathyroid function. Nephrol Dial Transplant 10:821-824.

106. Horl, WH 1995 Is it necessary to treat metabolic acidosis in chronic renal insufficiency? Nephrol Dial Transplant 10:1542-1543.

107. Kleeman, CR 1994 The role of chronic anion gap and/or nonanion gap acidosis in the osteodystrophy of chronic renal failure in the predialysis era: A minority report. Miner Electrolyte Metab 20:81-96.

108. Bushinsky, DA 1995 The contribution of acidosis to renal osteodystrophy. Kidney Int 47:1816-1832.

109. Oettinger, CW, Oliver, JC 1993 Normalization of uremic acidosis in hemodialysis patients with a high bicarbonate dialysate. J Am Soc Nephrol 3:1804-1807.

110. Harris, DCH, Yuill, E, Chesher, DW 1995 Correcting acidosis in hemodialysis: Effect on phosphate clearance and calcification risk. J Am Soc Nephrol 6:1607-1612.

111. Sebastian, A, Harris, ST, Ottaway, JH, Todd, KM, Morris, RC, Jr 1994 Improved mineral balance and skeletal metabolism in postmenopausal women treated with potassium bicarbonate. N Engl J Med 330:1776-1781.

112. Barzel, US 1995 The skeleton as an ion exchange system: Implications for the role of acid-base imbalance in the genesis of osteoporosis. J Bone Miner Res 10:1431-1436.

113. Bichara, M, Mercier, O, Borensztein, P, Paillard, M 1990 Acute metabolic acidosis enhances circulating parathyroid hormone, which contributes to the renal response against acidosis in the rat. J Clin Invest 86:430-443.

114. Goodman, WG, Belin, TR, Salusky, IB 1996 In vivo assessments of calcium-regulated parathyroid hormone release in secondary hyperparathyroidism. Kidney Int 50:1834-1844.

115. Kraut, JA, Mishler, DR, Singer, FR, Goodman, WG 1986 The effects of metabolic acidosis on bone formation and bone resorption in the rat. Kidney Int 30:694-700.

116. Torres, A, Lorenzo, V, Hernandez, D, Rodriguez, JC, Concepcion, MT, Rodriguez, AP, Hernandez, A, De Bonis, E, Darias, E, Gonzalez-Posada, JM, Losada, M, Rufino, M, Felsenfeld, AJ, Rodriguez, M 1995 Bone disease in predialysis, hemodialysis, and CAPD patients: Evidence of a better bone response to PTH. Kidney Int 47:1434-1442.

117. Kifor, O, Moore, FD, Wang, P, Goldstein, M, Vassilev, P, Kifor, I, Hebert, SC, Brown, EM 1996 Reduced immunostaining for the extracellular Ca2+-sensing receptor in primary and uremic secondary hyperparathyroidism. J Clin Endocrinol Metab 81:1598-1606.

118. Gogusev, J, Duchambon, P, Hory, B, Giovannini, M. Goureau, Y, Sarfati, E, Drueke, TB 1997 Depressed expression of calcium receptor in parathyroid gland tissue of patients with hyperparathyroidism. Kidney Int 51:328-336.

14 Diagnosis and Treatment of Osteoporosis Associated with Immunosuppressive Therapy

Maria A. Rodino, M.D.

Elizabeth Shane, M.D.

Introduction

Immunosuppressive therapy is used to manage a variety of medical conditions. Common examples include hematologic malignancies; pulmonary diseases associated with chronic inflammation like asthma, emphysema, and cystic fibrosis; and autoimmune disorders such as systemic lupus erythematosus (SLE), rheumatoid arthritis, polymyalgia rheumatica, and myasthenia gravis, to name only a few. In addition, immunosuppressive therapy is essential in the management of the expanding population of organ transplant recipients. The armamentarium of immunosuppressive agents currently available includes glucocorticoids, the cyclosporines and tacrolimus, azathioprine and mycophenolate mofetil, and methotrexate. Unfortunately, several of these agents have deleterious effects on the skeleton. Glucocorticoids are well-known to cause osteoporosis (1-3). In addition, the cyclosporines (4,5) and methotrexate (6) have also been shown to adversely affect bone and mineral metabolism. This chapter will review the pathogenesis, diagnosis and management of osteoporosis associated with immunosuppressive therapy.

Pathogenesis of Bone Loss Associated with Immunosuppressive Therapy

Glucocorticoids. Glucocorticoids have both direct and indirect effects on bone and mineral homeostasis which have been recently reviewed (1-3). They directly inhibit bone formation by decreasing recruitment of osteoblasts to bone-forming surfaces and inhibiting osteoblastic synthesis of both type I collagen and non-collagenous proteins of bone. There is experimental evidence that glucocorticoids directly stimulate bone resorption as well. Although the precise mechanism of this effect is unknown, induction of interleukin-6 (IL-6) receptors on osteoclasts may be, in part, responsible. The net effect of these direct actions, uncoupling of bone formation and resorption, is rapid and often clinically significant bone loss. In addition to these specific effects on bone, glucocorticoids indirectly contribute to bone loss by inhibiting pituitary secretion of gonadotropins (decreased gonadal androgens and estrogens), adrenocorticotropic hormone (decreased adrenal androgens and estrogens), and growth hormone (decreased skeletal growth factors). In addition, glucocorticoids decrease intestinal absorption of calcium and increase urinary excretion of calcium, resulting in negative calcium balance which may promote secondary hyperparathyroidism and thereby increase bone resorption. Finally, the myopathy and muscle weakness that frequently accompany glucocorticoid treatment may also contribute to bone loss by reducing the normal forces on bone produced by muscle contraction.

Cyclosporine A. Cyclosporine A (CsA) is a small fungal peptide that inhibits T cell function. It is most commonly used to prevent rejection after organ transplantation. In animal studies, administration of CsA in doses higher than or comparable to those used after transplantation is associated with severe cancellous bone loss (4, 5) accompanied by increases in both bone resorption and formation. The effects of CsA on the rat skeleton appear to be mediated, at least in part, by increased expression of interleukin-1 (IL-1), a cytokine that stimulates bone resorption. These effects are partially reversible after CsA is discontinued and are blocked by drugs that inhibit bone resorption. In rats, CsA causes gonadal dysfunction which may also contribute to bone loss.

In the majority of post-transplant regimens, CsA is used in conjunction with pharmacologic doses of glucocorticoids. Therefore, it has been difficult to determine whether CsA has specific effects on bone and mineral metabolism in humans. However, certain data suggest that CsA may stimulate bone formation, an effect opposite to that usually observed with glucocorticoids. Serum osteocalcin, usually reduced in patients receiving glucocorticoids alone, has been reported to be elevated in renal (7, 8), cardiac (9) and liver (10) transplant recipients receiving both drugs. It remains possible, however, that elevated osteocalcin levels in transplant recipients reflect CsA-induced nephrotoxicity and associated decreased renal clearance of this small molecule.

Tacrolimus (FK506). Tacrolimus is a fungal macrolide used most commonly after liver transplantation. Its immunosuppressive actions are similar to, although more potent than, those of CsA. This has permitted the use of lower doses of glucocorticoids in patients managed with tacrolimus. In animal studies, bone loss associated with tacrolimus is of even greater magnitude than that observed with CsA. (11). As with CsA, tacrolimus is generally used in conjunction with glucocorticoids, and therefore its independent effects in humans have not been well defined. However, recent data indicate that the amount of bone loss is similar in cardiac (12) and liver (13) transplant recipients treated with tacrolimus or CsA.

Azathioprine and Mycophenolate Mofetil. Azathioprine, a derivative of mercaptopurine, is frequently used in conjunction with glucocorticoids and CsA after organ transplantation. In addition, it may be useful in the management of chronic active hepatitis, glomerulonephritis, myasthenia gravis, scleroderma and other autoimmune diseases. Long term studies of the effects of azathioprine on bone are not available. Short term studies in rats show no effect on bone volume, but do document an increase in osteoclast number (5). Human studies are not available.

Mycophenolate mofetil is a new immunosuppressive agent which inhibits B and T cell lymphocyte proliferation and is being used increasingly to replace azathioprine in transplantation immunotherapy. Animal studies suggest this drug does not affect bone mass (14). Human studies are not available.

Methotrexate. Methotrexate is a folate antagonist used in high doses to treat certain malignancies. In low doses, it is an effective and widely used treatment for rheumatoid and certain other inflammatory arthritides. Methotrexate, administered to rats in doses comparable to those received by patients on low dose weekly methotrexate, causes cancellous bone loss. The mechanism of the bone loss appears to be uncoupling of bone formation and resorption as supported by decreased serum osteocalcin and increased urinary hydroxyproline and confirmed by histomorphometric studies (15). Severe osteoporosis has been reported in patients with rheumatoid arthritis or psoriasis treated with low dose methotrexate, but these patients have had other risk factors for osteoporosis (16). A recent 3-year study of patients with rheumatoid arthritis failed to show any difference in the rate of lumbar spine and femoral neck bone loss between methotrexate-treated patients and controls (17). However, if the methotrexate-treated patients received concomitant glucocorticoid therapy, they sustained significantly more bone loss (17).

Clinical Features of Bone Loss Associated with Immunosuppressive Therapy

Glucocorticoid-induced Osteoporosis. In 1932, Harvey Cushing first described bone loss as a complication of excess endogenous cortisol production in patients with ACTH-secreting pituitary adenomas (18). Today, exogenous glucocorticoid therapy is the most common cause of secondary osteoporosis. It is estimated that bone loss and/or fractures are present in 30-50% of patients treated with glucocorticoids for longer than 6 months (1, 2). Although such patients may have sustained bone loss related to immobilization or their underlying disease, most recent prospective studies have found that steroid-treated patients with rheumatoid arthritis and other collagen-vascular diseases such as giant cell arteritis and SLE, asthma, and sarcoidosis have more bone loss than disease-matched controls (1, 2).

Glucocorticoid-induced bone loss is most rapid during the first 6 months of therapy. Areas of the skeleton rich in trabecular or cancellous bone (ribs, vertebrae, and distal ends of long bones) are most severely affected, and are also the most common sites for fracture. Postmenopausal women may be at greater risk for fracture than other groups, perhaps because glucocorticoid-related bone loss is superimposed upon that already sustained because of aging and estrogen deficiency.

Dosing of glucocorticoids depends on the nature, severity and responsiveness of the disease. Patients may require more than 100 mg or less than 5 mg daily to control their illness. It is generally accepted that virtually all patients taking 10 or more mg daily of prednisone (or its equivalent) sustain significant bone loss regardless of age, race, gender or menopausal status. Doses between 7.5 and 10 mg per day of prednisone have also been shown to cause demineralization, particularly when administered for long periods of time. It is not clear whether there is a threshold glucocorticoid dose below which bone loss does not occur, since a single small dose (2.5 mg) of prednisone may affect the circadian rhythm of serum osteocalcin, suppressing the typical nocturnal rise (19). Even alternate-day glucocorticoid regimens (20) and inhaled steroids have been reported to cause bone loss (21).

Transplantation Osteoporosis. Transplant recipients are typically managed with "triple" immunosuppressive therapy. Such regimens virtually always include glucocorticoids, cyclosporine A or FK506, and either azathioprine or mycophenolate mofetil. A typical patient may receive 500 mg of methylprednisolone intraoperatively and 300-375 mg during the next 24 hours. Oral prednisone, 50-100 mg daily, is begun the second post-operative day, tapered to 30 mg by two weeks, 5 to 10 mg by 6 months and 0-10 mg by one year after transplantation. Rejection is usually treated with high dose oral or intravenous steroids. Transplant recipients usually remain on at least 5-10 mg of prednisone indefinitely, although in recent years, greater effort is made to taper these patients off glucocorticoids completely.

When the above doses of prednisone are given together with either CsA or FK506, rapid bone loss ensues (4, 22). Both lumbar spine and proximal femur are affected. Average rates of bone loss in transplant recipients range from 3% to 12%, with the majority occurring during the first 6 to 12 months. In many cases, immunosuppressant-induced bone loss is superimposed upon an already compromised skeleton. Most patients undergoing kidney transplantation have some form of renal osteodystrophy including hyperparathyroidism (with or without osteitis fibrosa), osteomalacia, osteosclerosis, or adynamic or aplastic bone disease (23). Patients awaiting lung transplantation are at risk for osteoporosis due to decreased mobility, hypoxia, malnutrition, vitamin D deficiency, tobacco use, and prior glucocorticoid therapy. In addition, cystic fibrosis, a common disease for which patients undergo lung transplantation, is often associated with osteoporosis and fractures (24). A recent cross-sectional study revealed that 45% of 55 patients awaiting lung transplantation had a BMD > 2 S.D. below age- and sex-matched controls (25). Similarly, at our institution, the majority of patients awaiting lung transplantation have either osteoporosis or low bone mass (26). Diseases for which patients commonly undergo liver transplantation, such as primary biliary cirrhosis, hemochromatosis, and steroid-treated, autoimmune chronic active hepatitis, may be associated with osteoporosis. In contrast to renal, hepatic, and respiratory failure, congestive heart failure has not been associated with a well-defined disorder of bone and mineral metabolism. However, mean bone mineral density has been reported to be lower in patients awaiting heart transplantation compared to age-matched normal individuals (27), and in another study, to young, normal individuals (28).

Fractures are also quite common following organ transplantation (4, 22) (**Table I**). In cardiac transplant recipients, the reported prevalence of vertebral fractures ranges from 18 to 50% (4, 22). In our own center, the incidence of vertebral fracture during the first year after transplantation was 35% (29). Post-menopausal women with low pre-transplant hip bone density were at greatest risk. However, men also fractured frequently, even when they had normal pre-transplant bone mass (29, 30). In liver transplant recipients, the incidence of fracture during the first post-transplant year ranges from 24 to 65%, the latter in women with primary biliary cirrhosis (4, 22). The reported incidence of fracture following lung transplantation is 25 to 37% (25, 31). Recent cross-sectional studies of fracture following renal transplantation vary from 7-11%, somewhat less perhaps due to the use of lower doses of immunosuppressants or to the fact that rejection is more easily detected in these patients (4, 22, 32, 33). Patients with Type I diabetes mellitus may have higher fracture rates (45%) after renal transplantation (33).

Diagnosis and Management of Osteoporosis Associated with Immunosuppressives

Before Immunotherapy. Since many patients who require immunosuppressive drugs already have pre-existing osteoporosis or low bone mass, a skeletal evaluation should be performed prior to or at the onset of therapy. The most important diagnostic studies to obtain are bone mineral density (BMD) (**Table II**) of the hip and spine. Patients with osteoporosis (T score > 2.5 standard deviations below normal peak bone mass) should begin therapy to increase bone mass. Moreover, since fractures occur at higher BMD in patients treated with glucocorticoids, it may also be reasonable to begin antiresorptive therapy in patients with osteopenia or low bone mass (T score between -1.0 and -2.5). Radiographs of the thoracic and lumbar spine should be obtained to diagnose prevalent vertebral fractures which are associated with increased risk of future fracture.

Biochemical evaluation should include serum calcium, intact parathyroid hormone, thyroid function tests, 25- hydroxyvitamin D and testosterone, since hypogonadism is common in men with chronic illnesses. Vitamin D deficiency and severe hypogonadism should be treated during the waiting period prior to transplantation or concomitant with the initiation of immunosuppressive therapy. Markers of bone formation (bone specific alkaline phosphatase and serum osteocalcin) and resorption (urinary pyridinium crosslink or N-telopeptide excretion) can also be measured, although they are primarily useful in the research setting.

After Immunosuppressive Therapy: General Measures

Whenever possible, efforts should be made to use the lowest effective dose of a short-acting immunosuppressive agent. An active life style with weight-bearing exercise may help reduce bone loss and maintain muscle strength, which, in turn,

Table I Fracture Incidence After Organ Transplantation

Kidney	3% to 10%
Liver	24% to 65%
Heart	18% to 36%
Lung	25% to 35%

Table II Prevention of Immunosuppressant-related Osteoporosis

Before Immunotherapy

1. Bone Mineral Density by DEXA
   T score < -2.5
   If T > 2.5, begin therapy for osteoporosis.

2. Lateral radiographs of thoracic and lumbar spine
   If prevalent fracture is present, begin therapy for osteoporosis.

3. Biochemical Evaluation
   Serum PTH, calcium, thyroid function tests, 25-hydroxy-vitamin D, testosterone.

4. Urinary markers (optional)
   N-telopeptide or pyridinium crosslinks
After Immunotherapy
General Measures
1. Use lowest possible effective dose of immunosuppressive agent
2. Provide 1500 mg daily of elemental calcium
3. Encourage mobilization and weight-bearing exercise, if possible
4. Treat hypogonadism

Specific Agents
1. Bisphosphonates
2. Calcitonin
3. Vitamin D metabolites
4. Hormone replacement therapy
5. Fluoride

may help prevent falls. A recent study suggests that resistance exercise training during the first few months following cardiac transplantation may help restore BMD in some patients (34). Since glucocorticoid-induced bone loss results in part from decreased intestinal calcium absorption and increased urinary calcium excretion, efforts should be made to optimize calcium balance with approximately 1500 mg elemental calcium per day unless contraindications exist (20).

After Immunosuppressive Therapy: Specific Agents

Since immunosuppressive therapy is often essential for survival, particularly in the organ transplant recipient, it is not always possible to use lower doses. Moreover, exercise and calcium supplementation alone are not adequate to prevent bone loss in many patients. Prevention of bone loss therefore requires the use of agents to help counteract the effects of immunosuppressive drugs on bone and mineral metabolism. These are categorized into drugs that inhibit bone resorption, such as bisphosphonates, calcitonin, and estrogen; those that stimulate bone formation, such as parathyroid hormone and sodium fluoride; and those for which the mechanism of action is not well-defined, such as testosterone and vitamin D.

Bisphosphonates. Bisphosphonates prevent bone loss by inhibiting bone resorption. Several of these agents have been shown to be effective in the prevention and treatment of glucocorticoid-induced bone loss (35-40). In a recent randomized, double-blind, placebo-controlled study of 141 men and women begun on high dose corticosteroid therapy (mean daily dose of prednisone = 20 mg) for a variety of rheumatologic conditions, 4 cycles of etidronate (400 mg/d for 14 days of every third month) prevented vertebral, femoral, and trochanteric bone loss (38). Alendronate, a more potent bisphosphonate, has been shown to prevent glucocorticoid-induced bone loss at the spine when given at doses of either 5 or 10 mg daily, and at the femoral neck and trochanter when given at a dose of 10 mg daily (39). In an open-label pilot study, pamidronate given intravenously every 3 months for 1 year caused an increase in bone mass in patients taking an average dose of 14 mg/d of prednisone (40).

Bisphosphonates have been demonstrated to prevent bone loss after transplantation as well. In a recent randomized study, bone loss was prevented in patients who received two intravenous infusions of pamidronate immediately and one month after renal transplantation (41). In a non-randomized study, cardiac transplant recipients were treated with a single intravenous infusion of 60 mg pamidronate within two weeks of transplantation followed by 4 cycles of oral etidronate (400 mg daily for 14 days every 3 months). Lumbar spine BMD declined by only 1.3% versus 7.4% in a group of historical controls (42). Bone loss at the femoral neck was also significantly reduced in the bisphosphonate-treated patients. The incidence of fracture one year after transplantation was 11% in the treated group compared to 35% in the untreated group (42). In contrast, cyclical etidronate, calcium, and 1αhydroxyvitamin D (1 mg daily) failed to prevent bone loss and fractures after liver transplantation (43). Clinical trials with alendronate are currently underway in organ transplant recipients.

Although bisphosphonates are promising agents for the prevention and therapy of immunosuppressant-related bone loss, they must be used with caution in certain clinical situations. Because they are renally excreted, bisphosphonates are not recommended in patients with moderate-to-severe renal insufficiency (serum creatinine > 3.0 mg/dl; creatinine clearance < 30 ml/min). Since both alendronate and pamidronate are associated with decreases in serum phosphorus and calcium, and increases in intact parathyroid hormone concentrations, these drugs could exacerbate hypophosphatemia or prolong the resolution of secondary hyperparathyroidism, common after renal transplantation. Finally, these drugs are not approved for use in pediatric populations where their use might affect skeletal growth.

Calcitonin. Calcitonin, another antiresorptive drug, has also been used to treat glucocorticoid-induced osteoporosis (44-46). Montemurro *et al.* studied 68 patients with sarcoidosis treated with prednisone and found that salmon calcitonin, given either by injection or intranasally, prevented bone loss at the lumbar spine (44). A recent randomized study comparing etidronate and injectable calcitonin after liver transplantation demonstrated a significant increase in vertebral BMD with both drugs (8.2% and 6.4%, respectively). No published data are available evaluating the efficacy of intranasal calcitonin in transplant recipients. However, our anecdotal experience with both injectable and intranasal calcitonin in the post-transplantation setting suggests that this drug may be relatively ineffective in preventing bone loss or fractures.

Estrogen. Many women requiring immunosuppressive therapy are either post-menopausal or pre-menopausal with hypothalamic amenorrhea related to their underlying illness. Moreover, both glucocorticoids as well as CsA and related compounds can inhibit gonadal steroid production. Post-menopausal and amenorrheic pre-menopausal women have rates of bone loss that exceed those of women with regular menses. Moreover, estrogens have been shown to reduce glucocorticoid-induced bone loss in post-menopausal women with asthma and rheumatoid arthritis (20, 49). Therefore, it is reasonable to offer hypoestrogenic women hormone replacement therapy. Estrogen has also been shown to prevent CsA-induced bone loss in animal studies (5). However, the extent to which hormone replacement alone may prevent bone loss after transplantation is unknown.

Analogues of Vitamin D. Vitamin D metabolites are commonly recommended in the management of both glucocorticoid and transplantation osteoporosis. The rationale for their use is based on the fact that these metabolites may counteract two important mechanisms of glucocorticoid-induced bone loss, namely, inhibition of intestinal calcium absorption and osteoblast function. In a study of 20 patients with rheumatoid arthritis treated with prednisone (daily dose, 5-15 mg), 1αhydroxuvota,om D_3 and calcitriol (1,25-dihydroxyvitamin D_3) significantly increased fractional calcium absorption and decreased serum parathyroid hormone concentrations (50). Moreover, calcitriol, at a daily dose of 0.6 μg, was shown to prevent lumbar spine bone loss in asthmatics begun on glucocorticoid therapy. The addition of calcitonin did not confer any additional benefit (51).

Vitamin D metabolites have been evaluated in transplant recipients as well. In one study, treatment with alphacalcidiol (0.5-1.0 mg daily) after cardiac transplantation, resulted in less bone loss at both the lumbar spine and femoral neck and fewer fractures than cyclic etidronate (52). Similarly, treatment with 0.5 μg daily of calcitriol for 2 years was effective in increasing lumbar spine and femoral neck BMD in 90 liver transplant recipients (53). In renal allograft recipients randomly selected to receive both 40 mg of calcidiol and 3 gm calcium carbonate daily, bone loss at the lumbar spine and femoral neck was prevented and the number of new vertebral fractures decreased compared to untreated controls (54).

Therapy with vitamin D and its metabolites is commonly associated with hypercalcemia and hypercalciuria. Thus, their use requires frequent monitoring of serum and urinary calcium. Calcitriol is the preferable analogue since it is the most polar form of vitamin D with the least accumulation in body fat, and most rapid resolution of toxic side effects.

Testosterone. Hypogonadism is common in men with chronic hepatic, renal, or cardiac disease. Moreover, both glucocorticoids and CsA suppress the hypothalamic-pituitary-gonadal axis often resulting in decreased serum testosterone levels. Hypogonadism is an established cause of osteoporosis in men. Therefore it is reasonable to consider testosterone therapy in men who are found to be hypogonadal prior to or during therapy with immunosuppressive agents. A recent randomized, crossover trial of hypogonadal men with glucocorticoid-treated asthma demonstrated a significant increase in lumbar spine but not hip BMD after one year of monthly testosterone injections (55).

In the case of organ transplant recipients, testosterone typically normalizes by 6 to 12 months after transplantation (22, 30). However, in our experience, approximately 25% of men evaluated one to two years after cardiac transplantation will have evidence of biochemical hypogonadism. There is general agreement that men who are truly hypogonadal should be treated with testosterone. However, there are no data on the effect of testosterone replacement on rates of bone loss after organ transplantation. It is not clear whether testosterone replacement is advisable to counter the generally transient decreases observed during the early months after transplantation.

The only absolute contraindication to testosterone therapy is prostatic cancer. However, there are a number of other potential risks of testosterone therapy, including acceleration of hyperlipidemia which may be particularly hazardous in patients already prone to atherosclerosis from hypertension, diabetes, glucocorticoid and CsA therapy. Other risks include prostatic hypertrophy and abnormal liver enzymes. Potential benefits of testosterone therapy include increased lean body mass, hemoglobin levels, and BMD.

Fluoride. Fluoride is one of the few drugs that can stimulate bone formation. As such, it is an appealing approach to disorders such as transplantation or glucocorticoid-induced osteoporosis, in which inhibition of osteoblast function may play a pathogenetic role. Disodium monofluorophosphate administration was associated with a 63% increase in trabecular BMD in patients with glucocorticoid osteoporosis (56). Disodium monofluorophosphate, elemental calcium and calcidiol was also associated with a significant increase in BMD in patients with established osteoporosis after cardiac transplantation, compared to patients receiving calcium and calcidiol alone (57). However, increases in BMD in response to fluoride therapy are not consistently associated with improvement in bone quality and stength, or reduction in fracture rates. Moreover, high doses (50-75mg) of sodium fluoride have troubling gastrointestinal side effects. The potential approval of slow-release fluoride in the United States, may, however, provide an alternative approach to therapy of glucocorticoid and transplantation osteoporosis.

Parathyroid Hormone The concept of administration of low-dose, intermittent subcutaneous injections of parathyroid hormone [PTH(1-34)] to patients with glucocorticoid-induced osteoporosis has become more attractive recently, as convincing experimental evidence for its anabolic properties has accumulated (58). Traditionally, PTH has been considered to be associated with bone loss, especially at cortical sites. However, it has become clear that low levels of PTH stimulate osteoblast activity and increase cancellous bone in human subjects while cortical bone and overall calcium balance remain stable. Moreover, Lane and colleagues have recently reported that intermittent PTH increased BMD and biochemical markers of bone formation in estrogen-treated women on chronic GC therapy (59). These data suggest that low-dose intermittent PTH may be useful in forms of osteoporosis characterized by low bone formation, such as high-dose glucocorticoid therapy. Although not currently approved for use in the United States, this agent is under active investigation and may prove to be a useful adjunct in the therapy of glucocorticoid-induced osteoporosis in coming years.

Conclusion

Most currently available immunosuppressive drugs have deleterious effects on the skeleton. Since immunosuppressive regimens typically include glucocorticoids, these have been most extensively studied in both humans and animal models. Glucocortiocoids interfere with bone and mineral metabolism by inhibition of bone formation, promotion of bone resorption, and suppression of skeletal growth factors and gonadotropins. In attempts to overcome immunosuppressant bone loss, drugs that inhibit bone resorption, such as bisphosphonates, appear to hold particular therapeutic promise.

References

1.   Lukert BP 1996 Glucocorticoid-induced osteoporosis. In: Marcus R, Feldman D, Kelsey J, eds. Osteoporosis. New York: Academic Press 801-820.

2. Lukert B, Kream BE 1996 Clinical and basic aspects of glucorticoid action in bone. In: Bilezikian JP, Raisz LG, Rodan GA, eds. Principles of Bone Biology. New York: Academic Press 533-548.

3. Canalis E 1996 Mechanisms of glucocorticoid action in bone: Implications for glucocorticoid-induced osteoporosis. J Clin Endocrinol Metab 81:3441-3447.

4. Shane E, Epstein E 1994 Immunosuppressive therapy and the skeleton. Trends Endocrinol Metab 4:169-175.

5. Epstein S 1996 Post-transplantation bone disease: the role of immunosuppressive agents on the skeleton. J Bone Miner Res 11:1-7.

6. Shane E 1996 Secondary causes of osteoporosis. In: Marcus R, Feldman D, Kelsey J, eds. Osteoporosis. New York: Academic Press 927-946.

7. Aubia J, Masramon J, Serrano, Lloveras J, Marinoso L 1988 Bone histology in renal transplant patients receiving cyclosporin. Lancet i:1048-1049.

8. Wilmink JM, Bras J, Surachno S, Heyst JLAM, Horst JM 1989 Bone repair in cyclosporin treated renal transplant patients. Transplant Proc 21:1492-1494.

9. Thiebaud D, Krieg MA, Gillard-Berguer D, Jacquet AF, Goy JJ, Burckhardt P 1996 Cyclosporine induces high bone turnover and may contribute to bone loss after heart transplantation. Eur J Clin Invest 26:549-555.

10. Hawkins FG, Leon M, Lopez MB, Valero MA, Larrodera I, Garcia-Garcia I, Loinaz C, Moreno Gonzalez E 1994 Bone loss and turnover in patients with liver transplantation. Hepato-Gastroenterol 41:158-161.

11. Cvetkovic M, Mann G, Romero D et al 1994 Deleterious effects of long term cyclosporine A, cyclosporine G, and FK506 on bone mineral metabolism in vivo. Transplantation 57:1231-1237.

12. Stempfle HU, Wehr U, Meiger B, Angermann CE, Rambeck WA, Gartner R 1996 Effect of FK506 (Tacrolimus) on trabecular bone loss shortly after cardiac transplantation. (Abstract) J Bone Miner Res 11;S127.

13. Apostlinas S, Sheiner P, Genyk Y, O'Rourke M, Wallenstein S, Luckey M 1997 Prospective comparison of bone loss with tacrolimus and cyclosporin A after organ transplantation. (Abstract) J Bone Miner Res 12: S402.

14. Dissanayake I, Goodman C, Bowman A, et al 1997 Mycophenolate mofetil; A promising new immunosuppressant which does not cause bone loss in the rat. (Abstract) J Bone Miner Res 1997.

15. May KP, West SG, McDermott MT, Huffer WE 1994 The effect of low-dose methotrexate on bone metabolism and histomorphometry in rats. Arthr Rheum 37:201-206.

16. Preston SJ, Diamond T, Scott A, Laurent MR 1993 Methotrexate osteopathy in rheumatic disease. Ann Rheum Dis 52: 582-585.

17. Buckley LM, Leib ES, Cartularo KS, Vacek PM, Cooper SM 1997 Effects of low dose methotrexate on the bone mineral density of patients with rheumatoid arthritis. J Rheumatol. 24:1489-1494.

18. Cushing H 1932 The basophil adenomas of the pituitary body and their clinical manifestations (pituitary basophilism). Bull Johns Hopkins Hosp 50:1,137.

19. Nielsen HK, Charles P, Mosekilde L 1988 The effect of single oral doses of prednisone on the circadian rhythm of serum osteocalcin in normal subjects. J Clin Endocrinol Metab 67:1025-1030.

20. American College of Rheumatology Task Force on Osteoporosis Guidelines 1996 Recommendations for the prevention and treatment of glucocorticoid-induced osteoporosis. Arthr Rheum 39:1791-1801.

21. Hanania NA, Chapman KR, Kesten S 1995 Adverse effects of inhaled corticosteroids. Am J Med 98:196-208.

22. Rodino MA, Shane E 1998 Osteoporosis after organ transplantation. Am J Med In Press.

23. Goodman WG, Coburn JW, Slatopolsky E, Salusky I 1996 Renal Osteodystrophy in Adults and Children. In: Favus MJ. ed. Primer on the Metabolic Bone Diseases and Disorders of Mineral Metabolism. Third Edition. Philadelphia: Lippincott-Raven 341-360.

24. Aris RM, Renner JB, Winders AD, Buell HE, Riggs DB, Lester GE, Ontjes DA 1998 Increased rate of fractures and severe kyphosis: sequelae of living into adulthood with cystic fibrosis. Ann Int Med 128: 186-193.

25. Aris RM, Neuringer IP, Weiner MA, Egan TM, Ontjes D 1996 Severe osteoporosis before and after lung transplantation. Chest 109:1176-1183.

26. Shane E, Silverberg SJ, Donovan D, et. al 1996 Osteoporosis in lung transplantation candidates with end-stage pulmonary disease. Am J Med 101:262-69.

27. Lee AH, Mull RL, Keenan GF, et al 1994 Osteoporosis and bone morbidity in cardiac transplant recipients. Am J Med 96:35-41.

28. Shane E, Mancini D, Aaronson K, Silverberg SJ, Seibel MJ, Addesso V, McMahon DJ 1997 Bone mass, vitamin D deficiency, and hyperparathyroidism in congestive heart failure. Am J Med 103:197-207.

29. Shane E, Rivas M, Staron RB, et al 1996 Fracture after cardiac transplantation: A prospective longitudinal study. J Clin Endocrinol Metab 81:1740-1746.

30. Shane E, Rivas M, McMahon DJ, et al 1997 Bone loss and turnover after cardiac transplantation. J Clin Endocrinol Metab 82:1497-1506.

31. Shane E, Papadopoulos A, Staron R, Addesso VA, Donovan DS, McGregor C, Schulman LL 1998 A prospective study of bone loss and fracture after lung transplantation. (Abstract) Am J Resp Crit Care Med.

32. Grotz WH, Mundinger A, Gugel B, Exner V, Kirste G, Schollmeyer PJ 1994 Bone fracture and osteodensitometry with dual energy x-ray absorptiometry in kidney transplant recipients. Transplantation 58: 912-915.

33. Nisbeth U, Lindh E, Ljunghall S, Backman U, Fellstrom B 1994 Fracture frequency after kidney transplantation. Transplantation Proc 26:1764.

34. Braith RW, Mills RM, Welsch MA, Keller JW, Pollock, ML 1996 Resistence exercise training restores bone mineral density in heart transplant recipients. J Am Coll Cardiol 28:6:1471-1477.

35. Reid IR, King AR, Alexander CJ, Ibbertson HK 1988 Prevention of steroid-induced osteoporosis with (3-amino, 1-hydroxypropylidine)-1, 1-bisphosphonate (APD). Lancet 143-146.

36. Mulder H, Struys A 1994 Intermittent cyclical etidronate in the prevention of corticosteroid-induced bone loss. Brit J Rheum 33: 348-350.

37. Diamond T, McGiugan L, Barbagalla S, Bryant C 1995 Cyclical etidronate plus ergocalciferol prevents glucocorticoid-induced bone loss in postmenopausal women. Am J Med 98:459-63.

38. Adachi JD, Bensen WG, Brown J, Hanley D, Hodsman A, Josse R, Kendler DL, Lentle B, Olszynski W, Ste-Maie L-G, Tenehouse A, Chines AA 1997 Intermittent etidronate therapy to prevent corticosteroid-induced osteoporosis. N Engl J Med 337: 382-387.

39. Saag K, Emkey R, Gruber B, Tesser J, Lane N, Yanover M, Dubois C, Freedholm D, Carofano W, Daifotis A 1997 Alendronate for the management of glucocorticoid-induced osteoporosis: results of a multi-center U.S. study. Arthr Rheum 40 (suppl), S136.

40. Gallacher SJ, Fenner JAK, Anderson K, Bryden FM, Banham SW, Logue FC, Cowan RA, Boyle IT 1992 Intravenous pamidronate in the treatment of osteoporosis associated with corticosteroid dependent lung disease: an open pilot study. Thorax 47: 932-936.

41. Fan S, Almond MK, Ball E, Evans K, Cunningham J 1996 Randomized prospective study demonstrating prevention of bone loss by pamidronate during the first year after renal transplantation. (Abstract). J Am Soc Nephrol 7:A2714.

42. Shane E, Thys-Jacobs S, Papadopoulos A, Addesso V, Mancini D, Seibel MJ, Silverberg SJ, Staron RB 1996 Antiresorptive therapy prevents bone loss after cardiac transplantation (CTX). (Abstract) J Bone Miner Res 11:635.

43. Riemens SC, Oostdijk A, van Doormaal J, et al. 1996 Bone loss after liver transplantation is not prevented by cyclical etidronate, calcium and alpha calcidiol. Osteoporosis Int 6:213-218.

246

44. Montemurro L, Schiraldi G, Fraioli P, Tosi G, Riboldi A, Rizzato G 1991 Prevention of corticosteroid-induced osteoporosis with salmon calcitonin in sarcoid patients. Calcified Tissue International 49:71-76.

45. Ringe JD, Wetzel D 1987 Salmon calcitonin in the therapy of corticosteroid-induced osteoporosis. Eur J Clin Pharmacol 33; 35.

46. Luengo M, Pons F, Martinez de Osaba MJ, Picado C 1994 Prevention of further bone loss by calcitonin in patients on long term glucocorticoid therpy for asthma: a two year follow-up study. Thorax 49:1099-1102.

47. Lukert B, Johnson BE, Robinson RG 1992 Estrogen and progesterone replacement reduces glucocorticoid-induced bone loss. J Bone Miner Res 7:1063-1069.

48. Ringe JD 1997 Active vitamin D metabolites in glucocorticoid-induced osteoporosis. Calcif Tiss Int 60:124-127.

49. Sambrook P, Birmingham J, Kelly P, Kempler S, Nguyen T, Pocock N, Eisman JA 1993 Prevention of corticosteroid osteoporosis - a comparison of calcium, calcitriol and calcitonin. N Engl J Med 328:1747-1752.

50. Van Cleemput J, Daenen W, Geusens P Dequeker J, Van de Werf F, Vanhaecke J 1996 Prevention of bone loss in cardiac transplant recipients. A comparison of biphosphonates and vitamin D. Transplantation. 61:1495-1499.

51. Neuhaus R, Lohmann R, Platz KP, Guckelberger O, Schon M, Lang M, Hierholzer J, Neuhaus P 1995 Treatment of osteoporosis after liver transplantation. Transplant Proc. 27:1227-1227.

52. Talalaj M, Gradowska L, Marcinowska-Suchowierska E, Durlik M, Gaciong Z, Lao M 1996Transplant Proc 28:3485-3487.

53. Reid IR, Wattie DJ, Evans MC, Stapleton JP 1996 Testosterone therapy in glucocorticoid-treated men. Arch Int Med 156:1173-1177.

54. Meunier PJ, Brancon D, Chavassieux P, Edouard C, Boivin C, Conrozier T, Macelli C, Pastoureau P, Delmas PD, Casez JP 1987 Treatment with fluoride, in Osteoporosis (C. Christiansen, J.S. Johansen, and B.J. Riis, Eds.), Osteopress, Copenhagen 824-828.

55. Meys E, Terreaux-Duvert F, Beaume-Six T, Dureau G, Meunier PJ 1993 Effects of calcium, calderol and monofluorophosphate on lumbar bone mass and parathyroid function in patients after cardiac transplantation. Osteoporosis Int 3: 329-332.

56. Dempster DW, Cosman F, Parisien M, Shen V, Lindsay R 1993 Anabolic actions of parathyroid hormone on bone. Endocrine Rev 14:690-709.

57. Lane NE, Thompson JM, Modin G, Sanchez S, Arnaud C 1997 Can parathyroid hormone treatment reverse steroid osteoporosis: preliminary results of biochemical markers and bone density. J Bone Miner Res 12 (Suppl 1)S130.

15 Cancer and Bone Disease

Mark S. Nanes, M.D., Ph.D.
Louisa Titus, Ph.D.

The Clinical Spectrum of Skeletal Metastases

Skeletal metastases cause extensive morbidity in half of all cancer patients (Coleman 87, 1). Thirty to 40% of patients who have bone metastases suffer from painful pathologic fractures that limit their independence during the period preceding death. In addition, 10-40% of cancer patients without skeletal lesions develop the humoral hypercalcemia of malignancy (HHM) (2, 3). Thus, the morbidity associated with the skeletal complications of malignancy is a frequent cause of pain and suffering, an antecedent to repeated hospitalization, and a contributor to increased health care costs. Our goal, as physicians and scientists, is to advance the understanding of skeletal pathophysiology in patients with malignancy so that metastases to bone are prevented, pain is reduced, and patient independence is maintained for as long as possible.

Cancers of the breast, lung, prostate, and multiple myeloma frequently affect bone and calcium homeostasis. Skeletal metastases from the solid tumors occur in almost 85% of cases (4, 5, 6). The increased prevalence of these cancers may account for a greater amount of biologic data on their skeletal pathophysiology compared to less common cancers. Much less is known about the biology of other tumor types, such as thyroid carcinoma, that also metastasize to bone. 20-40% of patients with small cell carcinoma of the lung and only 5% of patients with gastric carcinoma present with skeletal metastases. Renal and bladder carcinomas are more likely to cause hypercalcemia alone, although metastatic disease to bone does occur. Kanis has noted that the proportion of patients with skeletal metastases may reflect the length of time between diagnosis and death rather than the predilection of a particular tumor type for metastasizing to bone (7). Nevertheless, some cancers express important cell surface attachment signals that target bone, angiogenic cytokines that promote vascularization, or cell surface receptors that confer a response to bone derived growth factors. This phenotype increases the potential of a tumor for metastasizing to and surviving in bone. A variety of factors have been discovered that promote cancer cell adhesion, increase the proliferation of metastatic cells, and disrupt normal skeletal remodeling (8). Once resident in the skeleton, tumor-derived humoral or paracrine factors (cytokines) produced by cancer cells stimulate osteoblasts and osteoclasts in an unregulated manor. Such "dysregulatory" factors uncouple the normal balance between bone resorption and formation, a disruption that tips the balance in one or the other direction. This familiar story has been greatly expanded during the last few years with the discovery of an increased number of cytokines, a better understanding of how they disrupt skeletal homeostasis, and new insights into the reasons that specific malignancies present with unique clinical presentations. The cancers most commonly affecting bone; myeloma, breast, and prostate; have become models for three distinct pathophysiologic mechanisms. Multiple myeloma causes principally lytic bone lesions due to increased numbers of bone resorbing osteoclasts. Conversely, prostate cancer causes radiographically sclerotic bone lesions due to increased osteoblast function. Breast cancer has an intermediate presentation with mixed sclerotic/lytic lesions. Here we will pursue the unique features of these malignancies that contribute to their clinical presentations. We will also discuss how advances in our understanding of the pathophysiology can lead to targeted clinical management.

What are the mechanisms responsible for the disturbances in calcium homeostasis observed in patients with tumors that have not metastasized to bone? The more remote effects of malignancy include humoral (blood borne) factors that disrupt normal mineral homeostasis in the kidney and intestine. These factors cause secondary effects on bone. For example, a putative phosphaturic substance may be produced by mesenchymal tumors that cause hypophosphatemic osteomalacia (9). The discovery that 1,25-dihydroxyvitamin D3, the active form of vitamin D, is produced by certain lymphomas and leukemias has now been confirmed in several reports showing that overproduction of this secosteroid promotes hyperabsorptive (gut) and hypericsorptive (bone) hypercalcemia (10, 11, 85). It should be kept in mind that bone disease also results from cancer treatment, particularly when glucocorticoids are used as part of chemotherapeutic regimens or when the production of gonadal steroids is inhibited by gonadotropin hormone releasing factor agonists or inhibitors of steroid synthesis. Thus, the spectrum of clinical bone disorders caused by cancer may include generalized osteoporosis, osteosclerosis, and osteomalacia.

In this chapter the mechanisms of skeletal metastases at the biologic level will be related to clinical presentation of specific malignancies. The emphasis in this review will focus on how new approaches for prevention, monitoring, and treatment of the skeletal complications of malignancy resulted from basic and clinical research and what therapeutic weapons physicians might expect to be available in the future.

Biology of Skeletal Metastases: Skeletal Metastatic Phenotype

The most common skeletal sites for metastases include the spine, pelvis, ribs, skull, proximal femora, and humeri. Traditionally, the radiographic appearance of bone metastases has been described as osteolytic, osteosclerotic, or mixed. The first two categories define predominantly osteoclastic or osteoblastic lesions; respectively. Histologically, all of these lesions are mixed to some extent because resorption and formation of bone are coupled events. Cancers metastasize to bone via the hematogenous route, although lymphatic spread and direct local invasion can occur. Joseph-Claude Anthelme Recamier first suggested the concept of tumor metastases in 1829 in a description of a breast cancer patient who developed a brain mass. The concept was gradually accepted over the next 70 years with the demonstration of the histologic similarity between primary tumors and metastatic lesions. The route of spread to bone was a controversial subject because tumor cells entering the venous circulation would be expected to be stopped by the lungs. They were, of course, found in the skeleton. Definitive proof for hematogenous spread of cancers came with an experimental approach still used today: the establishment of metastases in tumor-inoculated animals. Of course we now readily accept the concept of metastases; however, there have been few explanations for the predilection of tumor cells for the skeleton. Early theories by Batson related the targeting of the axial skeleton to blood flow through the vertebral plexus, a retrograde route that would avoid the prerequisite of crossing from venous to arterial circulation through the lungs (12). More recent information suggests that unique properties of the tumor cells, and also of the site of invasion, contribute to the establishment of a metastatic lesion. For a malignant cell to journey from the primary tumor to a distant site there must be vascularization of the primary tumor, embolization, endothelial attachment, and invasion (13, 14). A cancer cell's propensity to metastasize to bone, per se, requires that the cell express the unique phenotype favoring attachment and growth in the bone microenvironment.

Early work revealed that extremely invasive tumors expressed receptors for the basement membrane protein laminin, which facilitated their attachment to bone endosteal surfaces (15). Tumor cells probably require many specialized receptors for attachment to bone endosteal surfaces including the integrin avb3 (vitronectin) that binds repetitive arginine-glycine-aspartate (RGD) sequences on numerous matrix proteins. RGD sequences in skeletal proteins such as fibronectin, osteopontin, and bone sialoprotein are attachment sites for bone resorbing osteoclasts and, as such, are ideal recognition signals for cancer cells (16-20). Indeed, culturing cells in the presence of synthetic RGD sequences can inhibit the attachment of breast cancer cells to bone in vitro (Van der Pluijm 96). These peptides are believed to compete for native avb3 receptors, thus blocking the attachment of cancer cells. Virtually all breast cancers metastatic to bone express the vitronectin receptor even if the primary tumor does not (21). Remarkable evidence has advanced this concept from a cell culture phenomenon to a potential in vivo approach that prevents skeletal metastases. Matsuura et al evaluated the role of another integrin, a4b1, which binds fibronectin and the cell adhesion molecule VCAM-1 (22). These investigators used a nude mouse model in which animals were inoculated with tumor cells (Chinese hamster ovary cells) genetically engineered to overexpress a4b1, after which the frequency of bone metastases could be monitored. Mice inoculated with control cells developed only pulmonary metastases while inoculation with the integrin expressing cells resulted in both pulmonary and bone lesions. Skeletal lesions could be prevented by administering an antibody against the a4 subunit of the integrin or against VCAM-1. These results were specific for a4b1 as they were not observed using cancer cells engineered to express a number of other integrins (avb3 was not studied). Similar studies using a tumor-inoculated nude mouse model revealed that the cell surface adhesion receptor E-cadherin protects against breast cancer metastases (23). Overall, the evidence suggests that tumor cell recognition of bone matrix proteins is an important attribute promoting skeletal metastases.

The expression of matrix protein by cancer cells may also contribute to the skeletal metastatic phenotype. A small but controlled prospective series has reported a positive relationship between the expression of bone sialoprotein, a matrix protein, by breast cancer cells and the probability of skeletal metastases (24). A larger retrospective evaluation found that bone sialoprotein expression occurred in 22% of tumors that metastasized to bone vs 7% of tumors that did not (25). Thus the expression of sialoprotein as well as its recognition through integrins favors metastases to bone. The property of a tumor cell allowing recognition of the bone surface seems easy to understand with regard to skeletal metastases. However, the mechanism by which expression of matrix proteins by tumor cells contributes to metastases is unclear. One possibility is that such expression represents a more differentiated phenotype that promotes survival of the tumor once it is established in bone.

Several additional markers have been identified in tumor cells that are associated with their propensity for skeletal metastases. A number of studies suggest that parathyroid hormone related protein (PTHrp) expression by breast cancer promotes metastases to the skeleton. This distant relative of PTH, originally identified as the cause of HHM in solid tumors, is expressed by tumors even if hypercalcemia is not a part of the clinical presentation. In a prospective study of breast cancer patients, immunohistochemical staining of the primary tumor for PTHrp predicted future skeletal metastases independently of other prognostic factors (26). Interestingly, the presence of PTHrp in human breast tumors is associated with the tissue micro-calcifications seen in mammography. Breast microcalcifications also develop in mice innoculated with a PTHrp expressing breast cancer (27). PTHrp expression is also more likely to occur in breast carcinoma metastatic to the skeleton than in the primary tumors or non-skeletal metastases (14, 28). PTHrp produced by cancer cells could act in a paracrine manor by stimulating bone cells, or through an autocrine mechanism that stimulates growth of cancer cells, as these cells often express their own receptors for PTH/PTHrp. Bioactive fragments of PTHrp may inhibit cancer cell growth while promoting invasion (29). Thus, the type of PTHrp fragment and the response of a particular cancer cell may contribute to skeletal invasiveness. Recently, Guise et al demonstrated that antibodies to PTHrp prevent the spread of breast cancer to bone in a cancer inoculated mouse model (30). The relationship between PTHrp expression and the development of skeletal metastases is independent of hypercalcemia in experimental mouse models, just as in patients. These important studies suggest that PTHrp promotes skeletal metastases by breast cancer and opens a fruitful area of research on the clinical prevention of bone metastases in breast cancer with PTHrp antibodies or receptor blocking peptides.

The importance of PTHrp expression in the skeletal metastatic phenotype of cancer is not limited to breast cancer. PTHrp expression in squamous cell carcinoma is the major cause of hypercalcemia in this malignancy. Iguchi et al found that inoculation of nude mice with a PTHrp expressing squamous cell carcinoma was followed by the formation of skeletal metastases which were blocked when the mice were treated with a PTHrp antibody (31). Virtually all prostate cancers expresses PTHrp, whether metastatic to bone or not (32, 33). PTHrp is not expressed in normal prostate tissue but its expression in benign prostatic hyperplasia is common (33). Thus, the accumulated evidence suggests that Koch's postulates are close to being fulfilled for both PTHrp and integrins for the skeletal metastatic potential of breast, and possibly squamous cell carcinoma (34). The attachment of cancer cells to bone endosteal surfaces may be followed by digestion of basement membrane type IV collagen via the action of tumor cell type IV collagenase, as this has been shown for metastases to soft tissues (35).

Local Disruption of Skeletal Remodeling

Once cancer cells become established in bone a complex series of events occurs that favors their survival, disrupts normal bone remodeling, and disturbs calcium homeostasis. Bone is remodeled in discrete units by resorbing osteoclasts and matrix synthesizing osteoblasts. This process has been reviewed elsewhere and is only briefly summarized here (8). The rate of bone loss or accretion reflects the sum of resorption and formation from many remodeling units. Although these remodeling units function asynchronously, the process of resorption and formation is tightly coupled within individual remodeling units. Such coupling assures that an excavated area will be almost (but not completely) replaced with new bone during a normal remodeling cycle. To achieve coupling, a complex communication between osteoblasts, osteoclasts, and the matrix microenvironment must occur by way of local or systemic growth factors, cytokines, and hormones. It is here, in the signaling process, that invading cancer cells are most likely to disrupt the balance of bone remodeling.

The arrival and attachment of cancer cells disrupts the resorption-formation balance in a direction that depends on the unique signals presented to the bone microenvironment. Several cytokines, growth factors, and prostaglandins have been suggested to influence bone cell activity. Interestingly, the source of these factors is not always the cancer tissue itself. Sources of regulatory factors may include activated invading mononuclear cells and growth factors liberated from the resorbing bone matrix. **Table 1** catalogues the growth factors and cytokines

252

that have been demonstrated to be produced by the cancer cells as evidenced by assay of the factor in cultured tumor cells or measurement of mRNA expression in situ. In some cases, secretion of one factor initiates a cascade in which a second or third regulatory factor is produced. Morinaga et al reported that breast and melanoma cancer cells cause the release of TGF-b, which, in turn stimulates osteoblasts to produce IL-11 (36). This paracrine production of IL-11 accelerates the recruitment of osteoclasts from their marrow progenitors. Experimental approaches designed to determine which factor initiates the cascade or is most important include methods to either block or constitutively express each cytokine so that the effect on bone can be measured. These experiments are difficult to do because specific blocking agents are not always available. Nevertheless, with the evidence collected to date a model can be constructed to explain the propensity of myeloma, breast, and prostate cancer to produce lytic, mixed, or blastic lesions in bone (**Figure 1**).

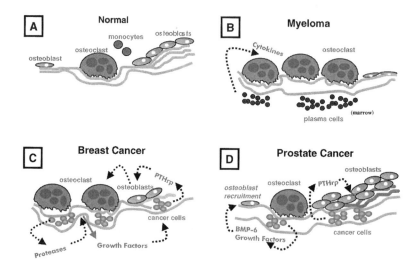

Figure 1: A model of cancer and bone disease is shown with emphasis on the differences between multiple myeloma, breast cancer, and prostate cancer. Panel A shows normal bone remodeling. Osteoclastic resorption is balanced by coupled osteoblastic formation. Panel B shows the effect of myeloma cells residing in marrow. These cells secrete cytokines responsible for the accelerated recruitment of osteoclasts from marrow progenitors and suppression of osteoblastic activity. Bone resorption occurs rapidly and is unchecked by formation. Panel C shows breast cancer cells which have survived in bone due to their skeletal metastatic phenotype. PTHrp production enhances survival of cancer cells in bone and stimulates osteoblasts to signal osteoclast recruitment. Proteases produced by cancer cells liberate skeletal matrix growth factors, which further stimulate cancer cell growth. Panel D shows the predominantly osteoblastic lesion of prostate cancer. The cancer cells express PTHrp, which enhance their survival in bone. These cells also secrete BMP-6, which stimulates osteoblast recruitment from stromal progenitors increasing bone formation. A more extensive list of the factors produced by these cancers is presented in **Table 1**.

The lytic lesions of multiple myeloma and the associated hypercalcemia are believed to occur from cytokine stimulated recruitment of osteoclasts from their marrow progenitors (37). Lymphotoxin (TNF-b) was the first cytokine identified as a product of cultured human myeloma cells. Lymphotoxin was shown to cause hypercalcemia when infused into mice (38). The production of lymphotoxin by myeloma cells may stimulate marrow stromal cells or osteoblasts to produce IL-6 which, in turn, acts on bone marrow precursors to accelerate differentiation toward the osteoclast pathway (39). Subsequent work also revealed IL-6 secretion by cultured myeloma cells, suggesting direct production (40). Interestingly, PTHrp production has not been described as a prominent feature of myeloma (41). Myeloma cells do produce IL-1, TGFb, and M-CSF, which contribute to the recruitment and activation of osteoclasts (42). These cytokines also inhibit osteoblast matrix protein synthesis (43, 44) and interfere with the osteoblast response to calciotropic hormones (45, 46). Thus, osteoblasts are unable to respond to the accelerated bone resorption with the normally coupled increase in bone formation. The resulting lesion is almost purely osteoclastic. This disruption in local signaling in the bone microenvironment causes a unique histology in which high numbers of resorbing osteoclasts rim lytic lesions with near absent osteoblastic activity. The suppression of osteoblastic activity accounts for the normal serum alkaline phosphatase, negative bone scans, and absence of sclerotic (bone forming) lesions on X-ray in multiple myeloma. The high rate of osteoclastic resorption liberates calcium and causes hypercalcemia and hypercalciuria since the flux of calcium from bone into blood exceeds the renal tubular threshold. Lymphotoxin may have a unique role in this model that distinguishes myeloma from other cancers in which coupled osteoblastic bone formation continues. Thus, from a clinical perspective, the reason for negative bone scans and normal alkaline phosphatase in myeloma is not only that the lesions are osteoclastic, but that osteoblasts have been thwarted.

Breast cancer patients present with bone lesions that are mostly osteolytic but these also have a sclerotic component on X-ray (63). This suggests that some coupled osteoblastic activity is occurring, unlike myeloma where the bone formation is blocked. PTHrp release in the bone microenvironment stimulates the release of interleukins that promote osteoclast recruitment, just as in myeloma. Thus, increased osteoclasts continuously resorb bone. However, recent work has revealed that PTHrp (and PTH) may actually have an anabolic function in bone. PTHrp binds the same PTH/PTHrp receptor as parathyroid hormone and stimulates osteoblast production of intracellular cAMP. Cyclic AMP stimulates increased transcription of the IGF-1 gene and IGF-1 promotes matrix protein production that mineralizes (64-70). Thus, IGF-1 may be one example of how PTHrp acts as an autocrine signal to increase bone formation. This action of PTHrp is different than the humoral effect known to cause HHM, where much higher levels of PTHrp from remote tumors have a predominant

Primary Cancer	Growth Factor/Cytokine	Reference
Breast	Parathyroid hormone related protein	28, 47, 43, 14, 34, 26
	Vascular endothelial growth factor, Acidic and Basic fibroblast growth factor	49
	Transforming growth factor-b	48, 49
	Platelet derived endothelial growth factor, Placenta growth factor, pleiotrophin	49
	Interleukins 6, 11, Oncostatin M, Leukemia inhibitory factor	50
	Midkine	51
	Insulin-like growth factor II	52
Lung	Parathyroid hormone related protein	53, 54
	Interleukins 1 and 6	53, 55
	Insulin-like growth factor I and II	56, 52
	Transforming growth factor-β	56
	Granulocyte colony stimulating factor	55
	Platelet derived endothelial growth factor	57
Prostate	Bone morphogenetic protein-6	58
	Parathyroid hormone related protein	33
	Vascular endothelial growth factor	59, 60
	Transforming growth factor-β	61
Multiple Myeloma	Lymphotoxin (TNF-β)	38
	Interleukin-1, Transforming growth factor-b, Macrophage colony stimulating factor	42
	Oncostatin M	62
	Interleukin-6	40

Table 1: Cytokines and growth factors expressed by breast, lung, prostate cancers, or multiple myeloma, as evidenced by measurement of mRNA or protein secretion.

effect on osteoclast recruitment. In skeletal breast cancer metastases, the overall rate of bone resorption exceeds this minimal anabolic effect of local PTHrp, thus, a predominantly osteolytic picture is observed. However, if osteoclastic resorption is prevented by administration of bisphosphonates, the relative rate of bone formation is increased and a lytic lesion can be replaced by a sclerotic one (71, 72). In addition, there is a conspicuous absence of lymphotoxin production by breast cancer cells. The absence of lymphotoxin or its secretion at much lower levels than observed in myeloma might also allow osteoblastic activity to continue, as discussed above. Some breast cancers have been shown to produce transforming growth factors that could also contribute to the behavior of these metastases (48).

Both squamous and small cell lung carcinoma skeletal metastases are osteolytic with a small osteoblastic component, similar to the lesions seen in breast cancer. PTHrp production is a common feature of these tumors (31). The mechanism of bone pathology due to production of cytokines in metastatic lung cancer is not well known but may be similar to that observed in breast cancer.

Human prostate cancers have been shown to produce bone morphogenetic protein 6 (BMP-6), a potent stimulator of osteoblast differentiation. Production of BMP-6 has been demonstrated in prostate cancer and prostate cancer cell lines, but not in benign prostatic hyperplasia (58). By secreting BMP-6, prostate metastases may stimulate the differentiation of mesenchymal precursors into osteoblasts with subsequent matrix protein production and mineralization (73). Active mineralization of these matrix proteins enhances the deposition of isotopic polyphosphates and the sensitivity of such scans for detection of metastatic prostate lesions. Similarly, alkaline phosphatase, which is produced by metabolically active osteoblasts, leaks into the blood stream where it can be used as an important biochemical marker. Lymphotoxin production by prostate cancers has not been described, thus, this stimulus to osteoclast recruitment is absent or diminished. The possibility that osteoclastogenesis is actually inhibited by prostate carcinoma is an interesting hypothesis that has not been tested. The expanding blastic lesions of metastatic prostate carcinoma are intensely painful but usually not associated with hypercalcemia or fracture. Interestingly, if the minimal osteoclastic activity is inhibited by administration of bisphosphonates, patients can actually become hypocalcemic, reflecting the greater degree of ongoing osteoblast function. Other mechanisms for prostate cancer metastases and osteoblastic activity have also been investigated. Invasive prostate tumors produce urokinase plasminogen activator, which may contribute to the skeletal metastatic and osteoblastic phenotype (74). The aminoterminus of this peptide stimulates osteoblast mitogenesis through a mechanism involving IGF-1. Indeed, this peptide can promote skeletal metastases in a mouse model (75, 76).

PTHrp probably targets prostate metastases to bone as it does in breast and lung. Almost all prostate cancers produce PTHrp. Interestingly, prostate specific antigen (PSA), a protease used as a marker for prostate cancer, can cleave PTHrp in vitro and abolish its ability to stimulate cAMP production by osteoblasts (77). The way in which this suggested action of PSA contributes to the clinical picture of osteoblastic lesions is not known.

Bone is a rich source of matrix associated growth factors that may accelerate the growth and spread of cancer cells. The release of TGF-b and other growth factors from lytic metastatic lesions provides cancer cells with a favorable microenvironment once they are established, and may contribute to the survival and proliferation of cancer cells in bone.

.

Detection of Skeletal Metastases: Scans

Technetium99m, (99mTc)-Sn compounds of polyphosphate and diphosphate bone scans, have been extremely useful for detection of skeletal metastases because these compounds are bone seeking. In this respect they are similar to the chemically related bisphosphonates currently used for treatment. These scans are sensitive and allow visualization of the entire skeleton. Factors that affect the uptake of these compounds in bone include local blood flow, capillary permeability, pH, and the rate of mineralization at the involved site (78). Tc99-bone scans continue to be the most useful way to detect skeletal metastases in cancers of the breast, lung, and prostate. These cancers are associated with osteoblastic activity within their sclerotic or sclerotic/lytic mixed lesions and will therefore deposit the Tc99-analog onto metabolically active areas in bone. As noted above, the lytic lesions of myeloma are not detected on bone scan because osteoblast bone formation is almost completely disabled. As discussed above, the cytokines produced by myeloma, including TNF-b, IL-1, and IL-6, actively suppresses osteoblastic activity while recruiting osteoclasts to the area (44, 45). Thus, osteoblast synthesis of matrix proteins is negligible and mineralization is impaired. For most cases of myeloma, radiographs are sufficient to evaluate skeletal lesions without the need for more expensive scans.

An important issue in the evaluation of skeletal metastases is the large number of false positive foci, up to 30%, on Tc99-polyphosphate scans. Plain radiographs and MRI are useful in distinguishing osteoporotic compression fractures or local inflammatory changes from metastatic invasion. MRI is superior to computed tomography for this purpose. Recently, Tc99-antigranulocyte bone marrow scintigraphy has become available for the evaluation of skeletal metastases. The use of this scan derives from the concept that metastasizing cancer cells first arrive in bone marrow prior to direct invasion of bone. Because Tc99-antigranulocyte scans measure an earlier stage in the spread of cancer, they may be useful in patients that have negative Tc99-polyphosphate scans 79-81). These techniques are costly. The clinical role Tc99-antigranulocyte bone marrow scintigraphy and other techniques such as bone Positron Emission Tomography, remains to be established by randomized clinical trials and long term follow up.

Careful cost/benefit analysis of screening bone scintigraphy in different cancers has not been done, thus, the decision to scan newly diagnosed patients rests on clinical judgement. The decision to screen depends on the aggressiveness of the type of cancer, the symptoms, and biochemical indices. For patients with myeloma, radiographs should be used when the patient develops local painful symptoms. For breast cancer patients, the decision to screen with Tc99-polyphosphate scans is more difficult. Since patients with stage I disease are unlikely to have distant metastases, bone scans should not be done in the absence of symptoms or metabolic signs of skeletal involvement (hypercalcemia, elevated alkaline phosphatase, or elevated biochemical markers of bone turnover). Patients with stage II-IV disease are more likely to have distant metastases and should have a screening bone scan (82).

Biochemical Markers for Screening

The use of biochemical markers of bone metabolism has been under investigation as an adjunct in the detection of skeletal metastases. Mean values for indices of bone resorption (hydroxyproline, pyridinoline and deoxypyridinoline, ICTP, and N- and C-terminal collagen cross-links) and bone formation (bone specific alkaline phosphatase, osteocalcin) are elevated in breast cancer patients with skeletal metastases. However, the diagnostic criteria using biochemical markers are uncertain because an extensive range of values has been observed and there is extensive overlap between groups with and without bone metastases (83). For breast cancer patients, biochemical screening with any of the tests noted above has been shown to miss up to 40% of those with bone metastases (the reader is referred to the extensive review by Vinholes 83 for references). Urine calcium excretion is a poor predictor of skeletal metastases and should not contribute to the decision to scan patients (84).

Once a screening bone scan is done for patients with prostate carcinoma, biochemical markers may help in determining which patients should be re-scanned at follow up. Most studies done to determine the efficacy of skeletal biochemical markers in prostate cancer compare one marker with another. Surprisingly, few studies have compared the positive predictive value of skeletal markers with that of PSA or prostatic acid phosphatase. Recent information suggests that the Prostate Specific Antigen (PSA) at the time of diagnosis is a useful predictor of skeletal metastases (85-87). A PSA<10 nearly excludes bone metastases with a negative predictive value of 98%. The positive predictive value of a PSA > 100 is 74% (88). It would seem reasonable to do a repeat bone scan for patients with rising prostate specific antigen, acid phosphatase, or increasing bone pain. The usefulness of bone specific alkaline phosphatase has also been demonstrated for diagnosis of skeletal metastases in prostate cancer (89, 90, 88). Other markers have been shown to be increased in groups of prostate cancer patients with skeletal metastases compared to those without metastases but diagnostic criteria have not been analyzed as extensively as for PSA and bone specific alkaline phosphatase (91-95).

Limited evidence suggests that biochemical markers of bone resorption and formation may be a useful adjunct in identifying skeletal metastases in patients with stage I breast cancer and prostate cancer. A definitive conclusion would require determination of positive and negative predictive values for each marker in these patients. It will be important to determine if the sensitivity and specificity of the biochemical markers differs in those patients with stage I breast cancer and those with more advanced disease. For prostate cancer patients, biochemical bone markers might be useful in combination with PSA in deciding who should have a bone scan. Biochemical testing could reduce costs in these groups.

Treatment: Pain

The goals for the treatment of skeletal metastases include control of pain, prevention of fractures, and management of HHM. Radiotherapy remains the cornerstone of treatment for metastatic bone pain. The mechanism through which radiotherapy controls bone pain is not known. Bone metastases produce pain by activating nociceptors in the periosteum. Thus, pain may occur when an osteoblastic lesion provides pressure to the periosteum or when the periosteum is stretched adjacent to a destructive osteoclastic lesion or frank pathologic fracture. Deformities in bone that result from local destruction or fracture also disturb adjacent nerve fibers, which enhance the magnitude of pain. Chemical mediators released in areas of skeletal metastases have also been suggested to contribute to bone pain. Potential mechanisms of action for radiotherapy include shrinkage of lesions, destruction of nociceptors, inhibition of chemical mediator release, and direct destruction of osteoblasts or osteoclasts. The rapidity of onset of radiotherapy, prior to tumor shrinkage or demonstrable changes in the size of lytic or blastic lesions, strongly supports an inhibitory effect on nociceptors or chemical mediator release. Radiotherapy in the form of external beam, hemibody radiation, or strontium89 (for prostate cancer) provides relief to more than half of treated patients within 48 hours. In addition, the extended duration of action and feasibility of re-treating relapses has made radiotherapy a first choice modality. Several studies have shown that radiation can be given as a single large dose rather than multiple smaller doses with the same efficacy and without an increase in side effects (96, 97). Such an approach decreases the frequency with which patients must be mobilized for therapy. The reader is referred to detailed reviews by Nielsen (98) and Mercadante (99).

Principles of analgesic use for treatment of bone pain have been described in detail (100). Patients should be treated with medications of increasing potency beginning with nonsteroidal antiinflammatory drugs followed by weak opiates and finally stronger opiates according to the World Health Organization Treatment Ladder. Non-steroidal antiinflammatory drugs may decrease the dose of opiates needed to control pain and should be continued, if tolerated, when opiates are begun. Appropriate adjustment of dose and frequency of opiates may allow control of baseline pain, and rapid acting/short duration opiates can be used to treat breakthrough pain. For optimum independence, patients may self administer shorter action opiates for treatment of breakthrough pain (101, 102). Unfortunately, discontinuation of analgesics more often occurs because of side effects than lack of efficacy.

The role of bisphosphonates in the management of skeletal metastases is increasing. Bisphosphonates, which are analogs of pyrophosphate, have been used clinically for 100 years (103). These compounds are composed of a P-C-P core structure with variable avidity for bone depending on the identity of one or two side chains on the carbon atom. All bisphosphonates inhibit bone resorption but they differ in potency. As can be seen in **Table 2**, the various compounds introduced for medical use may have up to a 1000-fold difference in potency (>10,000 in animal and in vitro studies) (103). In addition to the overall inhibition of bone resorption, etidronate also inhibits mineralization of bone, a feature greatly reduced in the more potent compounds. This has led to the replacement of etidronate in clinical practice by clodronate, and pamidronate, and more recently by even more potent compounds. Interestingly, the ranking of bisphosphonate potency in vitro is the same as in vivo (**Table 2**).

Bisphosphonate	*in vivo* *rat* Assay (log ED50)	*In vivo* Clinical Potency (human studies)	*in vitro* Inhibition of tumor cell adhesion to breast cancer
Etidronate	4	Least	Least
Clodronate	3.2		
Neridronate	1.9		
Pamidronate	1.9		
Alendronate	1.0		
Ibandronate	0.2		
Risedronate	0.2		
Zoledronate	-1.2	Most	Most

Table 2: Relative in vivo and in vitro potency of bisphosphonates. Column 1: Inhibition of bone resorption in thyroparathyroidectomized rats. Column 2: treatment of osteoporosis or of skeletal metastases. Column 3: inhibition of breast cancer cell adhesion to devitalized bone. The ranking of potency is the same in human and animal studies although the magnitude of the difference from etidronate (least) to zoledronate (most) is less in humans (adapted from van der Pluijm 97 and Fleisch 103).

Bisphosphonates are deposited in areas of bone resorption and taken up by osteoclasts. The uptake of bisphosphonates by osteoclasts causes changes in their specialized ruffled border that contacts the bone surface, decreases the expression of bone resorbing enzymes, and reduces osteoclast generation of protons. Thus, the localized acidic and enzymatically active environment between the osteoclast and bone is neutralized. Ultimately osteoclasts exposed to bisphosphonates undergo apoptosis (104). Thus, bisphosphonates would be expected to be most beneficial in predominantly osteoclastic bone lesions, particularly in the treatment of hypercalcemia. Bisphosphonates also inhibit the elaboration of osteoclast recruiting signals by direct action on osteoblasts. In this way, formation/resorption coupling is blocked leaving the balance in favor of formation. A number of studies have now demonstrated a role for bisphosphonates in preventing the establishment and progression of metastases, relieving pain, and preventing fractures (105-12, 72). In addition to the known efficacy of bisphosphonates in treating the hypercalcemia associated with cancer, the response rates for pain control, reduction in calciuria, fracture prevention, and reduction in progression of skeletal metastases ranged from 26-89% (113). Pamidronate infusions (90 mg iv, monthly) delays the onset of new skeletal complications in women with stage IV breast cancer, decreases bone pain, and is well tolerated (72). Bisphosphonates are deposited in metabolically active areas of bone where resorption by osteoclasts is inhibited. Thus, the mixed lytic/sclerotic lesions of breast and lung cancer are effectively treated with bisphosphonate therapy. The efficacy of bisphosphonates in myeloma might seem surprising since these compounds are similar to those used for bone scintigraphy, which is negative in myeloma. One explanation for bisphosphonate action is that deposition of very small amounts in bone is sufficient to inhibit osteoclast action, or that direct uptake by osteoclasts without deposition of the compounds in bone is sufficient to cause apoptosis and cell death. Bisphosphonates may also have a direct inhibitory effect on osteoblasts, however, there is no evidence that blastic lesions are prevented in patients with prostate cancer and the pain relief observed after pamidronate infusion is transient (114).

The efficacy of bisphosphonates for bone pain may depend on the dose, frequency, and potency of the compound used. For pamidronate, intravenous infusions of 60 mg/month may be more effective than 30 mg every 2 weeks (115). Overall, the efficacy of bisphosphonates in different clinical studies can be related to the potency of the compounds used (71, 115). As noted above, this relationship mirrors the ranking of potency of bisphosphonates in the prevention of cancer cell attachment to bone in vitro (20). Newer bisphosphonates such as zoledronate, which is many times more potent than etidronate, have great potential for providing significant prevention and control of the sequelae of skeletal metastases but long term-controlled studies will be needed to establish the routine use of bisphosphonates in cancer patients.

There is now evidence that bisphosphonates may be useful for primary prevention of skeletal metastases. Kanis et al recently reported the results of bisphosphonate therapy in patients with recurrent breast cancer who did not have skeletal metastases at the time of enrollment into the study (111). Although the drug did not decrease the total number of women that developed skeletal metastases, patients treated with 1600 mg/day oral clodronate for 3 years had 50% fewer skeletal metastases, 29% fewer vertebral deformities, and a 75% reduction in nonvertebral fracture. These results, along with the well-established safety profile of bisphosphonates, argue for an increased use of these compounds in breast cancer patients.

Hypercalcemia

The complication of hypercalcemia is commonly encountered in cancer patients. The hypercalcemia of malignancy may occur in patients with skeletal metastases because of the release of calcium from rapidly expanding osteolytic lesions or from humoral factors produced by tumors that have not metastasized to bone. PTHrp production by cancer is the most common mechanism causing the hypercalcemia of malignancy (116). PTHrp, which has a role in regulating embryologic endochondral bone formation, circulates in low concentrations in otherwise healthy individuals. When produced in excess by malignancies, PTHrp achieves high levels in the blood and binds the PTH/PTHrp receptor in osteoblasts. Osteoblasts release signals that promote osteoclastogenesis and bone resorption in response to PTHrp. Patients with HHM have hypercalcemia, phosphate wasting, and elevated nephrogenous cAMP, similar to patients with primary hyperparathyroidism. Unlike the action of PTH, PTHrp production by tumors does not stimulate 1,25-dihydroxyvitamin D3 production by the renal proximal tubule (117). This remarkable difference between endogenous PTH and PTHrp was first reported by Stewart in 1980 and remains an unsolved mystery in calcium biology. Infusion of PTHrp into normal animals does elevate 1,25-dihydroxyvitamin D3, thus there is something unique about PTHrp production by tumors that suppresses renal 1,25-dihydroxyvitamin D3 secretion. The histology of bone in patients with HHM is different from that observed with primary hyperparathyroidism, highlighting the difference between tumoral PTHrp effects and PTH. In the latter, bone resorption and formation are coupled so the anabolic action of PTH is observed along with the classic lesions of osteitis fibrosa cystica (OFC) intermingled with osteoclastic resorption. In contrast, these anabolic components are relatively reduced in HHM for unknown reasons. Infusion of PTHrp in normal animals can cause OFC. Since malignancies that produce PTHrp are not associated with OFC, they must produce additional humoral factors that suppress osteoblast activity (118). Whether any of the cytokines produced by skeletal metastases also operate humorally is unknown. The cytokines that act as paracrine factors in the microenvironment of metastatic lesions do not usually achieve very elevated concentrations in blood.

Patients presenting with a serum calcium >12 mg/dl (corrected for albumin) may have symptoms of polyuria, memory loss, dehydration, and weakness. As levels of calcium exceed 13-14 mg/dl mental clouding occurs and obtundation is

262

observed with levels > 15 mg/dl. Hypercalcemia inhibits the action of antidiuretic hormone in the renal collecting duct, which leads to excessive free water loss and dehydration. Dehydration causes further elevation of serum calcium concentration and ultimately obtundation. The initial goal of treatment in patients with hypercalcemia of any cause is rehydration and volume expansion with isotonic saline. Saline diuresis, and its associated calciuresis, can then be done to lower serum calcium concentration. The desired effect is achieved with isotonic saline infusion at a rate producing a urine output of 2 liters/24 HR. Only after intravascular volume expansion is complete should a loop diuretic be added to promote calciuresis. If a loop diuretic is added prior to achieving a urine output > 2 liters/24 HR, dehydration ensues and the serum calcium rises.

Intravenous pamidronate (60-90 mg/24 HR) is now the treatment of choice for severe hypercalcemia. The dose used depends on the severity of the hypercalcemia, renal function, and magnitude of dehydration. Patients should be rehydrated prior to administering pamidronate since a rise in serum creatinine occurs in 10-15% of those treated. Pamidronate will lower serum calcium by 48 hours and continues to be effective for 14 days, making biweekly infusions a reasonable approach to long term management. Intravenous pamidronate may cause pyrexia peaking at 24 hours and lasting 48-72 hours. Salmon calcitonin, 4-8 IU/kg, remains a useful drug in the first 48 hours of treatment as the effects of saline diuresis will not achieve a nadir in serum calcium for 48 hours and bisphosphonate therapy has a similar delay in effectiveness. Patients become refractory to calcitonin within the first few days after which it can be discontinued. Oral bisphosphonates are inferior to intravenous pamidronate in dehydrated severely hypercalcemic patients and should not be used for this purpose. Once the acute crisis has been treated, maintenance of eucalcemia with oral bisphosphonates is possible but patients must remain hydrated. Common mistakes in treating the hypercalcemia of malignancy include insufficient hydration, administration of loop diuretics prior to hydration, and prescribing oral loop diuretics in already dehydrated outpatients. Plicamycin therapy, which is toxic, has been replaced by bisphosphonates and has no further role in the management of HHM.

For some patients, unique mechanisms of hypercalcemia require special interventions. Up to 2/3 of patients with lymphoma have elevated circulating levels of 1,25-dihydroxyvitamin D3. In lymphoma and some other hematologic malignancies, the production of 1,25-dihydroxyvitamin D3 presumable occurs because of unregulated cholecaciferol-1a-hydroxylase activity by malignant lymphocytes ( ). Treatment of these patients with glucocorticoids (prednisone 60 mg a day po), along with volume expansion and saline diuresis, will lower serum calcium, after which the glucocorticoids can be tapered to the lowest dose that maintains eucalcemia.

Fractures

The treatment goal for fractures is to maintain mobility and prevent paraplegia. As with any surgical intervention, the risks must be weighed against the potential benefits of the procedure. Patients with pathologic fractures are often debilitated and nutritionally compromised; however, the orthopedic surgeon may be able to provide fixation of fractures that temporarily provide relief of nerve compression, stabilization, and continued mobility.

Monitoring the Response to Therapy

Both x-rays and Tc99-polyphosphate scans can be used to monitor the response to chemotherapy, x-irradiation, or bisphosphonates. In some cases, lesions become smaller, develop a sclerotic component indicative of healing, or exhibit a reduction in density in the case of blastic lesions.

Recent reports have suggested that biochemical markers of bone metabolism can be used to monitor therapy of skeletal metastases. Overall, markers of bone resorption or formation have been used to follow the response to treatment in clinical trials of bisphosphonates. Several reports have reported a transient decrease in urine pyridinolines or deoxypyridinolines following bisphosphonate treatment of patients with skeletal metastases from breast cancer (119, 120, 84, 121). A more recent study using a serum assay for pyridinolines correlated levels of this marker with the patient's metastatic burden in bone (122). Other resorption markers such as urine hydroxyproline also fall after treatment with bisphosphonates (84). Variable results have been reported for changes in formation markers, including alkaline phosphatase and osteocalcin, after treatment (83).

In multiple myeloma, treatment with bisphosphonates causes a fall in pyridinolines (123, 124). Less is known about markers of formation, which would not be expected to be as useful in myeloma. In contrast, patients with prostate cancer, who have elevated levels of formation markers, show a decrease in osteocalcin following treatment (125). Surprisingly, resorption markers also fall after treatment of prostate cancer (126, 92). As a research tool, markers have provided important information; however, their usefulness in treatment decisions for individual patients has not been extensively evaluated. These studies need to determine the positive and negative predictive value of biochemical markers as indicators of the response to therapy, and the contribution that markers might make in determining the need for repeated bisphosphonate therapy. NTx™ assays of type I collagen cross-link degradation products and C-telopeptide degradation products (Crosslaps™) show a greater decrease than other markers after treatment of HHM with pamidronate (121). Clearly, biochemical markers have no place in monitoring an individual patient's response to treatment of HHM. In clinical management, serum calcium remains the best measure.

Future Targets of Therapy

Currently, the prevention and treatment of bone metastases is limited to treatment of the primary tumor (chemotherapy, radiation), radiation therapy of metastatic lesions, and bisphosphonates. It is likely that availability of more potent bisphosphonates will provide better pain control, reduction in pathologic fractures, and long term control of HHM. However, most therapies for treatment of the skeletal complications of malignancy are directed at inhibition of osteoclast activity. Clearly, efforts must be made to capitalize on new information regarding the role of integrins and PTHrp expression in the establishment of skeletal metastases. Inhibition of cancer cell attachment to bone with integrin antagonists, particularly those directed against avb3 and a4b1, is an important research and development target for treatment of human disease. Similarly, antagonist peptides that block the PTH/PTHrp receptor are available and could be an additional modality in treating the skeletal complications of malignancy. Other targets include inhibitors of cytokine production or action, including receptor antagonists and soluble receptors that inactivate cytokines in the bone microenvironment. Many of these have been studied in animal models but not in human disease. Finally, efforts must be made to enhance bone formation in myeloma patients by identifying agents that stimulate osteoblast matrix production or inhibit the suppressive effects of lymphotoxin. Theoretically, administration of BMP-6, a cause of blastic lesions in prostate cancer, could potentially benefit patients with myeloma. In the near future, attacking cancer cells at every level of their action in bone should result in more successful treatment, a reduction in complications, and a decrease in the suffering of patients.

References

1.   Coleman RE, Rubens RD 1987 The clinical course of bone metastases from breast cancer. Br J Cancer 55:61-66.

2.   Muggia FM 1990 Overview of cancer related hypercalcemia: Epidemiology and etiology. Semin Oncol 17(suppl. 5):3-9.

3.   Mundy GR 1991 Mechanisms of osteolytic bone destruction. Bone 12(suppl. 1):S1-S6.

4.   Abrams J, Doyle LA, Aisner J 1988 Staging, prognostic features and special considerations in small cell lung cancer. Semin Oncol 15:261-277.

5.   Nielsen OS, Munro AJ, Tannock IF 1991 Bone metastases: pathophysiology and management policy. J Clin Oncol 9:509-524.

6.   Gittes RF 1991 Carcinoma of the prostate. N Engl J Med 324:236-245.

7. Kanis JA 1996 Rationale for the use of bisphosphonates in breast cancer. Acta Oncol 35:61-67.

8. Parfitt AM 1995 Bone remodeling, normal and abnormal: a biological basis for the understanding of cancer-related bone disease and its treatment. Can J Oncol 5:1-10.

9. Wilkins GE, Granleese S, Hegele RG, Holden J, Anderson DW, Bondy GP 1995 Oncogenic osteomalacia: evidence for a humoral phosphaturic factor. J Clin Endocrinol Metab 80: 1628-1634.

10. Breslau NA, McGuire JL, Zerwekh JE, FrenkelEP, Pak CYC 1984 Hypercalcemia associated with three patients with lymphoma. Ann Int Med 100:101.

11. Rosenthal N, Insogna KL, Godsall JW, Smaldone L, Waldron JA, Stewart AF 1985 Elevations in circulating 1,25-dihydroxyvitamin D3 in three patients with lymphoma associated hypercalcemia. J Clin Endocrinol Metab 60:29.

12. Batson OV 1940 The function of the vertebral veins and their role in the spread of metastases. Ann Surg 112:138-149.

13. Liotta LA 1986 Tumor invasion and metastases--role of the extracellular matrix. Cancer Res 46:1-7.

14. Kohno N, Kitazawa S, Fukase M, Sakoda Y, Kanbara Y, Furuya Y, Ohashi O, Ishikawa Y, Saitoh Y 1994 The expression of parathyroid hormone-related protein in human breast cancer with skeletal metastases. Surg Today 24:215-220.

15. Nakai M, Mundy GR, Williams RJ, Boyce B, Yoneda T 1992 A synthetic antagonist to laminin inhibits the formation of osteolytic metastases by human melanoma cells in nude mice. Cancer Res 52:5395-5399.

16. Davies J, Warwick J, Totty N, Philip R, HelfrichM, Horton M 1989 The osteoclast functional antigen, implicated in the regulation of bone resorption, is biochemically related to the vitronectin receptor. J Cell Biol 109:1817-1826.

17. Helfrich MH, Nesbitt SA, Dorey EL, Hoerton MA 1992 Rat osteoclasts adhere to a wide range of RGD (Arg-Gly-Asp) peptide-containing proteins, including the bone sialoproteins and fibronectin, via a beta 3 integrin. J Bone Miner Res 7:335-343.

18. Ross FP, Chapel J, Alvarez JI, Sander D, Butler WT, Farach-Carson MC, MintzKA, Robey PG, Teitelbaum SL, Cheresh DA 1993 Interactions between bone matrix proteins osteopontin and bone sialoprotein and the osteoclast integrin alpha v beta 3 potentiate bone resorption. J Biol Chem 268:9901-9907.

19. Van der Pluijm G, Mouthaan H, Baas C, de Groot H, Papapoulos S, Löwik C 1994 Integrins and osteoclastic resorption in three bone organ cultures: differential sensitivity to synthetic Arg-Gly-Asp peptides during osteoclasts formation. J Bone Miner Res 9:1021-1028.

20. Burger R, Wendler J, Antoni K, Helm G, Kalden JR, Gramatzki M 1994 Interleukin-6 production in B-cell neoplasias and Castleman's disease: evidence for an additional paracrine loop. Ann Hematol 69:25-31.

21. Liapis H, Flath A, Kitazawa S 1996 Integrin alpha V beta 3 expression by bone-residing breast cancer metastases. Diagn Mol Pathol 5:127-135.

22. Matsuura N, Puzon-McLaughlin W, Irie A, Morikawa Y, Kakudo K, Takada Y 1996 Induction of experimental bone metastasis in mice by transfection of integrin alpha 4 beta 1 into tumor cells. Am J Pathol 148:55-61.

23. Mbalaviele G, Dunstan CR, Sasaki A, Williams PJ, Mundy GR, Yoneda T 1996 E-cadherin expression in human breast cancer cells suppresses the development of osteolytic bone metastases in an experimental metastasis model. Cancer Res 56:4063-4070.

24. Bellahcene A, Kroll M, Liebens F, Castronovo V 1996 Bone sialoprotein expression in primary human breast cancer is associated with bone metastases development. J Bone Miner Res 11:665-670.

25. Bellahcene A, Menard S, Bufalino R, Moreau L, Castronovo V 1996 Expression of bone sialoprotein in primary human breast cancer is associated with poor survival. Int J Cancer 69:350-353.

26. Bundred NJ, Walls J, Ratcliffe WA 1996 Parathyroid hormone-related protein, bone metastases and hypercalcaemia of malignancy. Ann R Coll Surg Engl 78:354-358.

27. Kurebayashi J, Kurosumi M, Sonoo H 1996 A new human breast cancer cell line, KPL-3C, secretes parathyroid hormone-related protein and produces tumours associated with microcalcifications in nude mice. Br J Cancer 74:200-207.

28. Coleman RE, Houston S, James I, Rodger A, Rubens RD, Leonard RC, Ford J 1992 Preliminary results of the use of urinary excretion of pyridinium crosslinks for monitoring metastatic bone disease. Br J Cancer 65: 766-768.

29. Luparello C, Birch MA, Gallagher JA, Burtis WJ 1997 Clonal heterogeneity of the growth and invasive response of a human breast carcinoma cell line to parathyroid hormone-related peptide fragments. Carcinogenesis 18:23-29.

30. Guise TA, Mundy GR 1996 Physiological and pathological roles of parathyroid hormone-related peptide. Curr Opin Nephrol Hypertens 5:307-315.

31. Iguchi H, Tanaka S, Ozawa Y, Kashiwakuma T, Kimura T, Hiraga T, Ozawa H, Kono A 1996 An experimental model of bone metastasis by human lung cancer cells: the role of parathyroid hormone-related protein in bone metastasis. Cancer Res 56:4040-4043.

32. Iwamura M, di Sant'Agnese PA, Wu G, Benning CM, Cockett AT, Deftos LJ, Abrahamsson PA 1993 Immunohistochemical localization of parathyroid hormone-related protein in human prostate cancer. Cancer Res 53:1724-1726.

46. Kuno H, Kurian M, Hendy GD, White J, Deluca H, Nanes MS 1994 Tumor necrosis factor-a regulates nuclear protein-DNA binding at the vitamin D response element of the rat osteocalcin gene. Endocrinology 134: 2524-2531.

47. Vargas SJ, Gillespie MT, Powell GJ, Southby J, Danks JA, Moseley JM, Martin TJ 1992 Localization of parathyroid hormone-related protein mRNA expression in breast cancer and metastatic lesions by in situ hybridization. J Bone Miner Res 7:971-979.

48. Luparello C, Ginty AF, Gallagher JA, Pucci-Minafra I, Minafra S 1993 Transforming growth factor-beta 1, beta 2, and beta 3, urokinase and parathyroid hormone-related peptide expression in 8701-BC breast cancer cells and clones. Differentiation 55:73-80.

49. Relf M, LeJeune S, Scott PA, Fox S, Smith K, Leek R, Moghaddam A, Whitehouse R, Bicknell R, Harris AL 1997 Expression of the angiogenic factors vascular endothelial cellgrowth factor, acidic and basic fibroblast growth factor, tumor growth factor beta-1, platelet-derived endothelial cell growth factor, placenta growth factor, and pleiotrophin in human primary breast cancer and its relation to angiogenesis. Cancer Res 57:963-969.

50. Crichton MB, Nichols JE, Zhao Y, Bulun SE, Simpson ER 1996 Expression of transcripts of interleukin-6 and related cytokines by human breast tumors, breast cancer cells, and adipose stromal cells. Mol Cell Endocrinol 118:215-220.

51. Miyashiro I, Kaname T, Shin E, Wakasugi E, Monden T, Takatsuka Y, Kikkawa N, Muramatsu T, Monden M, Akiyama T 1997 Midkine expression in human breast cancers: expression of truncated form. Breast Cancer Res Treat 43:1-6.

52. Quinn KA, Treston AM, Unsworth EJ, Miller MJ, Vos M, Grimley C, Battey J, Mulshine JL, Cuttitta F 1996 Insulin-like growth factor expression in human cancer cell lines. J Biol Chem 271:11477-11483.

53. Ichinose Y, Iguchi H, Ohta M, Katakami H 1993 Establishment of lung cancer cell line producing parathyroid hormone-related protein. Cancer Lett 74:119-124.

54. Stuart-Harris R, Ahern V, Danks JA, Gurney H, Martin TJ 1993 Hypercalcaemia in small cell lung cancer: report of a case associated with parathyroid hormone-related protein (PTHrP). Eur J Cancer 29A:1601-1604.

55. Rizzoli R, Feyen JH, Grau G, Wohlwend A, Sappino AP, Bonjour JP 1994 Regulation of parathyroid hormone-related protein production in a human lung squamous cell carcinoma line. J Endocrinol 143:333-341.

56. Fischer JR, Darjes H, Lahm H, Schindel M, Drings P, Krammer PH 1994 Constitutive secretion of bioactive transforming growthfactor beta 1 by small cell lung cancer cell lines. Eur J Cancer 30A:2125-2129.

57. Giatromanolaki A, Koukourakis MI, Comley M, Kaklamanis L, Turley H, O'Byrne K, Harris AL, Gatter KC 1997 Platelet-derived endothelial cell growth factor (thymidine phosphorylase) expression in lung cancer. J Pathol 181:196-199.

46. Kuno H, Kurian M, Hendy GD, White J, Deluca H, Nanes MS 1994 Tumor necrosis factor-a regulates nuclear protein-DNA binding at the vitamin D response element of the rat osteocalcin gene. Endocrinology 134: 2524-2531.

47. Vargas SJ, Gillespie MT, Powell GJ, Southby J, Danks JA, Moseley JM, Martin TJ 1992 Localization of parathyroid hormone-related protein mRNA expression in breast cancer and metastatic lesions by in situ hybridization. J Bone Miner Res 7:971-979.

48. Luparello C, Ginty AF, Gallagher JA, Pucci-Minafra I, Minafra S 1993 Transforming growth factor-beta 1, beta 2, and beta 3, urokinase and parathyroid hormone-related peptide expression in 8701-BC breast cancer cells and clones. Differentiation 55:73-80.

49. Relf M, LeJeune S, Scott PA, Fox S, Smith K, Leek R, Moghaddam A, Whitehouse R, Bicknell R, Harris AL 1997 Expression of the angiogenic factors vascular endothelial cellgrowth factor, acidic and basic fibroblast growth factor, tumor growth factor beta-1, platelet-derived endothelial cell growth factor, placenta growth factor, and pleiotrophin in human primary breast cancer and its relation to angiogenesis. Cancer Res 57:963-969.

50. Crichton MB, Nichols JE, Zhao Y, Bulun SE, Simpson ER 1996 Expression of transcripts of interleukin-6 and related cytokines by human breast tumors, breast cancer cells, and adipose stromal cells. Mol Cell Endocrinol 118:215-220.

51. Miyashiro I, Kaname T, Shin E, Wakasugi E, Monden T, Takatsuka Y, Kikkawa N, Muramatsu T, Monden M, Akiyama T 1997 Midkine expression in human breast cancers: expression of truncated form. Breast Cancer Res Treat 43:1-6.

52. Quinn KA, Treston AM, Unsworth EJ, Miller MJ, Vos M, Grimley C, Battey J, Mulshine JL, Cuttitta F 1996 Insulin-like growth factor expression in human cancer cell lines. J Biol Chem 271:11477-11483.

53. Ichinose Y, Iguchi H, Ohta M, Katakami H 1993 Establishment of lung cancer cell line producing parathyroid hormone-related protein. Cancer Lett 74:119-124.

54. Stuart-Harris R, Ahern V, Danks JA, Gurney H, Martin TJ 1993 Hypercalcaemia in small cell lung cancer: report of a case associated with parathyroid hormone-related protein (PTHrP). Eur J Cancer 29A:1601-1604.

55. Rizzoli R, Feyen JH, Grau G, Wohlwend A, Sappino AP, Bonjour JP 1994 Regulation of parathyroid hormone-related protein production in a human lung squamous cell carcinoma line. J Endocrinol 143:333-341.

56. Fischer JR, Darjes H, Lahm H, Schindel M, Drings P, Krammer PH 1994 Constitutive secretion of bioactive transforming growthfactor beta 1 by small cell lung cancer cell lines. Eur J Cancer 30A:2125-2129.

57. Giatromanolaki A, Koukourakis MI, Comley M, Kaklamanis L, Turley H, O'Byrne K, Harris AL, Gatter KC 1997 Platelet-derived endothelial cell growth factor (thymidine phosphorylase) expression in lung cancer. J Pathol 181:196-199.

58. Bentley H, Hamdy FC, Hart KA, Seid JM, Williams JL, Johnstone D, Russell RG 1992 Expression of bone morphogenetic proteins in human prostatic adenocarcinoma and benign prostatic hyperplasia. Br J Cancer 66:1159-1163.

59. Boden SD, Hair G, Titus L, Racine M, McCuaig K, Wozney JM, Nanes MS 1997 Glucocorticoid-induced differentiation of fetal rat calvarial osteoblasts is mediated by bone morphogenetic protein-6. Endocrinology 138:2820-2828.

60. Jackson MW, Bentel JM, Tilley WD 1997 Vascular endothelial growth factor (VEGF) expression in prostate cancer and benign prostatic hyperplasia. J Urol 157:2323-2328.

61. Barrack ER 1997 TGF beta in prostate cancer: a growth inhibitor that can enhance tumorigenicity. Prostate 31:61-70.

62. Gu ZJ, Costes V, Lu ZY, Zhang XG, Pitard V, Moreau JF, Bataille R, Wijdenes J, Rossi JF, Klein B 1996 Interleukin-10 is a growth factor for human myeloma cells by induction of an oncostatin M autocrine loop. Blood 88:3972-3986.

63. Janicek MJ, Hayes DF, Kaplan WD 1994 Healing flare in skeletal metastases from breast cancer. Radiology 192:201-204.

64. Kream BE, Rowe DW, Gworek SC, Raisz LG 1980 Parathyroid hormone alters collagen synthesis and procollagen mRNA levels in fetal rat calvaria. Proc Natl Acad Sci USA 77:5654-5658.

65. McCarthy TL, Centrella M, Canalis E 1989 Parathyroid hormone enhances the transcript and polypeptide levels of insulin-like growth factor I in osteoblast-enriched cultures from fetal rat bone.Endocrinology 124:1247-1253.

66. McCarthy TL, Centrella M, Canalis E 1989 Regulatory effects of insulin-like growth factors I and II on bone collagen synthesis in rat calvarial cultures. Endocrinology 124:301-309.

67. McCarthy TL, Centrella M 1993 Regulation of IGF activity in bone. Adv Exp Med Biol 343:407-414.

68. McCarthy TL, Thomas MJ, Centrella M, Rotwein P 1995 Regulation of insulin-like growth factor I transcription by cyclic adenosine 3',5'-monophosphate (cAMP) in fetal rat bone cells through an element within exon 1: protein kinase A-dependent control without a consensus AMP response element. Endocrinology 136:3901-3908.

69. Canalis E, Centrella M, Burch W, McCarthy TL 1989 Insulin-like growth factor I mediates selective anabolic effects of parathyroid hormone in bone cultures. J Clin Invest 83:60-65.

70. Canalis E, McCarthy TL, Centrella M 1990 Differential effects of continuous and transient treatment with parathyroid hormone related peptide (PTHrp) on bone collagen synthesis. Endocrinology 126:1806-1812.

71. Body JJ, Coleman RE, Piccart M 1996 Use of bisphosphonates in cancer patients. Cancer Treat Rev 22:265-287.

72. Hortobagyi GN, Theriault RL, Porter L, Blayney D, Lipton A, Sinoff C, Wheeler H, Simeone JF, Seaman J, Knight RD 1996 Efficacy of pamidronate in reducing skeletal complications in patients with breast cancer and lytic bone metastases. Protocol 19 Aredia Breast Cancer Study Group. N Engl J Med 335:1785-1791.

73. Van Veldhuizen PJ, Sadasivan R, Cherian R, Wyatt A 1996 Urokinase-type plasminogen activator expression in human prostate carcinomas. Am J Med Sci 312:8-11.

74. Koutsilieris M, Frenette G, Lazure C, Lehoux JG, Govindan MV, Polychronakos C 1993 Urokinase-type plasminogen activator: a paracrine factor regulating the bioavailability of IGFs in PA-III cell-induced osteoblastic metastases. Anticancer Res 13:481-486.

75. Achbarou A, Kaiser S, Tremblay G, Ste-Marie LG, Brodt P, Goltzman D, Rabbani SA 1994 Urokinase overproduction results in increased skeletal metastasis by prostate cancer cells in vivo. Cancer Res 54:2372-2377.

76. Cramer SD, Chen Z, Peehl DM 1996 Prostate specific antigen cleaves parathyroid hormone-related protein in the PTH-like domain: inactivation of PTHrP-stimulated cAMP accumulation in mouse osteoblasts. J Urol Aug;156(2 Pt 1):526-531.

77. Wang DC, Kottamasu SR, Karvelis KC 1996 Scintigraphy in metabolic bone disease. In Primer on the metabolic bone diseases and disorders of mineral metabolism. Third ed. Murray J. Favus editor. New York. Lippincott-Raven.

78. Soderlund V 1996 Radiological diagnosis of skeletal metastases. Eur Radiol 6:587-595.

79. Limouris GS, Voliotopoulos V, Stavraka A, Vlahos L 1997 99mTc-antigranulocyte bone marrow scintigraphy of breast and prostate skeletal metastases. Anticancer Res 17:1615-1618.

80. Ryan PJ, Fogelman I 1997 Bone scintigraphy in metabolic bone disease. Semin Nucl Med 27:291-305.

81. Gold RH, Bassett LW 1986 Radionuclide evaluation of skeletal metastases: practical considerations. Skeletal Radiol 15:1-9.

82. Vinholes J, Coleman R, Eastell R 1996 Effects of bone metastases on bone metabolism: implications for diagnosis, imaging and assessment of response to cancer treatment. Cancer Treat Rev 22:289-331.

83. Body JJ, Dumon JC, Gineyts E, Delmas PD 1997 Comparative evaluation of markers of bone resorption in patients with breast cancer-induced osteolysis before and after bisphosphonate therapy. Br J Cancer 75: 408-412.

84. Perachino M, Di Ciolo L, Barbetti V, Puppo P 1996 Procollagen type I carboxyterminal extension peptide in serum: a reliable marker of bone metastatic disease in newly diagnosed prostate cancer? Eur Urol 29:366-369.

85. Akimoto S, Akakura K, Shimazaki J 1996 Clinical usefulness of serum carboxyterminal propeptide of type I procollagen and pyridinoline cross-linked carboxyterminal telopeptide of type I collagen in patients with prostate cancer. Jpn J Clin Oncol 26:157-163.

86. Wolff JM, Bares R, Jung PK, Buell U, Jakse G 1996 Prostate-specific antigen as a marker of bone metastasis in patients with prostate cancer. Urol Int 56:169-173.

87. Wolff JM, Boeckmann W, Effert PJ, Handt S, Jakse G 1996 Clinical use of prostate-specific antigen and prostate-specific antigen density in the staging of patients with cancer of the prostate. Eur Urol 30:451-457.

88. Lorente JA, Morote J, Raventos C, Encabo G, Valenzuela H 1996 Clinical efficacy of bone alkaline phosphatase and prostate specific antigen in the diagnosis of bone metastasis in prostate cancer. J Urol 155:1348-1351.

89. Chen SS, Chen KK, Lin AT, Chang YH, Wu HH, Hsu TH, Chang LS. The significance of serum alkaline phosphatase bone isoenzyme in prostatic carcinoma with bony metastasis. Br J Urol 1997 Feb;79(2):217-220

90. Ikeda I, Miura T, Kondo I 1996 Pyridinium cross-links as urinary markers of bone metastases in patients with prostate cancer. Br J Urol 77:102-106.

91. Hosoya Y, Arai K, Honda M, Sumi S, Yoshida K 1997 Serum levels of the carboxy-terminal propeptide of type I procollagen and the pyridinoline cross-linked carboxy-terminal telopeptide of type I collagen as markers of bone metastases in patients with prostate carcinoma. Eur Urol 31:220-223.

92. Westerhuis LW, Delaere KP 1997 Diagnostic value of some biochemical bone markers for the detection of bone metastases in prostate cancer. Eur J Clin Chem Clin Biochem 35:89-94.

93. Plebani M, Bernardi D, Zaninotto M, De Paoli M, Secchiero S, Sciacovelli L 1996 New and traditional serum markers of bone metabolism in the detection of skeletal metastases. Clin Biochem 29:67-72.

94. Bates T 1992 A review of local radiotherapy in the treatment of bone metastases and cord compression. Int J Radiat Oncol Biol Phys 23:217-221.

95. Nanes MS, Kuno H, Demay MB, Kurian M, Hendy GN, DeLuca HF, Titus L, Rubin J 1994 A single upstream element confers responsiveness to 1,25(OH)2D3 and tumor necrosis factor-a in the rat osteocalcin gene. Endocrinology 134:1113-1120.

96. Nielsen OS 1996 Palliative treatment of bone metastases. Acta Oncol 35 (Suppl 5):58-60.

97. Mercadante S 1997 Malignant bone pain: pathophysiology and treatment. Pain 69:1-18.

98. Twycross RG 1995 Management of pain in skeletal metastases. Clin Orthop 312:187-196.

99. Portenoy RK 1996 Adjuvant analgesic agents. Hematol Oncol Clin North Am 10:103-119.

100. Mercadante S 1994 Prevalence, causes and mechanisms of pain in home-care patients with advanced cancer. Pain Clin 7:131-136.

101. Fleisch H 1997 Bisphosphonates in bone diseases. From laboratory to the patient. Third ed. New York: The Parthenon Publishing Group.

102. Hughes DE, Wright KR, Uy HL, Sasaki A, Yoneda T, Roodman GD, Mundy GR, Boyce BF 1995 Bisphosphonates promote apoptosis in murine osteoclasts in vitro and in vivo. J Bone Miner Res 10:1478-1487.

103. Martoni A, Guaraldi M, Camera P, Biagi R, Marri S, Beghe F, Pannuti F 1991 Controlled clinical study on the use of dichloromethylene diphosphonate in patients with breast carcinoma metastasizing to the skeleton. Oncology 48:97-101.

104. Ernst DS, MacDonald RN, Paterson AH, Jensen J, Brasher P, Bruera E 1992 A double-blind, crossover trial of intravenous clodronate in metastatic bone pain. J Pain Symptom Manage 7:4-11.

105. Lahtinen R, Laakso M, Palva I, Virkkunen P, Elomaa I 1992 Randomised, placebo-controlled multicentre trial of clodronate in multiple myeloma. Lancet. 340(8827):1049-1052.

106. Paterson AHG, Powles TJ, Kanis JA, McCloskey E, Hanson J, Ashley S 1993 Double-blind controlled trial of oral clodronate in patients with bone metastases from breast cancer. J Clin Oncol 11: 59-65.

107. Van Holten-Verzantvoort AT, Kroon HM, Bijvoet OLM, Cleton FJ, Beex LV, Blijham G, Hermans J, Neijt JP, Papapoulos SE, Sleeboom HP, et-al 1993 Palliative pamidronate treatment in patients with bone metastases from breast cancer. J Clin Oncol 11: 491-498.

108. Conte PF, Latreille J, Mauriac L, Calabresi F, Santos R, Campos D, Bonneterre J, Francini G, Ford JM 1996 Delay in progression of bone metastases in breast cancer patients treated with intravenous pamidronate: results from a multinational randomized controlled trial. The Aredia Multinational Cooperative Group. J Clin Oncol 14: 2552-2559.

109. Kanis JA, Powles T, Paterson AH, McCloskey EV, Ashley S 1996 Clodronate decreases the frequency of skeletal metastases in women with breast cancer. Bone 19: 663-667.

110. Diener KM 1996 Bisphosphonates for controlling pain from metastatic bone disease. Am J Health Syst Pharm 53: 1917-1927.

111. Blomqvist C, Elomaa I 1996 Bisphosphonate therapy in metastatic breast cancer. Acta Oncol 35 (Suppl. 5): 81-83.

112. Kylmala T, Tammela T, Risteli L, Risteli J, Taube T, Elomaa I 1993 Evaluation of the effect of oral clodronate on skeletal metastases with type 1 collagen metabolites. A controlled trial of the Finnish Prostate Cancer Group. Eur J Cancer 29A: 821-825.

113. Coleman RE, Purohit OP, Vinholes JJ 1996 The future of bisphosphonates in cancer. Acta Oncol 35 (Suppl. 5): 23-29.

114. Stewart AF, Horst R, Deftos LJ, Cadman EC, Lang R, Broadus AE 1980 Biochemical evaluation of patients with cancer-associated hypercalcemia: evidence for humoral and nonhumoral groups. N Engl J Med 303:1377-1383.

115. Mundy GR 1997 Malignancy and the Skeleton. Horm Met Res 29:120-127.

116. Walls J, Bundred N, Howell A 1995 Hypercalcemia and bone resorption in malignancy. Clin Orthop 312: 51-63.

117. Vinholes J, Guo CY, Purohit OP, Eastell R, Coleman RE 1997 Evaluation of new bone resorption markers in a randomized comparison of pamidronate or clodronate for hypercalcemia of malignancy. J Clin Oncol 15:131-138.

118. Walne AJ, Jenkins PJ, James IT, Plowman PN 1997 Pyridinium crosslinks in the monitoring of patients with bone metastases from carcinoma of the breast. Clin Oncol R Coll Radiol 9:30-34.

119. Roux C, Ravaud P, Cohen Solal M, de Vernejoul MC, Guillemant S, Cherruau B, Delmas P, Dougados M, Amor B 1994 Biologic, histologic and densitometric effects of oral risedronate on bone in patients with multiple myeloma. Bone. 15: 41-49.

120. Peest D, Deicher H, Fett W, Harms P, Braun HJ, Planker M, Kindler U, Klinkenstein C, Schafer E, Schumacher K, Siecke H 1996 Pyridinium cross-links in multiple myeloma: correlation with clinical parameters and use for monitoring of intravenous clodronate therapy--a pilot study of the German Myeloma Treatment Group (GMTG). Eur J Cancer 32A: 2053-2057.

121. Clarke NW, Holbrook IB, McClure J, George NJ. Osteoclast inhibition by pamidronate in metastatic prostate cancer: a preliminary study. Br J Cancer 1991; 63:420-423

122. Takeuchi S, Arai K, Saitoh H, Yoshida K, Miura M 1996 Urinary pyridinoline and deoxypyridinoline as potential markers of bone metastasis in patients with prostate cancer. J Urol 156:1691-1695.

123. van Zaanen HC, Koopmans RP, Aarden LA, Rensink HJ, Stouthard JM, Warnaar SO, Lokhorst HM, van Oers MH 1996 Endogenous interleukin 6 production in multiple myeloma patients treated with chimeric monoclonal anti-IL6 antibodies indicates the existence of a positive feed-back loop. J Clin Invest 98:1441-1448.

124. Powell GJ, Southby J, Danks JA, Stillwell RG, Hayman JA, Henderson MA, Bennett RC, Martin TJ 1991 Localization of parathyroid hormone-related protein in breast cancer metastases: increased incidence in bone compared with other sites. Cancer Res 51:3059-3061.

125. Lokhorst HM, Lamme T, de Smet M, Klein S, de Weger RA, van Oers R, Bloem AC 1994 Primary tumor cells of myeloma patients induce interleukin-6 secretion in long-term bone marrow cultures. Blood 84:2269-2277.

126. Strang P 1996 Analgesic effect of bisphosphonates on bone pain in breast cancer patients. Acta Oncol 35 (Suppl. 5): 50-57.

127. Van der Pluijm G, Vloedgraven H, van Beek E, van der Wee-Pals L, Löwik C, Papapoulos S 1996 Bisphosphonates inhibit the adhesion of breast cancer cells to bone matrices in vitro. J Clin Invest 98:698-705.

128. Gudgeon CA, Werner ID, Dent DM 1996 A re-evaluation of isotope screening for skeletal metastases in node-negative breast cancer. S Afr Med J 86:166-169.

129. Centrella M, McCarthy TL, Canalis E 1988 Tumor necrosis factor alpha inhibits collagen synthesis and alkaline phosphatase activity independently of its effect on deoxyribonucleic acid synthesis in osteoblast-enriched bone cell cultures Endocrinology 123:1442-1448.

130. Ferrer FA, Miller LJ, Andrawis RI, Kurtzman SH, Albertsen PC, Laudone VP, Kreutzer DL 1997 Vascular endothelial growth factor (VEGF) expression in human prostate cancer: in situ and in vitro expression of VEGF by human prostate cancer cells. J Urol 157:2329-2333.

131. Inoue M, Minami M, Fujii Y, Matsuda H, Shirakura R, Kido T 1997 Granulocyte colony-stimulating factor and interleukin-6-producing lung cancer cell line, LCAM. J Surg Oncol 64:347-350.

132. Kohn EC, Liotta LA 1995 Molecular insights into cancer invasion: strategies for prevention and intervention. Cancer Res 55:1856-1862.

133. Jaques G, Rotsch M, Wegmann C, Worsch U, Maasberg M, Havemann K 1988 Production of immunoreactive insulin-like growth factor I and response to exogenous IGF-I in small cell lung cancer cell lines. Exp Cell Res 176:336-343.

134. Hoskin PJ 1995 Radiotherapy in the management of bone pain. Clin Orthop 312:105-119.

135. Morinaga Y, Fujita N, Ohishi K, Tsuruo T 1997 Stimulation of interleukin-11 production from osteoblast-like cells by transforming growth factor-beta and tumor cell factors. Int J Cancer 71:422-428.

16 Common Diseases Which May Complicate the Osteoporosis Phenotype

Michael Davies, M.D.

INTRODUCTION

Osteoporosis is the commonest condition to affect the bony skeleton producing considerable morbidity and mortality to those who sustain fractures. The majority of those affected are post-menopausal women and elderly people of both sexes. Although the majority of sufferers of osteoporosis are otherwise healthy people, a variety of diseases are associated with osteoporosis and sometimes treatment instituted for a particular disease impacts upon the skeleton. It is important to determine where possible those factors which either produce or exacerbate osteoporosis. It is only by understanding how a disease might affect the skeleton that prevention and possible treatment strategies can be developed.

Primary Hyperparathyroidism

Primary hyperparathyroidism (PHP) is a relatively common endocrine disturbance predominantly affecting post-menopausal women. Although originally believed to be an uncommon condition causing renal stones as well as hyperparathyroid bone disease, the advent of multichannel biochemical autoanalysers led to the routine measurement of serum calcium and to the discovery of far more mild forms of PHP. In the nineties, therefore, the majority of cases of PHP are relatively mild with a few, if any, symptoms, and there is much debate about the significance of the hyperparathyroid state to the development of osteoporosis. Indeed, in certain circumstances, parathyroid hormone (PTH) can be anabolic to bone and has been used to treat women with post-menopausal osteoporosis (1). Classical hyperparathyroid bone disease (osteitis fibrosa cystica) presents with bone pain and sometimes fractures through brown tumors. Radiographs of the digits show subperiosteal bone resorption and immunoassayable PTH (iPTH) values are extremely high. This presentation is relatively uncommon and is seen in two clinical situations. Firstly, the serum calcium is either normal or slightly raised and the hyperparathyroid state is complicated by vitamin D deficiency. The osteitis fibrosa is "cured" by vitamin D treatment which allows full biochemical expression of the hyperparathyroid state leading to an increase in serum calcium and obvious hypercalcemia. At the same time, iPTH values fall although they remain elevated (2). Secondly, osteitis fibrosa cystica is seen in severe often life threatening hypercalcemic states associated with large parathyroid tumors where first aid measures to correct electrolyte imbalance are followed by urgent parathyroidectomy.

Aside from these two clinical situations, what are the effects of PHP upon the skeleton and what, if anything, should be done?

PTH secretion is not autonomous in many patients with PHP, but responds to calcium chelation and calcium infusion (3). There is also anecdotal evidence of the normal pulsatile secretion of PTH occurring in PHP (4). However, most patients have PTH values higher than the normal reference range. The pulsatile release of PTH could therefore be anabolic to the skeleton, whilst the prolonged supranormal amounts of iPTH detectable in patients with PHP could be catabolic to bone. Finally, since most patients with PHP are post-menopausal women, there will be subjects in whom estrogen deficiency is impacting the skeleton. Inevitably, some women with post-menopausal osteoporosis will have coexistent PHP. It is necessary, therefore, to assess a large number of patients with PHP and compare them to age and sex matched controls to appreciate the effects of sustained hyperparathyroidism upon the skeleton.

Biochemical Markers of Bone Turnover. Biochemical markers of osteoblastic and osteoclastic activity are increased in the hyperparathyroid state, in keeping with the known effects of PTH on bone cells. Evidence for increased osteoblastic activity can be found by showing increases in the serum levels of bone specific alkaline phosphatase and osteocalcin. Mean urinary pyridinoline and deoxypyridinoline excretion are also increased in PHP, reflecting increased bone resorption and are more specific for osteoclastic bone resorption than hydroxyproline excretion.

Bone Histomorphometry. Analysis of bone biopsy specimens obtained from the iliac crest after *in vivo* labelling of the bone with tetracycline shows increases in bone turnover, which even in mild cases of PHP may be increased two-to three-fold (5). States of high bone turnover are considered to be detrimental to the skeleton, exacerbating remodeling imbalance and accelerating bone loss. Indeed, present treatment strategies for osteoporosis are principally aimed at reducing bone resorption and thus bone turnover. Because of increased bone turnover, osteoporosis and easy fracture might be increasingly common in untreated PHP. However, despite a substantial increase in bone remodeling histomorphometric analysis of bone shows that trabecular bone volume is maintained in PHP (5). In some studies mean trabecular bone volume is actually increased (5) and shows greater compressive strength (6). Furthermore, although individual trabecula become thinner with age the number of trabeculae and their separation does not change with time whereas the normal ageing process is characterised by loss of trabecular numbers and greater separation (5). Finally, trabecular connectivity is also maintained (7). Analysis of cortices from iliac crest biopsies does show thinning (5) and increased porosity (8). Doom *et al* (8) found a positive correlation between circulating levels of PTH and the degree of cortical porosity.

Bone Densitometry. There have been conflicting data from studies of bone densitometry which use varying methods for trying to assess bone mass. Some techniques look specifically at trabecular bone (QCT lumbar spine) whilst others look at both cortical and trabecular bone e.g. DXA, DPA spine. Assessing the appendicular skeleton can measure predominantly cortical bone. Since PTH excess appears to affect cortical bone more than trabecular bone it is perhaps not surprising that there have been conflicting messages about the impact of hyperparathyroidism upon the skeleton. QCT of the lumbar spine has shown less reduction in BMD than forearm BMD using single photon absorptiometry (9). Silverberg *et al* (10) who used DPA of the lumbar spine and hip and SPA of the forearm showed BMD at the radius to be less than 80% of age and sex matched controls whilst lumbar spine BMD was within 5% of the expected mean and the hip 90% of the expected mean. Because of the increase in bone turnover, there is an increase in remodeling space with a greater proportion of younger undermineralised osteons compared with normals. There will, therefore, be some reduction in bone mass using densitometric analysis, which will not be observed using bone histomorphometry. The accumulated evidence suggests that in mild PHP trabecular bone mass is preserved but cortical bone mass is reduced by up to 1SD. Such a change might be expected to double the risk of fracture, particularly at cortical sites. One might therefore see an increase in long bone fractures but no change to the prevalence of vertebral fractures.

In a large study of men and women with PHP, Larsson *et al* (11) found no evidence for an increase in hip fractures. Both Dauphine *et al* (12) and Kochersberger *et al* (13) found an increased prevalence of vertebral fractures in women with PHP, but others have failed to confirm the findings (14). In a recent paper, however, Silverberg *et al* (15) have reported a subset of patients with PHP in whom spinal bone mass is reduced in contrast to the majority of cases. Whether these subjects are patients with coexistent spinal osteopenia and PHP is not clear. If one combines information obtained from studies of the effects of pulsatile PTH administration to humans, the effects of PTH in patients with varying degrees of autonomous hyperparathyroidism and studies in experimental animals, it is reasonable to conclude that a mild excess of PTH preserves trabecular bone but leads to loss of cortical bone. More severe excesses of PTH may prejudice both cortical and trabecular bone.

Management. Patients with PTP and osteopenia or osteoporosis on BMD should be offered parathyroidectomy. There is often a dramatic and sustained improvement in BMD following successful surgery (16). In post-menopausal women, estrogens reduce markers of increased bone turnover as well as serum and urinary calcium. Norethindrone produces the same beneficial effects. In a cohort of women treated for 2 years forearm BMC increased by 1.9%/year (17). There are, however, no long term studies on the efficacy of HRT on the skeleton in post-menopausal women with PHP and osteoporosis.

Bisphosphonates should not be used as first line treatment for osteoporosis in this group of patients but can be used following surgery or in those subjects unfit for surgery. The most appropriate treatment for the skeleton following successful surgery is calcium supplementation with or without 800IU vitamin D per day. This should enhance bone healing but once increments in BMD have ceased then, if indicated, HRT or bisphosphonates can be introduced.

Some patients with PHP are given or choose to take a low calcium diet. It is an inappropriate way of managing this disease and may prejudice the skeleton. No restrictions to dietary calcium should be made.

Novel medical treatments for PHP may become available using agents which have a calcimimetic effect by stimulating the calcium sensing receptor and suppressing PTH secretion. By reducing the effects of PTH on various tissues they may provide an alternative to surgery by effectively acting as a means of producing medical parathyroidectomy (18).

Hyperthyroidism

Thyroid hormones are necessary for normal growth and development of the skeleton. Osteoblasts possess receptors for thyroid hormone and are believed to be the primary target cell for the action of thyroid hormone on bone. Thyroid hormones increase alkaline phosphatase and osteocalcin production by osteoblast like cells and insulin like growth factor 1 (IGF1) production also increase when fetal rat bone is treated with thyroid hormone. IGF1 increases osteoblast number and differentiation as well as collagen synthesis. In isolated osteoclasts thyroid hormone has no effect, but when mixed bone cells are added to the culture, osteoclastic activation occurs. It appears, therefore, that the effect of thyroid hormones on osteoclastic bone resorption is an indirect one, acting via the osteoblast or other cell type. In humans, states of thyroid hormone excess are accompanied by increases in serum levels of alkaline phosphatase and osteocalcin reflecting increased osteoblastic activity. There is also an increase in the urinary excretion of hydroxyproline and collagen crosslinked fragments reflecting increased osteoclastic activity. Markers of bone resorption are increased more than markers of bone formation, indicating a remodeling imbalance in favor of bone loss (5). Bone histomorphometry indicates that the primary effect of thyroid hormone on bone is to increase the number of new bone remodeling units, increasing both remodeling activity and remodeling space. The number of osteoclasts and resorption sites is increased and in concert with this there is hyperosteroidosis and mineralisation rates are increased. Remodeling imbalance results from a decrease in the duration of the remodeling cycle (normally up to 200 days) as a result of a reduction in the time scale of bone formation. In a detailed analysis of resorption and formation rates, Eriksen et al (19) found an increase in resorption (3.8 versus 1.1mmday) and a decrease in formation time (109 days versus 150 days) despite evidence that initially formation rates were rapid. There is, therefore, a net increase in bone resorption with release of calcium into the extracellular fluid. This leads to a reduction in serum PTH levels and a lowering of the serum concentration of 1,25 dihydroxyvitamin D_3 (20). These changes will result in a decrease in calcium absorption from the gut, an increase in urine calcium and negative calcium balance. Despite these homeostatic mechanisms overt hypercalcemia is sometimes seen in severe thyrotoxicosis.

Bone Mineral Density and Fractures. Patients with thyrotoxicosis have evidence of a reduced bone mineral density when compared with controls (2) and fracture rate may be increased in such patients. However, a past history of thyrotoxicosis is a risk factor for hip fractures (22) and individuals with a past history of thyrotoxicosis have been shown to fracture at an earlier age than subjects with a life-long euthyroid state (23). These data suggest that a remodeling deficit occurs in states of hyperthyroidism which cannot be fully reversed by return to a euthyroid state. Although longitudinal studies of bone density show improvements with correction of hyperthyroidism (24) there is some evidence that women with a past history of thyrotoxicosis and who are euthyroid have less bone than life-long euthyroid controls (25).

A reduction in BMD is seen in women given supraphysiological doses of thyroid hormone to suppress thyroid stimulating hormone (TSH) in thyroid cancer. A meta-analysis of reports in such cases suggests that treatment with supraphysiological doses of thyroxine accelerates post-menopausal bone loss by 1% per annum (26). The accumulated evidence indicates that an excess of thyroid hormone is detrimental to the skeleton, but unless this excess is long standing for several years it is unlikely to cause sufficient bone loss per se to cause osteoporotic fractures. However, in those individuals at increased risk of osteoporosis the thyrotoxic state, either overt or occult, will further prejudice the skeleton.

Bone mineral density improves with corrections of the thyrotoxic state but in view of the nature of bone remodeling, all the skeletal deficit may not be replaced. The data of Solomon et al (23) showing earlier fractures in women with previous thyrotoxicosis compared with life-long euthyroid controls supports this view.

The effect of thyroid hormone replacement therapy on bone mineral density is more contentious (27) with varying effects on BMD reported. Guo et al (28) have shown that bone turnover in post-menopausal women on thyroxine is related to serum TSH levels and reducing the dose of thyroxine in those with suppressed TSH is followed by a reduction in bone turnover and an increase in BMD.

Management of the Skeleton. Bisphosphonates have been shown to protect the skeleton from the effects of thyroid hormone in the experimental animal. Normal male subjects given thyroid hormone show an increase in urinary hydroxyproline and pyridinoline crosslink excretion (29) which is abolished by pretreatment with intravenous pamidronate. Estrogen treatment also offers protection to post-menopausal women receiving suppressive doses of thyroxine.

Patients with thyrotoxicosis should be made and maintained in a euthyroid state as quickly as possible. Post-menopausal women should be offered bone densitometry, especially if they have a history of previous fracture. Estrogens or bisphosphonates should be considered for those individuals with established osteoporosis. In those patients requiring doses of thyroid hormone to suppress TSH, BMD should be assessed and those with a low BMD or evidence of excessive bone loss considered for estrogen or bisphosphonate treatment. The efficacy of thyroid replacement therapy should be monitored to ensure TSH levels are not suppressed. Osteoporotic subjects with a history of past or present thyrotoxicosis should be made and maintained euthyroid and treated conventionally for their osteoporosis. Once a euthyroid state is produced, the response to treatment for osteoporosis should be similar to those osteoporotic women with no history of thyroid disease.

Vitamin D Deficiency and Osteoporosis

Vitamin D is available from two sources. The most important and only strictly physiological source is cholecalciferol (vitamin D_3) produced photochemically in the skin from the provitamin , 7 dehydrocholesterol. Vitamin D ingested with food is of secondary importance, the diet being a poor source of vitamin D in the absence of fortification. The recommended daily dietary intake of vitamin D is 400IU or 10µg/day where the diet is the only source of the vitamin. This level of supplementation has been shown to maintain the main circulating storage form of the vitamin, 25 hydroxyvitamin D (25(OH)D) at around 10ng/ml (30). Such a degree of vitamin D nutrition is sufficient to protect against the classic vitamin D deficiency disease, osteomalacia. In the United States the fortification of milk with vitamin D at 400IU/quart has done much to eradicate vitamin D deficiency, but in Europe there is less fortification and the population is therefore more dependent upon cutaneous synthesis which at more Northern latitudes occurs only during summer months and explains the seasonal variation in the serum concentration of 25 hydroxyvitamin D_3 (25OHD$_3$).

Both endogenously produced vitamin D_3 and the calciferols (cholecalciferol and ergocalciferol) provided in the diet must undergo metabolic transformation in the body before acquiring biological activity. Both are hydroxylated in the liver to 25(OH)D which is further hydroxylated in the kidney to the active metabolite 1,25 dihydroxyvitamin D $(1,25(OH)_2D)$. This second hydroxylation step is enhanced by the presence of parathyroid hormone, hypophosphatemia and hypocalcemia.

Dietary vitamin D is absorbed as a lipid soluble molecule along with fat. Impairment of fat absorption will predictably be associated with malabsorption of dietary vitamin D and will lead to a poorer state of vitamin D nutrition, particularly when dietary vitamin D plays a significant role in vitamin D nutrition.

The mucosa of the small intestine is a major target tissue for $1,25(OH)_2D$ which actively promotes calcium absorption. $1,25(OH)_2D$ binds to its specific intranuclear receptor (vitamin D receptor, VDR) and modulates gene expression. Calcium binding proteins are synthesised as a result of this genomic action leading to an increase in calcium absorption. Non-genomic actions may also produce calcium flux via a membrane receptor.

The role of $1,25(OH)_2D_3$ in bone physiology is complex and not fully understood partly because of the difficulties in extrapolating data from *in vitro* studies in cell systems to the intact animal. $1,25(OH)_2D_3$ promotes the differentiation of osteoclasts from mononuclear precursors and modulates osteoblast differentiation and activity, increasing alkaline phosphatase activity stimulating osteocalcin and osteopontin secretion but inhibiting type I collagen and bone sialoprotein. Polymorphisms of the vitamin D receptor itself may affect the responses to $1,25(OH)_2D_3$ and have been implicated in the development of osteoporosis through changes in bone mineral density (31).

The role of vitamin D in the development or exacerbation of osteoporosis.
Deficiency of vitamin D ultimately leads to osteomalacia and is associated with serum 25(OH)D levels below 5ng/ml. There is almost invariably an accompanying state of secondary hyperparathyroidism. Vitamin D replete individuals must be regarded as people in whom the state of vitamin D nutrition is not deleterious to the skeleton. Additionally, any change in vitamin D nutrition by the provision of supplemental vitamin D would not be accompanied by any changes in skeletal health or alterations of parathyroid function or calcium metabolism.

Between states of deficiency and repletion with vitamin D exist states of vitamin D insufficiency which can be defined as a level of vitamin D nutrition which is insufficient to maintain normal calcium metabolism without a degree of secondary hyperparathyroidism. As a result of suboptimal vitamin D nutrition and secondary hyperparathyroidism, remodeling imbalance is exacerbated and bone mineral density is reduced (32).

Plasma 25(OH)D levels decline with age by about 50% and the main reason for this appears to be a reduction in the cutaneous synthesis of the vitamin primarily arising from reduced solar exposure. There is, however, some evidence that the ageing skin is less efficient at vitamin D production because of thinning of the skin and reduction in the content of 7 dehydrocholesterol. Some studies have also shown a reduced capacity to absorb vitamin D by the gut. These factors coupled with declining food intake help to explain the poorer state of vitamin D nutrition in many elderly.

The consequences of vitamin D insufficiency arise as a result of the induction of secondary hyperparathyroidism. If the supply of 25(OH)D is insufficient to maintain an adequate amount of $1,25(OH)_2D$ then calcium absorption will fall and there will be a small reduction in ionised calcium sufficient to stimulate PTH secretion. The increase in PTH stimulates the renal 1α-hydroxylase and may be sufficient to restore the serum $1,25(OH)_2D$ and thus calcium absorption and ionised calcium to normal. Introduction of additional vitamin D will not only increase serum 25(OH)D but also $1,25(OH)_2D$ as a result of background secondary hyperparathyroidism. The loop is then completed by a further increase in calcium absorption, a tendency for the serum ionised calcium to rise with suppression of the previously raised PTH secretion, leading to a restoration of normal levels of calciotropic hormones and a reduction in bone turnover.

The optimum level of 25(OH)D is not known but values quoted range from 12ng/ml to 32ng/ml (33). The numbers of individuals at risk of vitamin D insufficiency will depend upon the cut off value for 25(OH)D. However, for a variety of reasons, it seems illogical to expect there to be a uniform cut off value for 25(OH)D between sufficiency and insufficiency. The level of 25(OH)D will be dependent upon renal function and the ability to generate $1,25(OH)_2D$ as well as the amount of $1,25(OH)_2D$ required for effective calcium absorption. The level of vitamin D nutrition required to protect against vitamin D insufficiency will therefore depend upon renal function, the ability of the gut to absorb calcium and the prevailing calcium intake. Thus the higher the calcium intake, the lower the level of vitamin D nutrition to prevent secondary hyperparathyroidism. If there is a primary problem with calcium absorption or a suboptimal level of dietary calcium, one might expect a degree of secondary hyperparathyroidism to increase serum $1,25(OH)_2D$ to compensate for the reduced calcium absorption. This situation is seen in some patients after partial gastrectomy and other causes of calcium malabsorption. It has recently been established that clinical states characterised by an increase in serum $1,25(OH)_2D_3$ such as primary hyperparathyroidism and malabsorptive states are associated with an increased rate of catabolism of 25(OH)D (34,35). There is a strong inverse relationship between the prevailing plasma concentration of $1,25(OH)_2D$ and the half life in serum of radiolabelled $25(OH)D_3$. When $1,25(OH)_2D$ levels are reduced by parathyroidectomy, withdrawal of $1,25(OH)_2D$ treatment or suppression of $1,25(OH)_2D$ levels by large calcium supplements, the clearance rate of 25(OH)D is prolonged (34,35). In the rat a low calcium diet increases the plasma clearance of 25(OH)D (36). These changes are accompanied by secondary hyperparathyroidism and raised $1,25(OH)_2D$ levels.

A state of vitamin D insufficiency may therefore arise from reduction in the amount of native vitamin D provided by the diet and endogenous synthesis or as a result of increased catabolism because of pre-existing hyperparathyroidism either primary or secondary with an increase, initially, of $1,25(OH)_2D$. Once a state of hyperparathyroidism occurs with an increase in serum $1,25(OH)_2D$ levels, the increased catabolism of 25(OH)D will itself produce or exacerbate states of vitamin D insufficiency and, of course, ultimately produce a state of vitamin D deficiency. It is therefore important to recognise that if the amount of calcium available for absorption is sub-optimal, secondary hyperparathyroidism may occur in the presence of an abundance of vitamin D. It is therefore important to consider not only vitamin D nutrition but also calcium nutrition when looking at the reasons for secondary hyperparathyroidism and changes in bone mass.

The efficiency of calcium absorption declines with age and at a time when food, and thus calcium, intake falls. In the experimental animal calcium uptake by isolated duodenal cells, the number of VDR and calbindin response to exogenous $1,25(OH)_2D$ all decline with age. VDR content of duodenal mucosa in humans declines by 30% between 20 and 80 years of age. It therefore follows that to effect an appropriate amount of absorption of calcium from the diet in the elderly an increase in the activity of PTH, $1,25(OH)_2D$ axis may be required. Many subjects have a suboptimal diet with respect to calcium content and this may be compounded by the age related changes in calcium absorption and availability of $1,25(OH)_2D$. A degree of secondary hyperparathyroidism should therefore be relatively common especially in the elderly and particularly in the northern latitudes, especially where fortification of food with vitamin D does not occur. The deleterious effects of calcium or vitamin D insufficiency upon the skeleton appears to arise from increase in serum PTH. Secondary hyperparathyroidism is believed to be a significant pathophysiological factor in senile or type II osteoporosis. Several studies have shown an increase in PTH with age with a weak but albeit significant negative correlation with serum 25(OH)D. Increasing serum 25OHD with vitamin D supplements reverses this secondary hyperparathyroidism. Studies in primary hyperparathyroidism suggest that the impact of parathyroid hormone is greater in cortical compared with trabecular bone (9) and it is believed that a similar mechanism may occur in Type II osteoporosis with an increase in bone turnover leading to bone loss at cortical sites.

Several studies have demonstrated significant relationships between vitamin D status, secondary hyperparathyroidism and bone mineral density in elderly and middle aged women. Chapuy et al (37) found increases in mean alkaline phosphatase, osteocalcin and collagen C telopeptide in healthy elderly women compared with young women. These changes correlated positively with serum PTH and negatively with hip bone mineral density. No relationships could be found between PTH and BMD or between 25OHD and BMD.

In elderly subjects the excretion of pyridinoline crosslinks was 2-to 3-fold higher in those with low 25(OH)D values and secondary hyperparathyroidism compared with vitamin D replete control (38). In a cross sectional study Khaw *et al* (39) showed a positive relationship between serum 25(OH)D and BMD of the spine and hip in a group of middle aged women (aged 45-65 years). Ooms *et al* (40) found low BMD values at the hip in subjects with a 25(OH)D value below a threshold of 12ng/ml; BMD was 5% higher in the femur for every 4ng/ml increase in 25(OH)D up to 12ng/ml. PTH was negatively related to BMD measured at both the radius and hip. Indeed a 25(OH)D of 4ng/ml was associated with a relative risk of hip fracture of 1.8. The relevance of some of these observations is borne out by the fact that some studies have shown an increase in PTH levels in elderly subjects with hip fracture (41).

It is important to recognise that a low BMD in an elderly person is a function of changes in remodeling imbalance over many years and the state of vitamin D nutrition can change quickly so that a failure to find correlations between calciotropic hormones and BMD should not necessarily be a surprise. It is perhaps of more relevance to look at the effects of interventional studies with vitamin D and calcium supplements upon calciotropic hormones, indices of bone turnover, bone mass and fracture.

Chapuy *et al* (42) were able to reduce serum PTH levels by 30% using calcium (1.2G) and vitamin D (20µg) daily to a group of elderly institutionalised subjects in France. These changes resulted in significant increases in serum 25(OH)D values and similar results were obtained Ooms *et al* in Holland using 10µg of vitamin D per day, PTH values falling by 15% (40). When a similar study was done in the United States supplements of vitamin D increased serum 25(OH)D but did not alter 1,25(OH)D or PTH levels. These individuals had states of vitamin D nutrition giving serum 25(OH)D values of 16ng/ml or greater (43). Even in healthy post-menopausal women daily supplements with 10µg vitamin D reduced winter bone loss and increased spinal BMD (44) and both Chapuy *et al* (42) and Ooms *et al* (40) showed increases in hip BMD of over 2% using calcium and vitamin D or vitamin D alone. There is an interesting distinction between these latter two papers. The average calcium intake in the placebo group was 500mg/day in Chapuy's study (42) but 860mg/day in Oom's study (40). The rate of bone loss in the placebo arm of the study of Chapuy *et al* was 3%/year. Intervention with 1.2G of elemental calcium and 20µg/day of vitamin D produced a 43% reduction in hip fractures and a 32% reduction in all non-vertebral fractures. Although there was no documented change in $1,25(OH)_2D$ levels this hormone was only measured in a subset or patients and only after 18 months of treatment. Changes in serum $1,25(OH)_2D_3$ occur shortly after correction of vitamin D insufficiency and might be expected to be resolved by 18 months consequent upon the observed reductions in PTH which fell by 46% and serum 25(OH)D values increased from a mean of 16ng/ml to 42ng/ml. The supplement of 1.2G of calcium increased dietary calcium from 500 mg to 1700 mg. In a more recent study Dawson-Hughes *et al* (45) treated an ambulant population of men and women of 65 years or older with 500 mg of calcium and 17.5ug vitamin D or placebo. Mean 25(OH)D values were 33ng/ml in the men and 25ng/ml in women, mean dietary calcium less than 800mg in both men and women, mean PTH 35-43pg/ml in the 4 groups of subjects. By European standards the subjects were vitamin D replete but dietary calcium was suboptimal. Calcium and vitamin D supplements produced significant increases in 25(OH)D with decrements in PTH and a reduction in non-vertebral fracture at 36 months, from 26 per 202 placebo group to

11 of 187 calcium and vitamin D group. There were small but significant reductions in bone loss in the group treated with calcium and vitamin D.

Studies using vitamin D supplementation alone have produced conflicting data. Heikinheimo *et al* (46) used an annual injection of 150,000 to 300,000 IU of vitamin D_2 in a group of approximately 800 men and women living in residential homes or their own homes over a 2-5 year period and found a significant reduction in long bone fractures in upper limbs and ribs but a non-significant reduction in hip fractures. The reduction in hip fractures was 22% but not significant because of sample size. Lips *et al* (47) using daily doses of 10µg of vitamin D_3 found no reduction in hip fractures in a cohort of over 2500 men and women aged over 70 years. There was however some reduction in PTH values and increases in hip BMD.

Chevalley *et al* (48) used vitamin D in both placebo and active treatment groups to ensure a vitamin D replete state and then gave calcium supplements to the active treatment group. There was a reduction in femoral bone loss in the active treatment group and a lower incidence of vertebral fractures. Recker *et al* (49) produced similar results in a 4 year study in women with a mean age of 73 years. No study has been performed using additional vitamin D to a group of calcium replete subjects.

There is convincing evidence for calcium and vitamin D insufficiency affecting bone loss and fracture via the effect of inducing secondary hyperparathyroidism and its deleterious effects, especially on cortical bone. Several intervention studies have shown the benefits of vitamin D either alone or in combination with calcium in suppressing secondary hyperparathyroidism, improving BMD and reducing long bone fractures. In these studies the groups will have been somewhat heterogenous since calcium intake and vitamin D nutrition varies from subject to subject. It is only possible to generalise on how to lessen the effects of calcium or vitamin D in sufficiency upon the skeleton. More detailed studies are needed looking at the specifics of calcium or vitamin D on the skeleton both alone and then in combination. No study has controlled vitamin D status and looked at variations in dietary calcium and vice versa. Studies in the United Stated often have vitamin D replete subjects, but even here there is evidence of increasing vitamin D insufficiency in the elderly. The recent Consensus Development Conference recommended a dietary intake of 1.5G elemental calcium daily in postmenopausal women and the elderly for prevention and treatment of osteoporosis (50). Additionally, to prevent or correct vitamin D insufficiency, supplementary vitamin D of up to 800IU/day may be given.

Introduction of calcium and vitamin D supplementation whilst of benefit to the skeleton may be insufficient to improve trabecular bone mass in those with established vertebral osteoporosis. In addition to calcium and vitamin D hormone replacement therapy (HRT), bisphosphonate may be given to improve trabecular bone mass and reduce spinal fracture. The efficacy of bisphosphonates have not been assessed in subjects who are calcium or vitamin D insufficient, but logically they could precipitate symptomatic hypocalcemia and would be less effective at filling in the remodeling space.

Intestinal Malabsorption and Osteoporosis

Osteoporosis is the commonest skeletal disease associated with intestinal malabsorption and arises for a number of reasons. The most important factor is the malabsorption of dietary calcium and to a lesser extent, vitamin D. Calcium malabsorption may be secondary to vitamin D deficiency, but is more often due to the primary disease process responsible for intestinal malabsorption. Since most of calcium absorption occurs in the small bowel, diseases with a predilection for the small bowel, e.g. Crohn's disease, celiac disease, by reducing the surface area for absorption causes calcium malabsorption. Colston *et al* (51) showed that in celiac disease malabsorption of calcium resulted from loss of enzymes and vitamin D regulated proteins (calbindin) normally found in mature enterocytes at the tips and in the mid portion of villi. The availability of calcium for absorption is also reduced by the presence of fat malabsorption,leading to the formation of calcium soaps. Even with an intact small bowel, calcium malaborption is seen in cholestatic liver disease. Calcium malabsorption might therefore be expected to trigger secondary hyperparathyroidism, which will lead to an elevation of serum $1,25(OH)_2D$ and may produce vitamin D deficiency as described earlier. States of secondary hyperparathyroidism may exist in patients with intestinal disease without overt evidence of intestinal malabsorption. These hyperparathyroid states may be sufficient to correct calcium malabsorption in certain instances but the skeleton can be subjected to the effects of an excess of PTH over many years. Diseases characterised by stearorrhoca are also associated with malabsorption of vitamin D and if the diet is the major source of the vitamin, deficiency of the vitamin D is to be expected. In addition to the direct effects of disturbed gut function upon vitamin D absorption it has been proposed that interruption to the enterohepatic circulation of 25(OH)D (52) can exacerbate other factors and lead to vitamin D deficiency. Studies done to support a conservative enterohepatic circulation of 25(OH)D have involved the use of bolus injections of radiolabelled 25(OH)D, often attached to a non-physiological vehicle (52). Under these circumstances the liver will rapidly metabolise and clear vitamin D sterols which may then be excreted in bile as more polar metabolites. Evidence that much unchanged 25(OH)D is excreted in bile is lacking. In the rat when radiolabelled vitamin D excretion products are collected from bile and administered orally to other animals, the metabolites are absorbed and reexcreted in bile (53). There is, however, no evidence that these compounds have any biological activity. It seems unlikely, therefore, that there is any gastrointestinal mechanism involved in conserving vitamin D. The converse probably applies with the liver and intestine being a major route for detoxifying and excreting vitamin D and its metabolites.

Intestinal malabsorption may produce osteoporosis by mechanisms other than derangements to calcium and vitamin D metabolism. Protein deficiency may adversely effect bone, and osteoblast function is known to be depressed by hypoalbuminemia. Negative energy balance leads to weight loss and eventually amonorrhoca from loss of estrogen. Vitamin K is a fat soluble vitamin, deficiency of which is not uncommon in patients with steatorrhoca. Whilst derangements of coagulation are well known, the potentially deleterious effects of vitamin K deficiency upon the skeleton have not been fully evaluated. Vitamin K is, however, an important factor for proteins found in bone matrix. Osteocalcin, matrix gia protein and protein S are generated by vitamin K dependent enzymes. Hodges et al (54) have reported low vitamin K levels in patients with hip fractures and Vermeer et al (55) have shown that the undercarboxylation of osteocalcin observed in many osteoporotics is reversed by modest doses of vitamin K. Ascorbic acid is also important for collagen synthesis and is a cofactor for several enzymes in the production of stable collagen polymer. Other micronutrients (Table I) are cofactors in the synthesis of bone matrix and may be deficient in patients with intestinal malabsorption.

Table I. Pathogenesis of Osteoporosis in Intestinal Malabsorption

Nutrient	Mechanism
Calcium	Malabsorption leading to ↑ PTH
Vitamin D malabsorption	Malabsorption also increased catabolism from calcium and ↑ $1,25(OH)_2D_3$ and ↑ PTH
Vitamin K dependent proteins	Osteocalcin, matrix gla protein and protein S - vit K
Ascorbic Acid	Essential for collagen cross links
Trace elements Zn Cu	Metallic cofactors for enzymes in synthesis of bone matrix
Protein function	Low albumin associated with depressed osteoblast
Calories	Low body mass leads to amenorrhoea and low E_2 status

Corticosteroids are commonly used in the management of inflammatory bowel disease and have many effects on the body which lead to bone loss. They impair calcium absorption, reduce sex hormone production, reduce osteoblast function, decrease type I collagen production, increase renal calcium excretion and increase bone resorption. In certain disease states steroid drugs, when used, amplify changes which are already damaging the skeleton e.g. calcium malabsorption, hypogonadism, depressed osteoblast function.

Post Gastrectomy Osteoporosis. Partial gastrectomy is performed less often today as the natural history and treatment of peptic ulcer disease changes. There remain many patients who underwent this surgery when it was fashionable and the effects upon the skeleton continue to be seen. Although both peptic ulcer disease and upper gastro-intestinal surgery were commoner in men, bone disease is commoner in women. Whilst osteoporosis might be expected to be more common, the majority of subjects with osteomalacia are also female. There is evidence for increased catabolism of vitamin D in some subjects with a previous gastrectomy (35) due to a combination of hyperparathyroidism and raised $1,25(OH)_2D$ levels. These circumstances presumably arise because of calcium malabsorption (56). The changes in calcium absorption documented in these subjects might be expected to increase bone turnover as a result of the induced secondary hyperparathyroidism and exacerbate remodeling imbalance. Additionally, calcium intake is often reduced because of loss of stomach volume and thus a reduced food intake. Steatorrhoea may further compromise calcium absorption.

Vertebral fractures occur more commonly in subjects with partial gastrectomy (57) and bone histology shows a spectrum of changes from frank osteomalacia to osteoporosis. Changes of hyperparathyroidism are also sometimes seen. Given the abnormalities of calcium and vitamin D metabolism seen in some patients with a history of previous partial gastrectomy, if the supply of vitamin D is sufficient, frank osteomalacia will not occur, but chronic secondary hyperparathyroidism will prove detrimental to the skeleton.

All patients should be assessed for present evidence of hyperparathyroidism and diminished BMD (assessed at both cortical and trabecular sites). Those with elevated PTH require large calcium supplements to suppress the secondary hyperparathyroidism (35). Additionally, those with established osteoporosis should receive either HRT or bisphosphonate therapy. Serum 25(OH)D should be measured in those patients with steatorrhoea or evidence of secondary hyperparathyroidism and sufficient vitamin D should be given to maintain 25(OH)D values in the normal range i.e. between 12 and 30ng/ml. This may require 25-100µg/day in those patients with normal fat absorption and be considerably higher in those with steatorrhoea. Response to treatment will require regular (circa ever 3 months) monitoring of serum PTH and 25OHD until a stable state is established.

Celiac Disease. Symptomatic bone disease is rare in celiac disease, but when sought, reduced BMD is not uncommon (58). The prevalence of celiac disease, assessed by endomysial antibodies, was found to be increased 10-fold in a group of asymptomatic osteoporotic subjects studied by Lindh *et al* (59). In adults in receipt of treatment for celiac disease, osteopenia is twice that expected with BMD reduced by 7-13% (60,61). Despite these findings there are no data showing increases in fractures in a celiac population. Children with treated celiac disease have been shown to achieve a normal adult bone mass, but adults found to have celiac disease treatment improved BMD but did not fully correct the skeletal deficit (62,63). These data suggest that in adults remodeling imbalance cannot be fully corrected. In a recent study by Selby *et al* evidence for continuing secondary hyperparathyroidism was found in a group of adult celiac patients treated with a gluten-free diet (64). These authors found differential reductions in BMD at cortical compared to trabecular sites, in keeping with a chronic excess of PTH presumably from reduced calcium absorption. This situation may be a consequence of covert or overt ingestion of gluten, or a failure of the small bowel mucosa to fully recover its absoptive capacity following gluten withdrawal.

Patients with celiac disease on treatment should be monitored for evidence of hyperparathyroidism and receive additional dietetic advice to avoid the covert ingestion of gluten. Calcium supplements should be given (1-2G/day) to suppress high PTH values and serial assessments of BMD made measuring both cortical and trabecular bone whenever possible. For subjects with osteoporotic BMD measurements which do not benefit from large calcium supplements over time, additional antiresponsive therapy should be given. This may be either HRT or bisphosphonate in post-menopausal women. Serum 25(OH)D and menaquinones should be measured in those individuals with evidence of osteoporosis and supplements given to correct any deficiency; however, in the author's experience, patients established on a gluten-free diet do not have problems with vitamin K deficiency.

Inflammatory Bowel Disease. Osteoporosis in ulcerative colitis is likely to be a consequence of corticosteroid use since the colon functions principally to conserve salt and water. A subset of patients do appear to respond to withdrawal of dairy products so that some patients with ulcerative colitis are kept in remission on milk-free diets. Such a regime may prove harmful to the skeleton, especially if systemic steroids are required periodically. Osteoporosis is more commonly seen in Crohn's disease, particularly when the small bowel is affected. Factors responsible for the development of osteoporosis include malabsorption of calcium and vitamin D, bile sequestrants, used to stop bile salts irritating the colon in terminal ileal disease, and the use of glucocorticoids in disease management. In severe cases, protein and calorie malnutrition and trace element loss may also affect the skeleton. Compston *et al* (65) found a reduced bone mass in 30% of an unselected group of patients with Crohn's disease and low 25(OH)D levels have been found in subjects with previous ileal resection (66). It is possible that the mechanisms described in celiac disease (34) and patients with partial gastrectomy (35) i.e. secondary hyperparathyroidism are present in these patients, but the concomitant use of glucocorticoids also accelerates bone loss. In addition to increased bone turnover, inflammatory bowel disease may be associated with low turnover osteoporosis. Histologically, this is characterised by thin osteoid scams, a low apposition rate, decreased collagen synthesis and impaired recruitment and activity of osteoblasts.

Patients should receive calcium and vitamin D supplements if 25(OH)D values are low and oral bisphosphonates should be given to those with osteoporosis or those receiving systemic glucocorticoids. Bisphosphonates do protect against steroid induced bone loss, but absorption may be a problem with patients in whom the small bowel is deceased. Cyclical intravenous pamidronate 30-60mg every 3 months has been beneficial for several patients with Crohn's disease and malabsorption (Davies unpublished observation). An alternative to bisphosphonate use may be nasal calcitonin. The efficacy of such experimental treatments should be assessed with yearly measurements of BMD. Patients on milk free diets should receive supplemental calcium to protect against the effects of a low calcium diet upon the skeleton. Low turnover osteoporosis is difficult to manage successfully and the presence of this disorder can only be determined by histological examination of bone biopsy samples.

Pancreatic Disease. Chronic pancreatic insufficiency causes steatorrhoea but unless complicated by cystic fibrosis or chronic alcoholism, rarely produces osteoporosis. Vitamin D deficiency and osteoporosis have both been described in cystic fibrosis, but this is such a debilitating condition that the etiology is likely to be multifactorial. In primary pancreatic insufficiency without other associated disease processes, the use of enzyme supplements, calcium and vitamin D to achieve normal 25(OH)D and PTH values should be sufficient to protect the skeleton. Where there are compounding factors such as diabetes, alcoholism or liver disease, assessment of BMD should be considered, and if frankly osteoporotic, specific antiresorptive treatments considered after correction of any vitamin D deficiency or secondary hyperparathyroidism.

Liver Disease. Chronic cholestatic liver disease produces intestinal malabsorption because of a lack of bile and bile salts. This results in both calcium and vitamin D malabsorption and may lead to vitamin D deficiency. Osteoporosis is common in patients with chronic liver disease partly because of the association of primary biliary cirrhosis with post-menopausal women, but also because these patients become chronically debilitated, a situation associated with low turnover osteoporosis. Rib fractures are common as are vertebral fractures which may be painful or painfree. Secondary hyperparathyroidism has been reported in subjects with coexistent vitamin D deficiency, but even when this is corrected, osteoporosis remains a problem. Calcium and vitamin D treatment will prevent high turnover hyperparathyroidism, but larger oral doses of vitamin D may be necessary because of malabsorption. Vitamin D metabolism is essentially normal in cholestatic liver disease (67) but may be impaired in alcoholic cirrhosis (68). Osteoporosis in alcoholics is complicated by the direct effects of alcohol on bone cells, undernutrition and hypogonadism.

HRT or bisphosphonates can be tried in hepatic osteodystrophy, but patients should undergo bone biopsy to assess for low turnover states, as these are less likely to respond to antiresorptive treatments. Trials of anabolic agents e.g. fluoride, PTH, or growth factors should be considered for those patients with low turnover osteoporosis which at the moment is difficult to manage. Despite claims for benefits to the underlying disease in 88 patients with primary biliary cirrhosis given urodeoxycholic acid, no improvement in the bone was seen (69).

It seems that patients with debilitating hepatic and bowel disease develop a form of osteopososis resulting from ill-understood derangements of osteoblast function. This is an area where identifying the process leading to defective osteoblast function could prove of immense benefit to the treatment of all forms of osteoporosis. Disentangling the mechanisms of deranged osteoblast function may lead to developments of anabolic agents to stimulate bone formation.

288

References

1. Lindsay R, Nieves J, Formica C, *et al* 1997 Randomised controlled study of effect of parathyroid hormone on vertebral bone mass and fracture incidence among post-menopausal women on estrogen with osteoporosis. Lancet 350:550-555.

2. Lumb GA, Stanbury SW 1974 Parathyroid function in human vitamin D deficiency and vitamin D deficiency in primary hyperparathyroidism. Am J Med 56:833-839.

3. Murray TM, Peacock M, Powell D, Monchik JM, Potts JT Jr 1972 Non-autonomy of hormone secretions in primary hyperparathyroidism. Clin Endocrinol 235-246.

4. Heath H III 1996 "Primary Hyperparathyroidism, Hyperparathyroid Bone Disease and Osteoporosis". In *Osteoporosis* Marcus R, Feldman D, and Kelsey J eds Academic Press San Diego 885-897.

5. Parisien M, Silverberg SJ, Shane E, de la Cruz L, Lindsay R, Bilezikian JP, Dempster DW 1990 The histomorphometry of bone in primary hyperparathyroidism: Preservation of cancellous bone structure. J Clin Endocrinaol Metab 70:930-938.

6. Mosekilde Le, Mosekilde L 1988 "Iliac crest trabecular bone compressive strength and ash weight is increased in moderate hyperparathyroidism". In *Bone-Morphometry* (Proceedings of the Fifth International Congress on Bone Morphometry, Niigata, Japan). Takahashi IIE, Ed. New York: Smith-Gordon 483.

7. Parisien M, Mellish RWE, Silverberg SJ, Shane E, Lindsay R, Bilezikian JP, Dempster DW 1992 Maintenance of cancellous bone connectivity in primary hyperparathyroidism: Trabecular strut analysis. J Bone Miner Res 913-919.

8. Van Doorn L, Lips P, Nettelenbos JC, Hackengt WHL 1989 Bone histomorphometry and serum intact PTH (1-84) in hyperparathyroid patients. Calcif Tissue Inter 44S:N36.

9. Adams JE, Whitehouse RW, Adams PH, Davies M 1990 The effects of primary hyperparathyroidism on trabecular and cortical bone mass. Calcif Tissue Res 46:144.

10. Silverberg SJ, Shane E, De La Cruz L, *et al* 1989 Skeletal disease in primary hyperparathyroidism. J Bone Miner Res 4:283-291.

11. Larsson K, Ljunghall S, Krusemo UB, Naessen T, Lindh E, Persson I 1993 The risk of hip fractures in patients with primary hyperparathyroidism: A population-based cohort study with a follow up of 19 years. J Intern Med 234:585-593.

12. Dauphine RT, Riggs BL, Scholz DA 1975 Backpain and vertebral crush fractures: An unemphasized mode of presentation for primary hyperparathyroidism. Ann Intern Med 83:365-367.

13. Kochersberger G, Buckley NJ, Leight GS, Martinez S, Studenski S, Vogler J, Lyles KW 1987 What is the significance of bone loss in primary hyperparathyroidism. Ann Intern Med 83:365-367.

14. Heath H III, Hogdson SF, Kennedy MA 1980 Primary hyperparathyroidism: Incidence, morbidity and economic impact in a community. N Engl J Med 302:189-193.

15. Silverberg SJ, Locker FG, Bilezikian JP 1996 Vertebral osteopenia: a new indication for surgery in primary hyperparathyroidism. J Clin Endocrinol Metab 81:4007-4012.

16. Silverberg SJ, Gratenberg F, Jacobs TP, 1995 Increased bone mineral density after parathyroidectomy in primary hyperparathyroidism. J Clin Endocrinol Metab 80:729-734.

17. Wishart J, Horowitz M, Need A, Chatterton B, Nordin BEC 1990 Treatment of post-menopausal hyperparathyroidism with norethindrone. Long term effects on forearm bone mineral content. Arch Intern Med 150:1951-1953.

18. Nemeth EF 1995 Ca^{2+} receptor-dependent regulation and cellular functions. News Physiol Sci 1995 10:1-5.

19. Eriksen FF, Mosekilde L, Melsen F 1985 Trabecular bone remodeling and bone balance in hyperthyroidism. Bone 6:421-428.

20. Bouillon R, Muls E, Demoor P 1980 Influence of thyroid function on the serum concentration of 1,25 dihydroxyvitamin D_3. J Clin Endocrinol Metab 51:793-797.

21. Linde J, Friis T 1979 Osteoporosis in hyperthyroidism estimated by photon absorptiometry. Acta Endocrinol 91:437-448.

22. Cummings SR, Nevitt MC, Browner WS, *et al* 1995 Risk factors for hip fracture in white women. Study of Osteoporotic Fractures Research Group. N Engl J Med 332:767-773.

23. Solomon BL, Wartofsky L, Burman KD. 1993 Prevalence of fractures in post-menopausal women with thyroid disease. Thyroid 3:17-23.

24. Rosen CJ, Alder RA 1992 Longitudinal changes in lumbar bone density among thyrotoxic patients after attainment of euthyroidism. J Clin Endocrinol Metab 75:1531-1534.

25. Grant DJ, McMurdo MET, Mole PA, Paterson CR 1995 Is previous hyperthyroidism still a risk factor for osteoporosis in post-menopausal women? Clin Endocrinol 43:339-345.

26. Faber J, Gallos AE 1994 Changes in bone mass during prolonged sub-clinical hyperthyroidism due to L-thyroxine treatment. A metaanalysis. Eur J Endocrinol 130:350-356.

27. Compston JE 1993 Thyroid hormone replacement therapy and the skeleton. Clin Endocrinol 39:519-520.

28. Guo CY, Weetman AP, Eastell R 1997 Longitudinal changes of bone mineral density and bone turnover in post-menopausal women on thyroxine. Clin Endocrinol 46:301-307.

29. Rosen HN, Moses AC, Gundberg C, *et al* 1993 Therapy with parenteral pamidronate prevents thyroid hormone induced bone turnover in humans. J Clin Endocrinol Metab 77:664-669.

30. Stanbury SW, Taylor CM, Lumb GA, Mawer EB, Berry J, Hann J, Wallace J 1981 Formation of vitamin D metabolites following correction of human vitamin D deficiency. Miner Electrolyte Metab 5:212-227.

31. Morrison NA, Qi JC, Tokita A, *et al* 1994 Prediction of bone density by vitamin D receptor alleles. Nature 367:284-287.

32. Chapuy MC, Meunier PJ. "Vitamin D Insufficiency in adults and the elderly". In *Vitamin D* Feldman D, Glorieux PH, Pike JW, eds Academic Press, San Diego, London, Sydney, Toronto 679-693.

33. Chapuy MC, Preziosi P, Maamer M, Arnaud S, Galan P, Hereberg S, Meunier PJ 1997 Prevalence of vitamin D insufficiency in an adult normal population. Osteoporos Int 7:439-443.

34. Clements MR, Davies M, Hayes ME, Hickey CD, Lumb GA, Mawer EB, Adams PH. 1992 The role of 1,25-dihydroxyvitamin D in the mechanism of acquired vitamin D deficiency. Clin Endocrinol 37:17-27.

35. Davies M, Heys SE, Selby PL, Berry JL, Mawer EB. 1997 Increased catabolism of 25 hydroxyvitamin D in patients with partial gastrectomy and elevated 1,25 dihydroxyvitamin D levels. Implications for metabolic bone disease. J Clin Endocrinol Metab 82:209-212.

36. Clements MR, Johnson L, Fraser DR 1987 A new mechanism for induced vitamin D deficiency in calcium deprivation 325:62-65.

37. Chapuy MC, Schott AM, Garnero P, Hans D, Delmas PD, Meunier PJ, 1996 Healthy elderly French women living at home have secondary hyperparathyroidism and high bone turnover in winter. J Clin Endocrinol Metab 81:1129-1133.

38. Brazier M, Kamel S, Maamer M, et al 1995 Markers of bone remodeling in elderly subjects. Effects of vitamin D insufficiency and its correction. J Bone Miner Res 10:1753-1761.

39. Khaw KT, Sheyd MJ, Compston J 1992 Bone density parathyroid hormone and 25 hydroxyvitamin D concentrations in middle aged women. Br Med J 305:273-277.

40. Ooms ME, Roos JC, Bezemer PD, Van Der Vijch WJF, Bouter LM, Lips P 1995 Prevention of bone loss by vitamin D supplementation in elderly women. J Clin Endocrinol Metab 80:1052-1058.

41. Comptson JE, Silver AC, Croucher PI, Brown RC, Woodhead JS 1989 Elevated serum intact parathyroid hormone levels in elderly patients with hip fracture. Clin Endocrinol 31:667-672.

42. Chapuy MC, Arlot ME, Duboeuf F, Brun J, Crouzet B, *et al* 1992 Vitamin D_3 and calcium to prevent hip fractures in elderly women. N Engl J Med 327:1637-1642.

43. Himmelstein S, Clemens TL, Rubin A, Lindsay R 1990 Vitamin D supplementation in elderly nursing home residents increases 25OHD but not 1,25(OH)$_2$D. Am J Clin Nutr 2:701-706.

44. Dawson-Hughes B, Dallal GE, Krall EA, Harris S, Sokoll LJ, Falconer G 1991 Effect of vitamin D supplementation on overall bone loss in healthy post-menopausal women. Ann Intern Med 115:505-512.

45. Dawson-Hughes B, Harris SS, Krall EA, Dalllal GE 1997 Effect of calcium and vitamin D supplementation on bone density in men and women 65 years of age or older. N Engl J Med 337:670-676.

46. Heikinheimo RJ, Inkovaara JA, Harju EJ, et al 1992 Annual injection of vitamin D and fractures of aged bones. Calcif Tissue Int 51:105-110.

47. Lips P, Graafinans WC, Ooms ME, Bezemer PD, Bouter LM 1996 Vitamin D supplementation and fracture incidence in elderly persons: a randomised placebo-controlled clinical trial. Ann Intern Med 124:400-406.

48. Chevalley T, Rizzoli R, Nydegger V, et al 1994 Effects of calcium supplements on femoral bone mineral density and vertebral fracture rate in vitamin D replete elderly patients. Osteoporos Int 4:245-252.

49. Recker RR, Hinders S, Davies KM, et al 1996 Correcting calcium nutritional deficiency prevents spine fractures in elderly women. J Bone Miner Res 11:1961-1966.

50. 1993 Consensus Development Conference: Diagnosis, Prophylaxis and Treatment of Osteoporosis. Am J Med 94:646-650.

51. Colston KW, MacKay AG, Finlayson C, Wu JCY, Maxwell JD 1994 Localisation of vitamin D receptor in normal human duodenum and in patients with celiac disease. Gut 35:1219-1225.

52. Arnaud SB, Goldsmith RS, Lambert PW, Go VLW 1975 25 hydroxyvitamin D$_3$. Evidence of an enterohepatic circulation in man. Proc Soc Exp Biol 149:570-572.

53. Glascon-Barre M 1986 Is there any physiological significance to the enterohepatic circulation of vitamin D sterols? J Am College Nutr 5:317-324.

54. Hodges SJ, Pilkington MJ, Stamp TCB, et al 1991 Depressed levels of circulating menaquinones in patients with osteoporotic fractures of the spine and femoral neck. Bone 12:387-389.

55. Vermeer C, Jie KSG, Knapen MHJ, et al 1995 Role of vitamin K in bone metabolism. Annu Rev Nutr 15:1-22.

56. Nilas L, Christiansen C, Christiansen J 1985 Regulation of vitamin D and calcium metabolism after gastrectomy. Gut 26:252-257.

57. Mellstrom D, Johansson C, Johnell O, et al 1993 Osteoporosis, metabolic aberrations and increased risk of vertebral fractures after partial gastrectomy. Calcif Tissue Int 53:370-377.

58. Walters JRF 1994 Bone mineral density in celiac disease. Gut 150-151.

59. Lindh E, Ljunghall S, Larsson K, Lavo B 1992 Screening for antibodies against gliadin in patients with osteoporosis. J Intern Med 231:403-406.

60. McFarlane J, Bhalla A, Morgan L, Reeves D, Robertson DAF 1992 Osteoporosis: A frequent finding in treated adult celiac disease. Gut 33:S48.

61. Butcher GP, Banks LM, Walters JRF 1992 Reduced bone mineral density in celiac disease – the need for densitometry estimations, Gut 33:S54.

62. Molteni N, Caraceni MP, Bardella MT, Ortolani S, Ganddlini GG, Bianchi P 1990 Bone mineral density in adult celiac patients and the effect of gluten free diet from childhood. Am J Gastroenterol 85:51-53.

63. Corazza GR, Disario A, Ceochetti L, et al 1995 bone mass and metabolism in patients with celiac disease. Gastroenterology 109:122-128.

64. Selby PL, Davies M, Warnes TW, Adams JE, Mawer EB 1995 Bone metabolism in celiac disease. J Bone Miner Res 10:S507.

65. Compston JE, Judd D, Crawley EO, et al 1987 Osteoporosis in patients with inflammatory bowel disease. Gut 28:410-415.

66. Driscoll RH, Meredith SC, Sitrin M, Rosenberg IH 1982 Vitamin D deficiency and bone disease in patients with Crohn's. Gastroenterology 83:1252-1258.

67. Krawitt EL, Grundman MJ, Mawer EB 1977 Absorption hydroxylation and excretion of vitamin D_3 in primary biliary cirrhosis. Lancet 2:1246-1249.

68. Mawer EB, Klass HJ, Warnes TW, Berry JL 1985 Metabolism of vitamin D in patients with primary biliary cirrhosis and alcoholic liver disease. Clin Sci 69:561-570.

69. Lindor KD, James CH, Crippin JS, Jorgenson RA, Dickson ER 1995 Bone disease in primary biliary cirrhosis. Does urodeoxycholic acid make a difference? Hepatology 21:389-392.

IV. The Future

17 Understanding and Manipulating Genes, Hormones and Bone Cells

Lawrence G. Raisz, M.D.

In view of the surprises in bone biology and osteoporosis research over the last two decades, one might consider predicting the future as a new definition of "chutzpah". However, it is worthwhile to consider how the many exciting new findings in our field might be applied in the future. This is likely to occur in three areas; (1) understanding and manipulating genes, (2) manipulating and modifying systemic and local hormones, and (3) manipulating and transferring bone cells. A large number of factors such as bone morphogenetic proteins (BMP's, reviewed by Drs. Gamer and Rosen in chapter 2) have been identified as regulators of bone cell function but have turned out to be multifunctional, affecting other mesenchymal tissues. On the other hand, knockout and over expression studies have provided surprising information on regulation of osteoblast and osteoclast function.

Understanding and Manipulating Genes

Assuming that osteoporosis is a polygenic disorder, the first goal must be to try to identify as many as possible the genes which determine variations in peak bone mass and bone loss in humans. Studies using a candidate gene approach have been somewhat disappointing. As pointed out by Dr. Adams in chapter 3 and Dr. Klein in chapter 4, studies in animal models which show large variations in bone mass are now underway in both mice and baboons. These could lead to the discovery of human homologs of the regulatory genes in animals. The close parallelism between the human and baboon genome makes this species particularly attractive; however, studies in mice can provide much information based on the rapidity with which different strains can be interbred and portions of the gene isolated. The most obvious outcome of genetic studies will be the ability to define a genotype which confers a high risk for osteoporosis. A less obvious, but exciting, possibility is that there will be subsets of osteoporotic patients who show genetic differences in the regulation or function of specific hormones and local factors. Such differences might allow us to reclassify osteoporosis on an etiologic basis and develop more focused therapeutic interventions.

Studies of the factors which regulate bone formation during development have identified a large number of genes that are important in the initiation and patterning of the cartilaginous template for the skeleton. Among these genes, the bone morphogenetic proteins (BMP's), PTH-related peptide (PTHrP) and the HOX and hedgehog genes appear to be particularly important. Variations in the expression of these genes might alter the mass and shape of the skeleton in such a way as to alter fracture risk. Particularly exciting is the discovery of the OSF-2/CBFA-1 gene, which codes for a transacting factor and is critical for the development of osteoblasts. This gene does not have major effects on differentiation of other tissues. Animals lacking this develop a cartilaginous skeleton with a relatively normal pattern, but fail to develop a bony skeleton. Heterozygotes develop the human counterpart of the disorder "cleidocranial dysplasia" with abnormalities of bone formation in the skull and clavicles. Whether this gene is only a differentiation switch for osteoblasts or has regulatory function remains to be explored.

At this point, gene therapy seems a distant and probably unlikely goal in primary osteoporosis, but is a possibility for the treatment of single-gene disorders of bone such as osteogenesis imperfecta in which collagen synthesis is abnormal. Methods for inserting genes for normal collagen or silencing the genes for defective collagen are being actively explored. One problem will be to develop a method to return the cells with "corrected" genes into the host so that they can make normal bone.

Manipulating and Modifying Hormones

Systemic Hormones. This approach has already seen substantial progress, particularly in the development of selective estrogen receptors modulators (SERM's), which can have a positive influence on bone, but do not stimulate the uterus or the breast. The future challenge will be to identify this difference in selectivity more precisely. It is presumably due to a difference in the interaction between the estrogen receptors, which have now been identified as being in two forms, $ER\alpha$ and $ER\beta$, and other transacting proteins. The identification of these pathways in bone cells could lead to the development of new agents which might not involve interaction with the estrogen receptor, but rather activation of the other transacting factors which take part in the SERM response.

The clinical application of the anabolic effect of intermittent parathyroid hormone injection is underway, but a better understanding of its mechanism might lead to more effective agents. One approach would be to develop agents which could cause pulsatile increases in endogenous PTH secretion, perhaps by acting on the parathyroid calcium receptor. Another possibility would be to develop peptidomimetics, which could be used orally and which acted on the PTH receptor. A peptidomimetic has already been made which mimics the ligand for the $\alpha_v\beta3$ receptor and inhibits bone resorption.

The growth hormone/insulin-like growth factor (GH/IGF) system could also be manipulated to treat osteoporosis. Oral stimulators of growth hormone release are being developed which might circumvent the requirement for injection, but selectivity for skeletal growth may be more difficult, not only because the GH/IGF system can increase bone resorption as well as bone formation.

Recent evidence in humans experimental animals suggests that androgens can stimulate bone formation. However, hirsutism and voice change in women and stimulation of the prostate in men are current drawbacks to androgen therapy. One possibility that should be explored is to find selective androgen receptor modulators (SARMs) which could increase bone and muscle strength without producing unwanted androgenic side effects. The effects on cardiovascular disease are less clear. Although efforts to separate the anabolic and masculinizing effects of androgens have been unsuccessful in the past, these have been focused largely on muscle and not bone.

Local Factors. It is highly likely that differences in the production or activity of cytokines and other local factors will be important in the pathogenesis of osteoporosis. Hence, manipulation of their production or activity could be a novel therapeutic approach. However, with the proliferation of information concerning cytokine effects on bone, it is impossible to predict which of these factors will be most important in pathogenesis or therapy. Important concepts have emerged from studies of cytokines on animal models, which may redirect our efforts. First, as noted by Drs. Titus and Names in the preceding chapter, it seems likely that the coordinated action of multiple cytokines will be involved in pathologic bone loss. Second, based on the discrepancies between studies of bioactivity and immunoactivity for specific cytokines, cofactors and binding proteins, including soluble receptors, may play an important role. Third, the identification of multiple cytokine receptors, which may mediate different cellular responses, opens up the possibility that differences in receptors, rather than in agonists or binding proteins, will be responsible for abnormalities in skeletal function.

The following examples illustrate these points, but many others can be found elsewhere in this volume. The importance of multiple cytokines is illustrated by the study of Kimble et al. showing that a combination of interleukin-1 receptor antagonist (IL-1RA) and tumor necrosis factor binding protein (TNFBP) can abrogate the bone loss that follows ovariectomy in rats. The role of binding proteins is suggested by recent studies showing that the decoy interleukin-1 receptor 2 (IL-1R2), which can decrease cytokine activity, may be reduced after ovariectomy in mice. This could represent a difference in a receptor or a binding protein since IL-1R2 can be either membrane bound or released into the extracellular fluid.

The IGF's are local as well as systemic growth factors. Moreover, their local activity is regulated by the production of binding proteins. IGF binding protein 4 (IGFBP-4) and IGFBP-5 are produced locally. IGFBP-4 inhibits IGF responses, while IGFBP-5 can bind IGF to the matrix, regulate its release and enhance its activity. Thus a potential future mechanism for altering local growth would be to decrease IGFBP-4 or increase IGFBP-5 production. In the case of IGFBP-5, the anabolic agents such as PTH and PGE_2 can not only stimulate synthesis, but also increase proteolysis, which would release IGF-1 from the matrix and enhance its local action.

The family of $TGF\beta$ and BMP's provides another opportunity for manipulation which has already been used in the repair of local skeletal defects. However, these relatively nonspecific growth factors may affect many other tissues. The most promising approach that might utilize these factors would be to increase their production selectively in bone cells. Based on the finding that OSF-2/CBFA-1 is a specific induction factor for osteoblasts, it is possible that new, more selective growth factors for bone will be discovered.

The powerful stimulation of bone formation that occurs with long-term administration of prostaglandin E_2 (PGE_2) suggests another area for exploration. While PGE_2 also stimulates bone resorption and has many systemic side effects, there are multiple receptors for prostaglandins of the E series. Hence, it is possible that the anabolic and resorptive responses could be mediated by different pathways. Since prostaglandins increase bone turnover and high turnover is associated with low bone mass, accelerated bone loss and increased fracture risk, it may even be that a decrease in local prostaglandin production in bone would benefit osteoporotic patients. The regulation of skeletal prostaglandin production is largely through the inducible prostaglandin G/H syntheses or cyclooxygenase (PGHS-2 or COX-2). COX-2 has been implicated as the critical enzyme in prostaglandin production in response to cytokines and hence probably plays a role in the bone loss that occurs around sites of inflammation. Recently COX-2 selective inhibitors have been developed which could be used not only to treat inflammatory bone loss, but to reduce bone turnover and decrease bone loss in osteoporotic patients.

Manipulating and Transferring Bone Cells

Recent studies have opened up the possibility that bone cells could be manipulated genetically or expanded outside the body and returned to the skeleton. The pioneering work of Friedenstein demonstrated that marrow fibroblasts could form bone in diffusion chambers implanted subcutaneously. Subsequently it was found that marrow stromal cells could form mineralized nodules in vitro. These processes involve the differentiation of precursor cells into osteoblasts. Friedenstein postulated that there were both "determined osteoprogenitor cells" (DOPC) among marrow stromal fibroblasts. The IOPC could differentiate not only into osteoblasts, but also into fibroblasts, chondrocytes, myocytes and adipocytes. The adipocyte pathway is of particular interest since the hematopoietic marrow is often replaced by fat. This

298

transformation occurs with aging and may be associated with a decrease in the number and function of osteoblasts. Adipogenesis may be mediated by the peroxisome proliferator activator receptor (PPAR), which is a member of the steroid receptor family. The $PPAR_\gamma$ receptor is found in stromal cells and can be activated by prostaglandin metabolites, thiazolidinediones, and high concentrations of nonsteroidal anti-inflammatory drugs such as indomethacin. Blocking activation of this receptor might decrease adipogenesis in the marrow and permit a greater number of cells to differentiate into osteoblasts. It is also possible that genes which regulate osteoblast differentiation directly such as the OSF-2/CBFA-1 gene may be activated to directly increase osteoblast formation.

Osteoblastic colonies from stromal cells in culture could theoretically be used to replenish a diminished osteoblastic population in patients. Human marrow stromal fibroblasts can produce bone when locally transplanted together with bone mineral into immunodeficient mice. This approach could be used to produce local increases in bone formation, but might not be helpful in generalized bone disease. While it has not yet been possible to seed skeletal tissue with osteoblast precursors injected into the circulation, such an approach would be needed to replace populations of abnormal bone cells in severe forms of osteogenesis imperfecta.

Conclusion

There is a vast array of possibilities for managing osteoporosis in the future. These possibilities range from extensions of current work on growth factors and cytokines to replacement or regeneration of cells of the osteoblast lineage. These are by no means the only important approaches. Further work on osteoblast and matrix biochemistry could lead to the development of new, more precise markers of bone resorption and formation. Studies on cell function and signal transduction could lead to new pharmacologic agents which inhibited bone resorption or stimulated bone formation. New imaging techniques or other physical methods could help us to assess bone quality as well as bone mass. The substantial progress of the last few decades has made it possible to ask these questions and develop strategies to answer them. The next few decades will be an exciting time.

References

1. Rogers L, Mahaney MC, Beamer WG, Donahue LR, Rosen CJ 1997 Beyond one gene-one disease: alternative strategies for deciphering genetic determinants of osteoporosis. Calcif Tiss Int 60:225-228.

2. Ralston SH 1997 Osteoporosis. Brit Med J 315:469-473.

3. Raisz IG, Rodan GA 1997 Embryology and cellular biology of bone. In "Metabolic Bone Disease", LV Avioli and SM Krane, eds. Academic Press, San Diego 1-22.

4. Wallis GA 1996 Bone growth: coordinating chondrocyte differentiation. Curr Biol 6:1577-1580.

5. Lee B, Thirunavukkarasu K, Zhou L, Pastore L, Baldini A, Hecht J, Geoffroy V, Ducy P, Karsenty G 1997 Missense mutations abolishing DNA binding of the osteoblast-specific transcription factor OSF2/CBFA1 in cleidocranial dysplasia. Nature Genet 16:307-310.

6. Rodan GA, Martin TJ 1981 Role of osteoblasts in hormonal control of bone resorption—A hypothesis. Calcif Tiss Int 33:349-351.

7. Yasuda H, Shima N, Nakagawa N, Yamaguchi K, Kinosaki M, Mochizuki S, Tomoyasu A, Yano K, Goto M, Murakami A, Tsuda E, Morinaga T, Higashio K, Udagawa N, Takahashi N, Suda T 1998 Osteoclast differentiation factor is a ligand osteoprotegerin/osteoclastoclastogenesis-inhibitory factor and is identical to TRANCE/RANKL. Proc Natl Acad Sci USA 95:3597-3602.

8. Lacy D, Timms E, Tan HL, Kelley MJ, Dunstan CR, Burgess T, Elliott R, Colombero A, Elliott G, Scully S, Hsu H, Sullivan J, Hawkins N, Davy E, Capparelli C, Eli A, Qian YX, Kaufman S, Sarosi I, Shalhoub V, Senaldi G, Guo J, Denaly J, Boyle WJ 1998 Osteoprotegerin ligand is a cytokine that regulates osteoclast differentiation and activation. Cell 93:165-176.

9. Brandsrom H, Jonsson KB, Ohlsson C, Vidal O, Ljunghall S, Ljunggren O 1998 Regulation of osteoprotegerin mRNA levels by prostaglandin E_2 in human bone marrow stroma cells. Biochem Biophys Res Commun 247:338-341.

10. Tsukii K, Shima N, Mochizuki S, Yamaguchi K, Kinosaki M, Yano K, Shibata O, Udagawa N, Yasuda H, Suda T, Higashio K 1998 Osteoclast differentiation factor mediates an essential signal for bone resorption induced by 1α,25-dihydroxyvitamin D_2, or parathyroid hormone in the microenvironment of bone. Biochem Biophys Res Commun 246:337-341.

11. Bryant HU, Dere WH 1998 Selective estrogen receptor modulators—An alternative to hormone replacement therapy. Proc Soc Exp Biol Med 217:45-52.

12. Cosman F, Lindsay R 1998 Is parathyroid hormone a therapeutic option for osteoporosis? A review of the clinical evidence. Calcif Tiss Int 62:475-480.

13. Engleman VW, Nickols GA, Ross FP, Horton MA, Griggs DW, Settle SL, Ruminski PG, Teitelbaum SL 1997 A peptifomimetic antagonist of the $\alpha_v\beta_3$ integrin inhibits bone resorption in vitro and prevents osteoporosis in vivo. J Clin Invest 99:2284-2292.

14. Rosen CJ, Conover C 1997 Growth hormone insulin-like factor-1 axis in aging—A summary of a national institutes of aging-sponsored symposium. J Clin Endocrinol Metab 82:3911-3919.

15. Raisz LG, Wiita B, Artis A, Bowen A, Schwartz S, Trahiotis M, Shoukri K, Smith J 1996 Comparison of the effects of estrogen alone and estrogen plus androgen on biochemical markers of bone formation and resorption in postmenopausal women. J Clin Endocrinol Metab 8:37-43.

16. Wang C, Swerdloff RS 1997 Androgen replacement therapy. Ann Med 29:365-370.

17. Raisz LG 1988 Local and systemic factors in the pathogenesis of osteoporosis. New Engl J Med 318:818-828.

18. Horowitz MC 1993 Cytokines and estrogen in bone: anti-osteoporotic effects. Science 260:626-627.

19. Bonewald LF, Mundy GR 1989 Role of transforming growth factor β in bone remodelling: a review. Conn Tissue Res 23:201-208.

20. Kimble RB, Matayoshi AB, Vannice JL, King VT, Williams C, Pacifici R 1995 Simultaneous block of interleukin-1 and tumor necrosis factor is required to completely prevent bone loss in the early postovariectomy period. Endocrinol 136:3054-3061.

21. Pilbeam C, Rao Y, Alander C, Voznesensky O, Okada Y, Sims J, Raisz LG, Lorenzo J 1997 Down regulation of mRNA expression for the "decoy" interleukin-1 receptor 2 by ovariectomy in mice. J Bone Miner Res 12:S433.

22. Hakeda Y, Kawaguchi H, Hurley M, Pilbeam CC, Abreu C, Linkhart TA, Mohan S, Kunegawa M, Raisz LG 1996 Intact insulin-like growth factor binding protein-5 (IGFBP-5) associates with bone matrix and the soluble fragment of IGFBP-5 accumulated in culture medium of neonatal mouse calvariae by parathyroid hormone and prostaglandin E_2. treatment. J Cell Physiol 166:370-379.

23. Pilbeam CC, Harrison JR, Raisz LG 1996 Prostaglandins and bone metabolism. In "Principles of Bone Biology", JP Bilezikian LG Raisz, GA Rodan, eds. Academic Press, San Diego, CA 715-729.

24. Vane JR, Bakhle YS, Botting RM 1998 Cyclooxygenases 1 and 2. Ann Res Pharmacol Toxicol 38:97-120.

25. Friedenstein AJ 1995 Marrow stromal fibroblasts. Calcif Tiss Int 56:S17.

26. Spiegelman BM 1998 PPAR-γ: Adipogenic regulator and thiazolidinedione receptor. Diabetes 47:507-514.

27. Thompson DL, Lum KD, Nygaard SC, Kuestner RE, Kelly KA, Gimble KA, Moore EE 1998 The derivation and characterization of stromal cell lines from the bone marrow of p53-/-mice: New insights into osteoblast into osteoblast and adipocyte differentiation. J Bone Miner Res 13:195-204.

28. Kuznetsov SA, Krebsbach PH, Satomura K, Kerr J, Riminucci M, Benayahu D, Robey PG 1997 Single-colony derived strains of human marrow stromal fibroblasts from bone after transplantation in vivo. J Bone Miner Res 12:1335-1347.

Index

Quantitative ultrasound, bone mineral density, 76
QUS. *See* Quantitative ultrasound

R

Radius
    body weight and, 99
    bone mass density, 93, 94
    calcium intake and, 97–98
    male osteoporosis, 184–185
    physical activity and, 102
Raloxifene, 158–159
    patient of choice, 159
Recombinant inbred strains, 38–41, *39*
Renal failure, 205
    renal osteodystrophy, 205
Renal osteodystrophy, 205–232
    acidemia, bone loss, 220, *220*
    acidosis
        correction of, 221–222
        effects on bone, 220–221
    adynamic bone disease, 218–219
        pathogenesis, 218–219
    calcitriol, 215–216
    calcium receptor agonests, 216
    classification, 207–209, 209t, *210–211*
    high-turnover bone disease, 207, 209–213
    hyperparathyroidism, in dialysis patient, 213–218
    low turnover bone disease, 207
    management of adynamic bone, 219–222
    mixed bone disease, 207
    pathogenesis, 205–207
    phosphorus control, 214–215
    renal failure, 205
    surgical therapy, high turnover bone disease, 216–218
Renal tubular calcium reabsorption, 143
Repetitive arginine-glycine-aspartate, 249
RGD. *See* Repetitive arginine-glycine-aspartate
Rheumatoid arthritis, 233
Risedronate, 145
    skeletal metastasis and, 259
Risk factors, 110–113
    amenorrheic athletes, 113
    smoking, 110–113
Running, bone mass and, 110
Selective estrogen receptor modulation, 158–159
    postmenopausal osteoporosis, 147–148

S

SERM. *See* Selective estrogen receptor modulation
Sex steroid levels, male osteoporosis, 185–186
Sexual maturation
    bone mass and, 90–95
    calcium intake, weight, physical activity, interaction of, 102–105
Sialoprotein, expression, 250
Sickle cell disease, 113
Signaling, bone morphogenetic proteins, 12–16, *13*
    model, *13*
Single gene mutations, 38
Single-photon absorptiometry, bone mineral density, 75
Skeletal metastases, 247–248
    phenotype, 248–251
Skeletal morphogenesis, molecular genetics of, 7–23
Skiing, bone mass and, 110
SLE. *See* Systemic lupus erythematosus
SMAD family, bone morphogenetic proteins signaling, 15
Smoking, 110–113
    postmenopausal osteoporosis, 139
Snow, precautions, 140
Sodium, postmenopausal osteoporosis, 139
Sodium fluoride, postmenopausal osteoporosis, 140, 147
SPA. *See* Single-photon absorptiometry
Stairway, as hazard, 175
Strength, of bone, 57–72, *68*
    appendicular bone girth, 59
    bone strain, response to, 65–67
    clinical predictor, 58
    collagen, tensile strength, 63
    epigenetic, genetic factors, in determining, 57–72
    ethnicity, fracture rate, 62
    fibrogenesis imperfecta ossium, 64
    fluoride poisoning, 63
    future developments, 67–68
    geometry, 60
    gross structural components, 58–62
    height, 59
    osteogenesis imperfecta, 64
    ultrastructural components, 63–65
    vitamin D receptor, osteoporosis, 65
    weight training, 62
Strength sports, bone mass and, 110
Strength training, with osteoporosis, 129t
Supplements, male osteoporosis, 193–195